The Role of Health Insurance in the Health Services Sector

NATIONAL BUREAU OF ECONOMIC RESEARCH
Universities-National Bureau Conference Series
No. 27

edited by
RICHARD
N.
ROSETT

The Role of Health Insurance in the Health Services Sector

A Conference of the Universities-
National Bureau Committee for
Economic Research

Distributed by
NEALE WATSON
ACADEMIC
PUBLICATIONS
New York

NATIONAL BUREAU OF
ECONOMIC RESEARCH
New York
1976

Library of Congress Cataloging in Publication Data

Main entry under title:
The role of health insurance in the health services sector.

(Universities-National Bureau conference series; 27)
Includes bibliographical references.
1. Insurance, Health—United States—Addresses, essays, lectures.
2. Medical economics—United States—Addresses, essays, lectures.
I. Rosett, Richard N., 1928–   II. Universities-National Bureau Committee for Economic Research.   III. Series.

HG396.R64   368.4'2'00973   76-8856

ISBN 0-87014-272-0

Relation of the National Bureau Directors to
Publications Reporting Conference Proceedings

Since the present volume is a record of conference proceedings, it has been exempted from the rules governing submission of manuscripts to, and critical review
by, the Board of Directors of the National Bureau.

(Resolution adopted July 6, 1948,
as revised November 21, 1949,
and April 20, 1968)

Funds for the economic research conference program of the
National Bureau of Economic Research are supplied by the
National Science Foundation

Contents

Preface

Conferences are sponsored by the Universities–National Bureau Committee for Economic Research in order to focus attention on major new areas of research. The economics of health easily satisfied the criteria for sponsorship. Though empirical and institutional studies of health economics can be found even in the earliest literature on economics, no major economic theorist concerned himself with any of the questions that are peculiar to the field until Kenneth Arrow published "Uncertainty and the Welfare Economics of Medical Care" in 1963. Since then, partly stimulated by rising public interest in national health insurance and partly attracted by the extremely interesting theoretical questions raised by Arrow, economists have increasingly turned their attention to health, applying sophisticated analysis to vast bodies of data newly made available by government agencies and various professional organizations and private survey centers.

Thus, when a committee was formed (consisting of Martin Feldstein, Michael Grossman, and myself) to organize a conference on an extremely important but narrowly defined topic in health economics, it was easy to find a dozen papers for which research was already in progress. Indeed, it would have been almost as easy to find twice that number, and many of the participants who served as discussants are themselves engaged in research that could appropriately have been included.

Michael Grossman and Martin Feldstein did much of the work of selection for the conference and therefore deserve a share of whatever credit or blame derives from it. Finally, Feldstein deserves an additional share for having had some part in the education of fully half the participants.

RICHARD N. ROSETT

The Role of Health Insurance in the Health Services Sector

PART ONE

The Market for Health Insurance

1

KENNETH ARROW
Harvard University

Welfare Analysis of Changes in Health Coinsurance Rates

SUMMARY

This is a study of the welfare implications of changes in the coinsurance rate of health insurance policies. Only efficiency aspects are studied; distributional problems are ignored.

The basic function of health insurance is the reduction of uncertainty; other things being equal, individuals prefer and are willing to pay for a reduction in their financial risks. To that extent, a reduction in the coinsurance rate would represent a welfare gain. However, given that illness has occurred, insurance constitutes a subsidy to one form of consumption and therefore implies an efficiency loss whose magnitude depends on supply as well as demand conditions.

To get a precise expression for the net welfare change associated with a change in the coinsurance rate, it is necessary to formulate the problem as a miniature general equilibrium model, with both supply and demand considerations made explicit. Account must be taken of the random factors in demand, the financing of health insurance (here assumed to be by lump-sum taxation), the elasticity

Part of Rand Corporation study for the Office of Economic Opportunity (R-1281-OEO). The author is indebted to Charles Phelps and John Stein for many helpful comments, especially with regard to implicit assumptions and to exposition. All opinions are those of the author and not necessarily of the Rand Corporation or the United States government.

of supply, and the determination of medical prices through supply and demand. For each coinsurance rate, there is an equilibrium price for medical services. Each individual, given his income net of the taxes needed to pay for health insurance, has a demand for medical services in each state of nature and therefore an expected utility, taking into account uncertainty about health and medical costs. In the study I evaluate the change in expected utility as the coinsurance rate changes (see especially theorems 1 and 3).

If the supply of medical services is totally inelastic, then a change in coinsurance rates has no efficiency effect whatsoever. The price of medical services charged by the seller changes just enough so that the coinsurance payment (the price to the buyer) remains constant; hence, there is no effect on demand or on financial risk. When supply is totally inelastic, changes in coinsurance rates affect only the distribution of income between suppliers of medical services and the rest of the population.

1. INTRODUCTION

In this paper I make the following assumptions:
1. The health status of an individual is a random variable whose distribution is independent of prices and income;[1] the individual aims to maximize his expected utility.
2. The utility depends on the amount of goods other than health care, the amount of health care, and the state of health.
3. The insurance offered reimburses the expenditure on health care by a fixed proportion.
4. Given this coinsurance rate, the individual freely chooses the amount of medical care he wants after knowing his health status.
5. The health insurance payments are financed by lump-sum taxes.

I ignore distributional considerations and assume a single person in the economy. The interaction between distribution and insurance needs separate analysis.

Involved in this study is an investigation of the gain or loss of welfare associated with a small change in the coinsurance rate. For this purpose, it is clearly necessary to consider both supply and demand. The rapid increase in the prices of medical services since the introduction of Medicare and Medicaid can possibly be interpreted as the response of a market with relatively inelastic supply to a sudden increase of demand; if medical supply were highly elastic, the consequences for demand and therefore for efficiency could well have been very different.

I have constructed a miniature general equilibrium model of the economy disaggregated only into medical and nonmedical service markets. On the supply side, the main issue is the transformation between medical and nonmedical services. The hypothesis of perfect elasticity of supply has been implicit in most previous work. The general case is treated here. The particular case in which the elasticity of supply is zero turns out to have a property that may be surprising at first glance, although it is not hard to see that it is true: welfare, and indeed the allocation of resources as a whole, is totally independent of the coinsurance rate. All a change in the rate does is to transfer purchasing power between the medical and other sectors of the economy.

The welfare gains and losses have been treated in a paper by Feldstein (1973), although the theoretical basis of the calculation is not set forth too exactly. He also considers the nonoptimal behavior of nonprofit institutions. I shall analyze Feldstein's results in another paper.

2. EXPLICIT FORMULATION OF THE MODEL

Let

s = state of health
x_{1s} = demand for goods other than health care by individual in state s
x_{2s} = demand for medical care in state s
x_1 = supply of goods other than medical care
x_2 = supply of medical care
$U(x_{1s}, x_{2s}, s)$ = utility in health state s if x_{1s}, x_{2s} is consumed in that state
p = price of medical care received by seller
q = price of medical care paid by buyer
T = lump-sum taxes needed to finance health insurance
y = income after taxes

Prices, taxes, and income are measured, with "other goods" as numeraire. To avoid distributional considerations, I assume that all individuals have identical endowments and identical utility functions. I further assume a very large population, with the state of health varying independently from individual to individual. Measure all quantity variables on a per capita basis. Then the aggregate demand for commodity i is $E(x_{is})$, which is nonstochastic and is, in equilibrium, equal to the supply, x_i.

(1) $E(x_{is}) = x_i$ $(i = 1, 2)$

I assume that the insurance policies specify

$r = q/p$ = coinsurance rate

but that the actual values of p and q are determined by market forces, to satisfy (1). The total cost of insurance (per capita) is then $(p - q) x_2$, or,

(2) $T = (1 - r)px_2$

The representative individual derives his income by selling x_1 units of goods other than medical care (more exactly, the resources that will produce x_1 units of other goods) and x_2 units of medical care, the former at a price equal to 1, the latter at price p. Hence,

(3) $y = x_1 + px_2 - T = x_1 + rpx_2 = x_1 + qx_2$

I assume that the individual's supply decisions are made on a purely economic basis; there are no net advantages or disadvantages to the production of medical services. If supply is inelastic, x_1 and x_2 are given, and p is determined by demand conditions. If medical services are produced perfectly elastically at price p, $x_1 + px_2$ is given to the individual and to society, p is determined by technological considerations, and the actual values of x_1 and x_2 are determined by demand conditions.

In the general imperfectly elastic supply case, the supply functions $x_1(p)$ and $x_2(p)$ are determined so as to maximize $x_1 + px_2$ subject to a transformation constraint. Since p is the marginal rate of transformation,

(4) $\dfrac{dx_1}{dp} + p\dfrac{dx_2}{dp} = 0$

Once the state s has occurred, the individual maximizes $U(x_{1s}, x_{2s}, s)$ subject to the constraint

(5) $x_{1s} + qx_{2s} = y$

(Strictly speaking, the budget constraint is a weak inequality, but in this case it is assumed to be binding.) The optimality conditions then are (5) and the equations,

(6) $\dfrac{\partial U}{\partial x_{1s}} = \lambda_s, \quad \dfrac{\partial U}{\partial x_{2s}} = \lambda_s q$

where λ_s is the marginal utility of income in state s.

The optimization defines, for each s, the demand functions $x_{1s}(q, y)$ and $x_{2s}(q, y)$. For given r, q and y are in turn functions of p, x_1, and x_2. The aggregate demands, $E(x_{is})$ $(i = 1, 2)$, are therefore also functions of these variables. The two equations (1) are not independent; if the equation for $i = 2$ is multiplied by q and added to that for $i = 1$,

$$E(x_{1s} + qx_{2s}) = x_1 + qx_2$$

but from (3) and (5), this reduces to the tautology, $E(y) = y$ (recall that y is not dependent on s). Hence, the equilibrium values of p, x_1, and r_2 are defined by one of the equations (1) together with the supply conditions. There is thus an equilibrium allocation of resources between medical care and other goods for each value of the coinsurance rate r, and I wish to evaluate these alternative equilibria. Ideally, I would like to optimize on r; as a minimum, I would like to determine whether an increase or a decrease in the coinsurance rate would increase welfare.[2]

The criterion of welfare is taken to be the expected utility of the representative individual. This respects his attitude to risk aversion; it also has the implication of respecting his tradeoff between medical care and other goods in any given state of health, a point that might be more arguable but will not be challenged here. Let W be the individual's welfare:

(7) $$W = E[U(x_{1s}, x_{2s}, s)]$$

The equilibrium magnitudes of the system are functions of r. In particular, for each s, x_{1s} and x_{2s} are functions of q and y, which in turn are determined, for fixed r, by p, x_1, and x_2. Hence, W is a function of r. I shall examine the effects of marginal changes in W; the spirit of this analysis is therefore very similar to Lesourne's (1975, Ch. 3, Sec. I).

3. THE GENERAL FORMULA FOR WELFARE EFFECTS: FIRST FORM

First, differentiate the budget equation (5) with respect to r.

$$\frac{dx_{1s}}{dr} + q\frac{dx_{2s}}{dr} = \frac{dy}{dr} - x_{2s}\frac{dq}{dr}$$

But from (3),

$$\frac{dy}{dr} = \frac{dx_1}{dr} + q \frac{dx_2}{dr} + x_2 \frac{dq}{dr}$$

so that

(8) $$\frac{dx_{1s}}{dr} + q \frac{dx_{2s}}{dr} = \frac{dx_1}{dr} + q \frac{dx_2}{dr} + (x_2 - x_{2s}) \frac{dq}{dr}$$

Now differentiate the welfare criterion (7) with respect to r.

$$\frac{dW}{dr} = E \left(\frac{\partial U}{\partial x_{1s}} \frac{dx_{1s}}{dr} + \frac{\partial U}{\partial x_{2s}} \frac{dx_{2s}}{dr} \right)$$

First substitute from (6) and then from (8):

$$\frac{dW}{dr} = E \left[\lambda_s \left(\frac{dx_{1s}}{dr} + q \frac{dx_{2s}}{dr} \right) \right]$$

$$= E \left[\lambda_s \left(\frac{dx_1}{dr} + q \frac{dx_2}{dr} + (x_2 - x_{2s}) \frac{dq}{dr} \right) \right]$$

Notice, however, that the magnitudes

$$\frac{dx_1}{dr}, \frac{dx_2}{dr}, \text{ and } \frac{dq}{dr}$$

are independent of the state of health and hence are not random variables. They can therefore be factored out of any expectation. The marginal effect of coinsurance rate on welfare therefore takes the form

(9) $$\frac{dW}{dr} = \left(\frac{dx_1}{dr} + q \frac{dx_2}{dr} \right) E(\lambda_s) - E \left[\lambda_s (x_{2s} - x_2) \right] \frac{dq}{dr}$$

The first term of (9) represents the welfare gain within each state s resulting from an increase in the coinsurance rate, which is a decrease in the subsidy to the consumption of medical services. The second term is the distinctive element that measures the welfare loss because of increased risk-bearing. With regard to the second term, notice that from (1), x_2 is the mean value of x_{2s}; hence, by the usual definition of a covariance,

(10) $$E \left[\lambda_s (x_{2s} - x_2) \right] = \sigma_{\lambda_s x_{2s}}$$

the covariance of medical services used with the marginal utility of income. I shall return to this term in Section 5.

At the moment, I use standard methods of second-best analysis (see, for example, the discussion in Lesourne, 1975, cited above) to restate the first factor in the first term of (9). This is the conventional measure of marginal welfare effect, and I give it the symbol

(11) $$W_0 = \frac{dx_1}{dr} + q\,\frac{dx_2}{dr}$$

Because of uncertainty and the fact that markets are therefore not perfect (in the sense that the full set of contingent markets is not available), there are two somewhat different expressions that can be found for W_0, the first of which is more useful econometrically and the second of which is more useful for theoretical analysis.

Since x_{2s} is a function of q and y, and with the aid of the definition of income (3),

(12)
$$
\begin{aligned}
\frac{dx_{2s}}{dr} &= \frac{\partial x_{2s}}{\partial q}\frac{dq}{dr} + \frac{\partial x_{2s}}{\partial y}\frac{dy}{dr} \\[2mm]
&= \frac{\partial x_{2s}}{\partial q}\frac{dq}{dr} + \frac{\partial x_{2s}}{\partial y}\left(\frac{dx_1}{dr} + q\,\frac{dx_2}{dr} + x_2\,\frac{dq}{dr}\right) \\[2mm]
&= \left(\frac{\partial x_{2s}}{\partial q} + x_2\,\frac{\partial x_{2s}}{\partial y}\right)\frac{dq}{dr} + \frac{\partial x_{2s}}{\partial y}\left(\frac{dx_1}{dr} + q\,\frac{dx_2}{dr}\right)
\end{aligned}
$$

Take expectations of both sides of (12). From (1),

$$E\left(\frac{dx_{2s}}{dr}\right) = \frac{dE\,(x_{2s})}{dr} = \frac{dx_2}{dr}$$

and therefore,

$$\frac{dx_2}{dr} = \frac{dq}{dr}\left[E\left(\frac{\partial x_{2s}}{\partial q}\right) + x_2\,E\left(\frac{\partial x_{2s}}{\partial y}\right)\right] + \left(\frac{dx_1}{dr} + q\,\frac{dx_2}{dr}\right)E\left(\frac{\partial x_{2s}}{\partial y}\right)$$

Now, from (4) and (11),

$$W_0 = \frac{dx_1}{dr} + q\,\frac{dx_2}{dr} = \frac{dx_1}{dr} + p\,\frac{dx_2}{dr} + (q-p)\,\frac{dx_2}{dr}$$

(13)
$$
\begin{aligned}
&= (q-p)\,\frac{dx_2}{dr} \\[2mm]
&= (q-p)\,\frac{dq}{dr}\left[E\left(\frac{\partial x_{2s}}{\partial q}\right) + x_2\,E\left(\frac{\partial x_{2s}}{\partial y}\right)\right] \\[2mm]
&\quad + (q-p)\,E\left(\frac{\partial x_{2s}}{\partial y}\right)W_0
\end{aligned}
$$

The expression

$$(14) \quad \bar{S}_{22} = E\left(\frac{\partial x_{2s}}{\partial q}\right) + x_2 E\left(\frac{\partial x_{2s}}{\partial y}\right)$$

resembles a Slutsky compensated derivative but, in fact, is not, nor is it the expectation of one. However, it can also be written

$$\bar{S}_{22} = \frac{\partial E\,(x_{2s})}{\partial q} + E\,(x_{2s})\,\frac{\partial E\,(x_{2s})}{\partial y}$$

If a demand curve for medical services is fitted to time series in the usual way, the dependent variable is $E\,(x_{2s})$, and therefore all the terms in the expression can be calculated from the econometric analysis.

Solve in (13) for W_0, using the abbreviation (14).

$$(15) \quad W_0 = \frac{(q - p)\,\bar{S}_{22}}{1 + (p - q)\,E\left(\dfrac{\partial x_{2s}}{\partial y}\right)}\,\frac{dq}{dr}$$

When there is some insurance, $q < p$; since medical services are a normal good, the denominator is certainly positive, and the sign of W_0 is opposite to that of $\bar{S}_{22}$ (if $dq/dr > 0$).

An alternative expression for $\bar{S}_{22}$ will strongly suggest that it must be negative. Let S_{22s} be the compensated effect of a change in the price of medical services for a given state s—that is, the derivative of x_{2s} with respect to q when the consumer remains on an indifference curve for that state.

$$S_{22s} = \frac{\partial x_{2s}}{\partial q} + x_{2s}\,\frac{\partial x_{2s}}{\partial y}$$

Then

$$\frac{\partial x_{2s}}{\partial q} + x_2\,\frac{\partial x_{2s}}{\partial y} = S_{22s} - (x_{2s} - x_2)\,\frac{\partial x_{2s}}{\partial y}$$

Taking expectations,

$$\bar{S}_{22} = E\,(S_{22s}) - E\left[(x_{2s} - x_2)\,\frac{\partial x_{2s}}{\partial y}\right]$$

Of course, for each s, $S_{22s} < 0$, so the first term is negative. The second term is the covariance between medical services and the marginal propensity to consume them (remember that this is the covariance across states of health for a given individual). This term can also, and perhaps more illuminatingly, be rewritten as follows:

Since

$$(x_{2s} - x_2)\frac{\partial x_{2s}}{\partial y} = \tfrac{1}{2}\frac{\partial (x_{2s} - x_2)^2}{\partial y}$$

(16)
$$E\left[(x_{2s} - x_2)\frac{\partial x_{2s}}{\partial y}\right] = \tfrac{1}{2}E\left[\frac{\partial (x_{2s} - x_2)^2}{\partial y}\right] = \tfrac{1}{2}\frac{\partial E[(x_{2s} - x_2)^2]}{\partial y}$$

$$= \tfrac{1}{2}\frac{\partial \sigma^2_{x_{2s}}}{\partial y}$$

$$\bar{S}_{22} = E(S_{22s}) - \tfrac{1}{2}\frac{\partial \sigma^2_{x_{2s}}}{\partial y}$$

The second term is rather unexpected; it represents the effect of income on the variance of health expenditure. It seems reasonable to assume that a higher income permits higher medical expenditures in more serious illnesses; hence, one would expect that the variance of medical expenditures would increase with income. Therefore, it is to be presumed *a fortiori* that $\bar{S}_{22}$ is negative and that $W_0 > 0$ when $q > p$. Phelps has taken the absolute values of the residuals from a regression of physician visits on a number of variables including income (see Newhouse and Phelps, 1973) and shown that the correlation with income is slightly negative, in contrast to this argument. However, the effect is small compared with the first term in (16), so that the negativity of $\bar{S}_{22}$ is not in question.

Remark 1   Clearly, when $q = p$ (no insurance at all), then W_0 vanishes completely.

Remark 2   If $dq/dr = 0$, then again $W_0 = 0$. Then by (11), the first term in (9) is 0 and so is the second term, so that $dW/dr = 0$. To bring this out more clearly, notice that the specific definition of r played no role in the analysis; any parameter of the insurance contract would have yielded the same formulas. In particular, r might have been replaced by q everywhere. That is, one could imagine an insurance system in which the government chose the buyer's price, rather than a coinsurance rate, and then let the forces of the market determine seller's price and from that the needed lump-sum taxes. The analysis would have proceeded along the same lines, except that dq/dr would have been replaced by the number 1. If

(17) $$W_0' = \frac{dx_1}{dq} + q\,\frac{dx_2}{dq}$$

then the analogue of (15) is

$$(18) \quad W'_0 = \frac{(q - p)\bar{S}_{22}}{V} \ , \text{ where } V = 1 + (p - q) E \left(\frac{\partial x_{2s}}{\partial y} \right)$$

and (15) itself becomes

$$(19) \quad W_0 = W'_0 \ \frac{dq}{dr}$$

From (9), (10), (11), (18), and (19), one can write Theorem 1.

Theorem 1   A general formula for the marginal effect of an increase in the coinsurance rate on expected welfare is

$$\frac{dW}{dr} = \left[W'_0 E(\lambda_s) - \sigma_{\lambda_s x_{2s}} \right] \frac{dq}{dr}$$

where

$$W'_0 = \frac{(q - p)\bar{S}_{22}}{V} \ , V = 1 + (p - q) E \left(\frac{\partial x_{2s}}{\partial y} \right)$$

and $\bar{S}_{22}$ is given by either of the following formulas:

$$\bar{S}_{22} = \frac{\partial E(x_{2s})}{\partial q} + E(x_{2s}) \frac{\partial E(x_{2s})}{\partial y}$$

$$= E(S_{22s}) - \tfrac{1}{2} \frac{\partial \sigma^2_{x_{2s}}}{\partial y}$$

and S_{22s} is the compensated effect of a change in the price of medical services within a given state. I shall argue in Section 5 that under plausible assumptions the covariance between marginal utility of income and medical services is positive.

It should be pointed out that the welfare effect in Theorem 1 is measured in utility terms and therefore in arbitrary units. Usually, welfare losses are measured in some convenient numeraire. In this case, there is no completely obvious numeraire. Goods other than medical services appear to be the obvious choice, but under conditions of uncertainty this is not a well-defined commodity; one has to distinguish among other goods in different states of health. The simplest numeraire appears to be the composite good consisting of one unit of "other goods" in every state of health. The marginal utility of this composite is $E(\lambda_s)$, and therefore the welfare loss measured in other goods is obtained by dividing dW/dr by $E(\lambda_s)$.

4. THE GENERAL FORMULA FOR WELFARE EFFECTS: TAKING EXPLICIT ACCOUNT OF SUPPLY FACTORS

In the formulas in Theorem 1 I ignored the fact that r was to be interpreted as the coinsurance rate; the formulas are valid for any shift in the insurance scheme or indeed in any other parameter. The specific effect of coinsurance rates is confined to the expression dq/dr, the effect of the coinsurance rate on the buyer's price of medical services. The evaluation requires supply considerations.

In the case of perfectly elastic supply, the seller's price, p, is given by the technology. Since $q = rp$,

(20) $$\frac{dq}{dr} = p$$

when supply is perfectly elastic. Then the expressions in Theorem 1 can be evaluated from demand considerations alone.

Theorem 2   When supply of medical services is perfectly elastic, production of a unit of medical services requires giving up p units of other goods. Then the marginal welfare effect of an increase in the coinsurance rates is

$$\frac{dW}{dr} = [W_0' E(\lambda_s) - \sigma_{\lambda_s x_{2s}}]p$$

where W_0' is defined in the statement of Theorem 1.

The welfare evaluations of medical insurance that have been made (for example, Feldstein, 1973; Pauly, 1968) have assumed perfect elasticity.

The imperfectly elastic case, at least in the short run, is much more realistic. Even in the long run, the production of both physicians and hospital services occurs under such special circumstances that perfect elasticity cannot be taken for granted.

Assume that the supplies of the two types of goods are functions of $p = q/r$; in particular, x_1 and x_2 are functions of p. Let

$$x_i' = \frac{dx_i}{dp} \; (i = 1, 2)$$

Differentiate the equation (1)

$$E(x_{2s}) = x_2(p)$$

with respect to r to solve for dq/dr.

$$(21) \quad E \left(\frac{\partial x_{2s}}{\partial q} \frac{dq}{dr} + \frac{\partial x_{2s}}{\partial y} \frac{dy}{dr} \right) = x_2' \frac{dp}{dr}$$

From (3)

$$\frac{dy}{dr} = (x_1' + qx_2') \frac{dp}{dr} + x_2 \frac{dq}{dr}$$

Any shift in supplies induced by a change in p must lie on the transformation surface; by (4),

$$x_1' + px_2' = 0$$

Hence, as before,

$$x_1' + qx_2' = (q - p)x_2'$$

From (21)

$$E \left(\frac{\partial x_{2s}}{\partial q} + x_2 \frac{\partial x_{2s}}{\partial y} \right) \frac{dq}{dr} = x_2' \left[1 + (p - q) E \left(\frac{\partial x_{2s}}{\partial y} \right) \right] \frac{dp}{dr}$$

or, with the notation defined in the statement of Theorem 1,

$$(22) \quad \bar{S}_{22} \frac{dq}{dr} = x_2' V \frac{dp}{dr}$$

From the identity $p = q/r$,

$$\frac{dp}{dr} = \frac{1}{r} \frac{dq}{dr} - \frac{q}{r^2}$$

Substitute in (22) and solve for dq/dr.

$$(23) \quad \frac{dq}{dr} = \frac{pVx_2'}{x_2' V - r\bar{S}_{22}}$$

From (23) the following observations emerge:
1. since $\bar{S}_{22} < 0$, $dq/dr < p$, if x_2' is finite;
2. if x_2' is infinite (perfect elasticity), $dq/dr = p$;
3. if $x_2' = 0$ (perfect inelasticity), $dq/dr = 0$;
4. as r approaches 0, dq/dr approaches p (this assumes that there is satiation in demand and some elasticity of supply, so that there is a finite equilibrium value of p).

Substituting (23) into Theorem 1, after some simplification, yields Theorem 3.

Theorem 3 Let $x_2(p)$ be the supply function of medical services. Then,

$$\frac{dW}{dr} = \frac{[(q - p)\bar{S}_{22}E(\lambda_s) - V\sigma_{\lambda_s r_{2s}}] px_2'}{Vx_2' - r\bar{S}_{22}}$$

where V and $\overline{S}_{22}$ are defined as in the statement of Theorem 1. The evaluation of this expression depends on econometric estimation of the demand and supply curves and on the evaluation of the covariance term.

5. COVARIANCE BETWEEN MARGINAL UTILITY OF INCOME AND MEDICAL SERVICES

To show that this covariance is positive, it suffices to indicate that both are increasing functions of the state of health. This presupposes that the states of health are measured in order of increasing severity of illness (poor health has a high index number). The desired result is derived from the following assumptions:

A.1.   For fixed levels of medical services and other goods, the marginal rate of substitution of other goods for medical services is an increasing function of the state of health.

A.2.   For fixed levels of medical services and other goods, the marginal utility of other goods does not decrease with the state of health.

A.3.   For a fixed state of health, the utility is jointly concave in medical services and other goods and twice continuously differentiable.

A.4.   For a fixed state of health and a fixed level of medical services, the marginal rate of substitution of other goods for medical services increases with an increase in the amount of other goods.

A.1 amounts to saying that the states of health are ordered in such a way as to make it true; the assumption is not tautological because it does assert that if the marginal rate of substitution increases from one state to another for one pair of values of medical services and other goods, it does so for all.

A.2 means that if an individual is initially given a fixed level of other goods and of medical services for all states of health, he would prefer to switch, if at all, to having the level of other goods rise with illness, if the switch can be made on an actuarially fair basis and if the level of medical services in any state is not subject to change. As Joseph Newhouse has pointed out to me, A.2 is not expected to hold for all states of health (see also Arrow, 1974, p. 5). Certainly, some states of health sharply reduce the value of other goods to the patient; he is too ill to enjoy the consumption and *ex ante* would have preferred to have shifted consumption of other goods to states of better health. In many states of ill health, however, other goods (such as domestic servants and other forms of service, or travel to less demanding climates) may be valued very highly. The result contained in Theorem 4 remains valid if A.2 holds only on the average or even if the marginal utility of other goods falls, but not too rapidly, as the state of health deteriorates.

A.3 is a usual statement of risk aversion. It means that given any two possible pairs (x_1^0, x_2^0) and (x_1^1, x_2^1) of other goods and medical services, the individual would prefer their average to an even chance of getting one or the other.

A.4 is self-explanatory.

I first derive expressions for the rates of change of medical services and of the marginal utility of income with respect to state of health and then show that, under the above assumptions, both are positive.

Differentiate the optimality conditions (6) and the budget equation (5) with respect to s, the state of health.

$$U_{11} \frac{dx_{1s}}{ds} + U_{12} \frac{dx_{2s}}{ds} + \left(-\frac{d\lambda_s}{ds}\right) = -U_{1s}$$

$$U_{21} \frac{dx_{1s}}{ds} + U_{22} \frac{dx_{2s}}{ds} + q\left(-\frac{d\lambda_s}{ds}\right) = -U_{2s}$$

$$\frac{dx_{1s}}{ds} + q\frac{dx_{2s}}{ds} = 0$$

where

$$U_{ij} = \frac{\partial^2 U}{\partial x_{is}\,\partial x_{js}}\,(i, j = 1, 2),\, U_{is} = \frac{\partial^2 U}{\partial x_{ix}\,\partial s}\,(i = 1, 2)$$

We can treat this system in the usual way as linear in the derivatives, dx_{1s}/ds, dx_{2s}/ds, and $-d\lambda_s/ds$. From the second-order conditions for a constrained optimum, the determinant, D, of the above system must be positive. Straightforward use of Cramer's rule yields

(24) $$\frac{dx_{2s}}{ds} = \frac{U_{2s} - qU_{1s}}{D}$$

(25) $$\frac{d\lambda_s}{ds} = \frac{U_{1s}(qU_{21} - U_{22}) + U_{2s}(U_{12} - qU_{11})}{D}$$

Since $q = U_2/U_1$, the numerator of (24) can be written

$$U_2 \left(\frac{U_{2s}}{U_2} - \frac{U_{1s}}{U_1} \right) = U_2 \frac{\partial \log (U_2/U_1)}{\partial s}$$

Since $U_2 > 0$ and, from A.1, U_2/U_1 is increasing in s,

$$\frac{dx_{2s}}{ds} > 0$$

Equivalently,

$$U_{2s} > qU_{1s}$$

From A.4,

$$U_{12} - qU_{11} = U_2 \left(\frac{U_{21}}{U_2} - \frac{U_{11}}{U_1} \right) = U_2 \frac{\partial \log (U_2/U_1)}{\partial s} > 0$$

From the last two relations, the numerator of (25) satisfies the inequality

$$U_{1s}(qU_{21} - U_{22}) + U_{2s}(U_{12} - qU_{11}) > U_{1s}(qU_{21} - U_{22}) + qU_{1s}(U_{12} - qU_{11})$$

$$= -U_{1s}(U_{11}q^2 - 2U_{12}q + U_{22}) \geqslant 0$$

since $U_{1s} \geqslant 0$ by A.2, and

$$U_{11}q^2 - 2U_{12}q + U_{22} \leqslant 0$$

by A.3.

Theorem 4 According to assumptions A.1–A.4, the marginal utility of income is positively correlated with medical expenditures. The covariance constitutes an offsetting risk adjustment to the marginal welfare change with respect to an increase in coinsurance.

In particular, Theorem 4 establishes that some insurance is better than no insurance. From Theorem 1 and from the fact that $V = 1$ when $r = 1$ (that is, $q = p$),

$$\frac{dW}{dr} = -\sigma_{\lambda_s x_{2s}} \frac{dq}{dr} < 0$$

if $dq/dr > 0$.

It appears that nothing further can be estimated on a theoretical basis except for the special case of inelastic supply discussed in the next section. It is not even excluded, so far as I can see, that complete insurance be optimal, although it is unlikely. In that case, $q = 0$; hence, the budget constraint tells us that $x_{1s} = y$, and x_{2s} is determined by the condition

$$\frac{\partial U_s}{\partial x_{2s}} = 0$$

Since medical care is always costly in terms of discomfort and time, we can suppose that the demand will be satiable. The solution to the last equation, when $x_{1s} = y$, will be denoted by x_{2s}^0. When $q = 0$, it is easy to calculate that $D = -U_{22}$. Hence (24) and (25) become

$$\frac{dx_{2s}^0}{ds} = -\frac{U_{2s}}{U_{22}}, \quad \frac{d\lambda_s}{ds} = U_{1s} - \frac{U_{2s}U_{12}}{U_{22}} = U_{1s} + U_{12}\frac{dx_{2s}^0}{ds}$$

The consumption of free medical services is certainly increasing with the state of health (measured to increase with increasing illness); indeed, since the state of health has so far appeared only ordinally, it is reasonable to identify x_{2s}^0 with s, so that $dx_{2s}^0/ds = 1$. Hence,

$$\frac{d\lambda_s}{ds} = U_{1s} + U_{12}, \quad \sigma_{\lambda_s x_{2s}} = \sigma_{\lambda_s s}$$

The relation between marginal utility of income and state of health when medical care is free depends on the cross-effects of state of health and of medical services on the marginal utility of other goods. It can be shown (see Appendix 1) that the covariance in question equals the variance of free medical services multiplied by an average value of the derivative $d\lambda_s/ds = U_{1s} + U_{12}$; in symbols,

$$\sigma_{\lambda_s s} = U\sigma_s^2$$

where U is a weighted average of the values of $U_{1s} + U_{12}$ for varying s.

The risk-aversion term may not vanish even for zero coinsurance. (Remember that this is a term in the *marginal* welfare effect; the risk-aversion welfare gain is of the first order in the coinsurance rate.) It is therefore conceivable that it outweighs the allocation term. In general, the values of U_{1s} and U_{12} should be small, so perfect insurance should not be optimal.

The calculation of $\sigma_{\lambda_s x_{2s}}$ can be made only by assuming specific forms for the utility function and the distribution of states of health. A specific example is developed in Appendix 2.

6. THE CASE OF PERFECTLY INELASTIC SUPPLY

In welfare economics we are accustomed to the argument that when supply is totally inelastic, changes in prices have no welfare effects. The argument may need to be reexamined here because of the presence of uncertainty in demand and the absence of contingent markets; but the conclusion remains valid. It does not seem to have been adequately emphasized in the literature on health insurance that *if the supply of medical care is perfectly inelastic, then there is no welfare effect at all from a change in the coinsurance rate*. There is, however, a rise in the price of medical services paid to the supplier; in a multiperson world this amounts to a redistribution of income to the suppliers of medical services.

This conclusion follows immediately by setting $x_2' = 0$ in Theorem 3. Notice that if x_1 and x_2 are both given, either of the equations (1) has only a single unknown, q; r, the coinsurance rate, does not enter, and income, y, is determined by q, from (3). The equilibrium buyer's price and income are the same for all values of r; in particular, the demands for medical services and for other goods in each state s is the same for all r, and therefore expected utility is independent of r.

The only variable that does change with changing r is p, since $p = q/r$. That is, the price of medical services rises as coinsurance rates fall. The pre-tax income of society is increasingly directed to medical services. To the extent that taxes to pay for medical services do not fall on medical income, there is a transfer of income to the suppliers of medical services. To illustrate, suppose that the cost of medical insurance is paid for by a proportional income tax at a rate t.

$$t = \frac{(p - q)x_2}{x_1 + px_2} = \frac{(1 - r)qx_2}{rx_1 + qx_2}$$

Then, the ratio of post-tax nonmedical incomes to their level with no insurance is

$$\frac{(1 - t)x_1}{x_1} = 1 - t = \frac{r(x_1 + qx_2)}{rx_1 + qx_2}$$

which decreases from 1 toward 0 as r decreases from 1 to 0. Correspondingly, the ratio of post-tax medical incomes to their no-insurance level is

$$\frac{(1 - t)px_2}{qx_2} = \frac{1 - t}{r} = \frac{x_1 + qx_2}{rx_1 + qx_2}$$

which rises from 1 as r decreases.

APPENDIX 1

Covariance of Marginal Utility of Income and Health

Theorem If X is a random variable and $f(X)$ is a function, then $\sigma_{f(X)X} = u\,\sigma_X^2$, where u is a weighted average of $f'(X)$.

Proof Let $g(x)$ be the density of X, a and b the limits of the range of X, $G(x)$ the cumulative distribution of X, and

$$H(x) = \int_a^x yg(y)dy$$

$$\sigma_{f(X)X} = E\left[f(X)X\right] - E(X)E\left[f(X)\right]$$

Integrating by parts,

$$E\left[f(X)X\right] = \int_a^b f(x)xg(x)dx = f(b)H(b) - f(a)H(a) - \int_a^b f'(x)H(x)dx$$

$$E\left[f(X)\right] = \int_a^b f(x)g(x)dx = f(b)G(b) - f(a)G(a) - \int_a^b f'(x)G(x)dx$$

By definition,

$$H(b) = E(X),\ H(a) = 0,\ G(b) = 1,\ G(a) = 0$$

Hence,

$$\sigma_{f(X)X} = \int_a^b f'(x)\left[E(X)G(x) - H(x)\right]dx$$

Let

$$W(X) = E(X)G(x) - H(x)$$

Then,

$$\sigma_{f(X)X} = \int_a^b f'(x)W(x)dx$$

This holds for any function $f(X)$. In particular, let $f(X) = X$, so that $f' = 1$.

$$\sigma_x^2 = \int_a^b W(x)dx$$

so that

$$\sigma_{f(X)X}/\sigma_x^2 = \int_a^b f'(x)w(x)dx$$

where

$$w(x) = W(x)\Big/\int_a^b W(x)dx$$

By construction,

$$\int_a^b w(x)dx = 1$$

To show that $u = \sigma_{f(X)X}/\sigma_X^2$ is a weighted average of $f'(X)$, it suffices to show that $w(x)$ is nonnegative, or, equivalently, that $W(x)$ is nonnegative.

Differentiating,

$$W'(x) = E(X)g(x) - xg(x) = g(x)[E(X) - x]$$

Hence, $W(x)$ is increasing for $x < E(X)$ and decreasing for larger values of x. It has a maximum at $x = E(X)$ and minimums at the extremes, $x = a$ and $x = b$. But $W(a) = 0$, $W(b) = E(X) - H(b) = E(X) - E(X) = 0$, so $W(x) > 0$ for all x, $a < x < b$.

In the text, X is interpreted as the state of health s (as measured by the consumption of medical services, x_{2s}^0, when free) and $f(X)$ is interpreted as the marginal utility of income, λ_s, with the derivative $d\lambda_s/ds = U_{1s} + U_{12}$.

APPENDIX 2

Covariance of Marginal Utility of Income and Medical Services for a Specific Utility Function and Distribution of States of Health

I seek here to illustrate how expressions might be found for the covariance term of Section 5 if assumptions are made about the nature of the utility function and the distribution of medical services for a given coinsurance rate.

Assume that

$$U(x_{1s}, x_{2s}, s) = -(1/c)e^{-cx_{1s}} + U_2(x_{2s}, s)$$

That is, I assume (1) that utility is additive in other goods and in medical services, and (2) the utility function for other goods has constant absolute risk aversion (this assumption is made by Feldstein, 1973). Assume further that the distribution of medical services for a given income and a given coinsurance rate is described by a gamma distribution (see Friedman, 1971),

$$\frac{a^b}{\Gamma(b)} e^{-ax_{2s}}(x_{2s})^{b-1}$$

Then, for any numbers m, n,

$$E(e^{-mX_{2s}}X_{2s}^{n}) = \frac{a^{b}}{\Gamma(b)} \int_{0}^{+\infty} e^{-mx_{2s}}x_{2s}^{n}e^{-ax_{2s}}x_{2s}^{b-1}dx_{2s}$$

$$= \frac{a^{b}}{\Gamma(b)} \int_{0}^{+\infty} e^{-(a+m)x_{2s}}x_{2s}^{n+b-1}dx_{2s}$$

Let

$$y = (a+m)x_{2s}$$

(2.1) $$E(e^{-mX_{2s}}X_{2s}^{n}) = \frac{a^{b}}{\Gamma(b)} \frac{1}{(a+m)^{n+b}} \int_{0}^{+\infty} e^{-y}y^{n+b-1}dy$$

$$= \frac{a^{b}\Gamma(n+b)}{\Gamma(b)(a+m)^{n+b}}$$

If $m = 0$, $n = 1$, we have

$$E(X_{2s}) = \frac{\Gamma(b+1)a^{b}}{\Gamma(b)a^{b+1}} = \frac{b}{a}$$

Since

$$\lambda_{s} = \frac{\partial U}{\partial x_{1s}} = e^{-cx_{1s}} = e^{-c(y-qx_{2s})} = e^{-cy}e^{cqx_{2s}}$$

with the aid of the budget constraint,

$$E(\lambda_{s}) = e^{-cy}E(e^{cqx_{2s}}) = \frac{a^{b}\Gamma(b)e^{-cy}}{\Gamma(b)(a-cq)^{b}} = \frac{a^{b}e^{-cy}}{(a-cq)^{b}}$$

from (2.1), with $m = -cq$ and $n = 0$.
   Then,

$$\sigma_{\lambda_{s}r_{2s}} = E(\lambda_{s}X_{2s}) - E(\lambda_{s})E(X_{2s})$$

$$= E(e^{-cX_{1s}}X_{2s}) - \frac{ba^{b-1}e^{-cy}}{(a-cq)^{b}}$$

$$= e^{-cy}E(e^{cqX_{2s}}X_{2s}) - \frac{ba^{b-1}e^{-cy}}{(a-cq)^{b}}$$

$$= e^{-cy}\left[\frac{a^{b}\Gamma(b+1)}{\Gamma(b)(a-cq)^{b+1}} - \frac{ba^{b-1}}{(a-cq)^{b}}\right]$$

$$= \frac{e^{-cy}ba^{b-1}cq}{(a-cq)^{b+1}}$$

where use is made of (2.1) with $m = -cq$ and $n = 1$.

This calculation is designed to show merely that manageable formulas are not impossible, even though at the cost of strong assumptions. The parameters a and b of the distribution of medical services demanded are in principle observable. The absolute risk aversion cannot be inferred from data on the demand for medical services but is at least inferrable for observed behavior in the presence of uncertainty—for example, the choice of stock portfolios. The assumption of constant absolute risk aversion is uncomfortable; it implies, for example, that the demand for risky assets does not increase with wealth. However, alternative assumptions, such as constant relative risk aversion, do not lead to simple formulas, though in any case they always lead to expressions that can be evaluated numerically.

NOTES

1. This assumption may be false if higher income leads to better living conditions or to preventive medicine, which decreases the probability of serious illnesses. In the present context, the income effects are those arising from changes in the coinsurance rate and could not reasonably loom large.
2. Of course, this is within the context of insurance schemes that are purely linear in medical costs. Indeed, actual insurance plans, with their deductibles followed by coinsurance, are nonlinear and need closer investigation.

REFERENCES

1. Arrow, K. J., "Optimal Insurance and Generalized Deductibles," *Scandinavian Actuarial Journal*, 1974, pp. 1–42.
2. Feldstein, M., "The Welfare Loss of Excess Health Insurance," *Journal of Political Economy*, 81 (March–April 1973), pp. 251–280.
3. Friedman, B. S., "A Study of Uncertainty and Health Insurance," Ph.D. dissertation, Massachusetts Institute of Technology, 1971.
4. Lesourne, J., *Cost-Benefit Analysis and Economic Theory* (Amsterdam: North-Holland, 1975).
5. Pauly, M., "The Economics of Moral Hazard," *American Economic Review*, 68 (June 1968), pp. 531–537.

1 | COMMENTS

William A. Brock
University of Chicago

Kenneth J. Arrow has constructed a miniature general equilibrium model that is, on the surface, especially tailored to answer welfare questions about coinsurance rates. Actually, however, a completely different interpretation can be given to the model that will yield additional insights.

Let $f(s)$ be the density function of states of health. Instead of thinking of

$$(1) \qquad W = E[u(x_{1s}, x_{2s}, s)] = \int u(x_{1s}, x_{2s}, s) f(s) ds$$

as the expected utility of the representative individual, think of it as a welfare function for a society composed of heterogeneous individuals with no uncertainty in which $f(s)$ equals the "*proportion*" of individuals of type s. W is a "natural" welfare function in the sense that it gives equal weight to equal numbers—that is, it is an equal treatment property. (See Arrow and Kurz [1970] for a discussion of welfare functions in growth theory in which the utility of future generations is weighted by their numbers in the social welfare function.) Given this interpretation, Arrow's work looks more like a standard welfare analysis of distortions. If there is only one type s, it *is* a standard distortions analysis and the results of Foster and Sonnenschein (1970) and Kawamata (1972) can be applied to yield theorems on the welfare effects of increased "coinsurance" rates for general n goods models. In most n goods cases, welfare decreases as distortion increases if there is some substitutability in production, and welfare remains the same if supply is perfectly inelastic.

The same can be said for the insurance interpretation of Arrow's model. If there is only one state of health in the world, there is nothing to insure—thus there is nothing to compensate the economy for the welfare loss resulting from the wedge imposed between the selling price and the buying price of medical services.

According to the principle of continuity, this result tells us that we need substantial variations (1) in the utility functions $u(x_{1s}, x_{2s}, s)$ and/or (2) in the density $f(s)$ before insurance has any chance of becoming worthwhile from a welfare point of view. Observations (1) and (2) are brought out fairly clearly in Arrow's Equation (9) and his Theorem 4.

Some diagrams will be useful. These diagrams depict the standard classroom presentation of the welfare analysis of distortions. *OAB* is the transformation frontier. For given $1 > r \equiv q/p =$ buying price/selling price, a distorted equilibrium E is depicted in Figure 1. Distorted equilibrium is a selling price p and a point E such that indifference curve *DF* is tangent to the line with slope $-1/q$ through E, the line through E with slope $-1/p$ is tangent to the transformation frontier, and $r = q/p$. It is intuitive from Figure 1 that E will

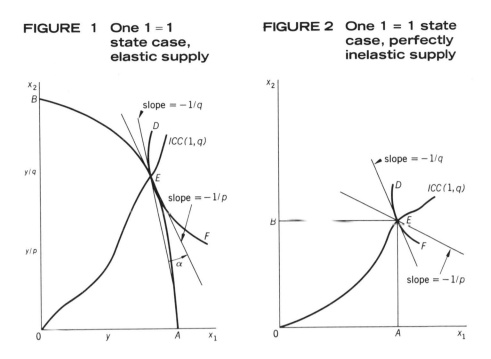

FIGURE 1 One 1 = 1 state case, elastic supply

FIGURE 2 One 1 = 1 state case, perfectly inelastic supply

change when r changes and that welfare will fall when the wedge α increases—i.e., when r decreases, the subsidy to the consumption of medical care increases. It is obvious from Figure 2 that since E does not change when r changes, welfare does not change in the perfectly inelastic supply case. Given r, find distorted equilibrium in Figure 2. Merely find q so that $ICC(1,q)$ passes through the corner point E of AEB and set p so that $r = q/p$. Here $ICC(1,q)$ denotes the income consumption curve of the representative individual as a function of prices $(1,q)$.

Basically, what Arrow has done in his paper is to extend the analysis of figures 1 and 2 to the case of heterogeneous individuals. That is, $ICC(1,q)$ is replaced by

(2) $\int_s ICC_s(1,q)f(s)ds$

where (2) is a vector integral function of q. It is just the vector sum of income consumption curves across s—each ICC_s weighted by $f(s)$. Arrow's analysis in Section 6 points out that W in (1) does not change when r changes for the case of perfectly inelastic supply. It is obvious that the equilibrium E does not change from Figure 2. It is *not* obvious at first glance, however, that W does not change since the *distribution* of demand across individuals may change. I.e., it is not clear that there is *only* one q such that

(3) $\int_s ICC_s(1,q)f(s) = E$

even though, as Arrow correctly points out, q appears only in the left-hand side of Equation (3). Something needs to be assumed to guarantee uniqueness of the solution q to (3). A sufficient condition for uniqueness is

$$\frac{d}{dq}\int_s x_{2s}(1,q)\, ds < 0$$

for q satisfying (3), plus an appropriate boundary condition (see Dierker [1972]). At any rate, r has *no* impact on welfare because r does not affect the *set* of equilibria defined by (3).

It is worth pointing out that distorted equilibrium may not be unique for nonlinear transformation frontiers even though utility is normal in both goods and only one state exists. Normality is sufficient for uniqueness if the transformation frontier is *linear*. (See Foster and Sonnenschein [1970] and Kawamata [1972] for a general discussion.) If equilibrium is not unique, Arrow's differential analysis may break down.

A general uniqueness theorem may be formed by writing the equations that define distorted equilibrium as

(4) $G(q,r) = 0$

Then follow Brock's argument (1973, p. 555). His argument is easily extended to general n goods models with a *vector* of distortions $r \in R^k$ by assuming Dierker's uniqueness condition (1972) for a fixed r_0 and assuming

(5) $$\frac{\partial G}{\partial q}$$

is non-singular on the set $\{q \,|\, G(q,r) = 0\}$ for each r. Just use (5) to prove that the number of equilibria is independent of r and use Dierker's condition for $r = r_0$ to obtain unique equilibrium for *all* r.

Thus, it appears that Arrow's analysis may be extended to n goods models with vectors of distortions. The concept of radial increase in distortion introduced by Foster and Sonnenschein (1970) will probably be needed here.

I think that I have said enough about the mathematics of Arrow's exercise. Let us now turn to the economics. The following points suggest natural lines for extending Arrow's analysis.

1. Arrow assumes only one coinsurance rate r for all states of health. It is natural to ask from the perspective gained by viewing Arrow's model as a model of people of type s if there are incentives for insurance companies to divide states into classes and offer different coinsurance rates for each class and be able to make a profit net of enforcement cost by so doing. Enforcement cost must be paid because a person may try to convince companies that he exists in a state of health that has a different coinsurance rate from the state that he is actually in. Since there is some sort of tradeoff between risk and distortion in Arrow's model, it is natural to perform such a subdivision of the set of states with corresponding coinsurance rates so as to maximize ex-

pected utility, taking into account the resource cost of the subdivision. Under what conditions can private enterprise solve this problem without government intervention? Extending Arrow's model to include such optimum partitioning of the set of states that I suggested above is likely to be important for policy purposes.

Let me expand on this point. Divide states of health into S_1, S_2, where S_1 denotes those states in which the consumption of medical care is very painful (involving radiation therapy, heart surgery, removal of sex organs, etc.) and where S_2 denotes those states in which consumption of medical services is less painful (corrective eyeglasses, minor dentistry, minor cosmetic surgery, treatment of baldness, nose jobs, sex therapy at Masters and Johnson, etc.). Quite clearly, one would want a higher coinsurance rate for S_2 states.

It seems to mo that a very interesting general theory could be built by *explicitly* modeling the amount of overconsumption in a given class of states as a function of the particular characteristics of the medical services—a Lancaster-Becker type of approach.

In a world in which the law of large numbers applies, it seems possible that private enterprise would solve the problem without government intervention subject to solving the difficulties pointed out by Rothschild and Stiglitz (1973) and Wilson (1973). Obviously, incentives will be set up to subdivide states of health in order to capture the efficiency losses, but equilibrium may not exist if differentiation generates lumpy costs (Rothschild and Stiglitz, 1973; Wilson, 1973). It may be that some kind of equilibrium may exist if the "cost" of subdividing sets of states is explicitly modeled.

2. Is the optimal choice of *r* in Arrow's problem *enforceable* in the sense that it will be sustained by a competitive insurance industry? Since it is probably not enforceable in this sense, will it be enforceable at reasonable administrative cost?

3. The model needs to be disaggregated into different classes of people if it is to be part of a "project to study the financing of medical care services for the poor and near-poor" (Arrow, 1973, p. iii). But this should be a relatively routine extension of Arrow's basic theory.

REFERENCES

1. Arrow, K. J., "Welfare Analysis of Changes in Health Coinsurance Rates," R-1281-OEO, The Rand Corporation, November 1973.
2. _____., and M. Kurz, *Public Investment, the Rate of Return, and Optimal Fiscal Policy* (Baltimore: The Johns Hopkins Press, 1970).
3. Brock, W. A., "Some Results on the Uniqueness of Steady States in Multi-Sector Models of Optimum Growth when Future Utilities Are Discounted," *International Economic Review,* 14 (October 1973), pp. 535–559.
4. Dierker, E., "Two Remarks on the Number of Equilibria of an Economy," *Econometrica*, 40 (1972), pp. 951–954.

5. Foster, E., and H. Sonnenschein, "Price Distortion and Economic Welfare," *Econometrica*, 38 (March 1970), pp. 281–297.
6. Kawamata, K., "Price Distortion and Potential Welfare," Ph.D. dissertation, University of Minnesota, 1972.
7. Rothschild, M., and J. Stiglitz, "Analysis of Equilibrium in Insurance Markets," Departments of Economics, Princeton and Yale universities, 1973.
8. Wilson, C., "An Analysis of Simple Insurance Markets with Imperfect Differentiation of Consumers," University of Rochester, December 1973.

Isaac Ehrlich

University of Chicago and
National Bureau of Economic Research

Professor Arrow's paper addresses the welfare implications of changes in health coinsurance rates in a rigorous and stimulating fashion. It formally restates the ubiquitous moral hazard argument within a general equilibrium setting in which the effects of changes in coinsurance rates on the demand for and the supply of medical care are considered simultaneously. The paper also systematically considers the effects of coinsurance rate changes on the presumed utility costs of risk-bearing under some restrictive assumptions concerning the relation between preferences for goods and medical care services and various states of health. Both analyses, rigorous throughout, are developed with admirable clarity and simplicity. In the course of this investigation Arrow develops an intuitively plausible, though generally unrecognized, proposition. He shows that if the supply of medical services is perfectly inelastic, then changes in coinsurance rates—indeed, any changes in the terms under which market health insurance is provided—would have no effects on welfare. As he has already taught us in his analysis of employer or co-worker discrimination,[1] the existence of discrimination under perfectly inelastic supplies of relevant factors may affect only the distribution of income among various groups in the economy without engendering any allocative effects. In this study Arrow has developed a similar proposition under conditions of uncertainty by demonstrating that when the supply of relevant goods is perfectly inelastic, the expected utility of a representative individual is unaffected by an increase in the wedge between buyer's and seller's price of medical care brought about by a reduction in the health coinsurance rate.

Yet I have a basic reservation concerning the generality of the analysis of welfare effects associated with changes in health coinsurance rates as developed in this paper. My reservation stems from the implicit assumption from which the welfare implications have been derived that there are no close substitutes or complements to market health insurance, or, put differently, that coverage of medical care expenditures via a market insurance contract is the only means of shifting related financial risks. But surely various alternative means of "insurance" are available that may reduce vulnerability to illness, its severity, or, in general, the burden of medical care expenditures associated with poor states of health. I call these means "self-insurance" and "self-protection."[2] Things like nonprescription drugs, health foods and diets, physical exercise, frequent (uninsured) medical check-ups or, in general, the effective practice of "preventive medicine" are illustrative. Indeed, there are even more general methods of risk-shifting or self-insurance, such as dependence on family members or friends to assume financial responsibilities and to provide some health care services in poor states of health, or the choice of specific occupations and residential locations in which specific health risks are relatively low. The base of the argument I wish to develop in connection with these alternative means of health insurance is that they, like insurance-induced consumption of medical care services, draw scarce resources away from the production of other goods and services. Preventive care may be quite costly in terms of time and other resource expenditures, and raising large families as a means of shifting financial risks seems an inferior method of insurance. Since the availability of market health Insurance does not eliminate expenditure of resources on self-insurance and self-protection, the relevant question from a welfare point of view is how changes in health coinsurance rates affect the *overall* allocation of resources to the general "health" sector encompassing both market- and self-insured health services and the transaction costs of insurance. In general, one may not be able to answer this question unambiguously without referring to the relative efficiency or inefficiency implicit in the provision of each form of insurance at the margin.

To illustrate the argument more pointedly I shall assume, merely for expositional convenience, that medical care outlays do not enhance utility directly, but rather are dictated as an objective medical requirement following the onset of poor states of health. Put differently, given the state of health, the demand for medical care services is perfectly inelastic.[3] Poor states of health are assumed to affect consumers' welfare mainly via their impact on the magnitude of the ensuing financial liabilities. These entail both direct costs of medical care and the opportunity costs of sick days, which are assumed to be monotonically related to expenditures on medical care (for simplicity, non-pecuniary costs are ignored). I shall also make the symmetrical assumption that preventive care and other means of self-insurance are not desired per se but only as means of shifting health risks, and that their sole impact is to reduce the extent of financial liabilities (medical care expenditures in particular) without affecting the probabilities that such states would occur.[4] That is to say, more self-insurance merely reduces the outlays on medical care services during poor states of health. Under these assumptions, an optimal allocation of resources between market-insured medical care (including transaction costs of insurance) and self-insurance services would equate the shadow price of transferring income between any two states of health via self-insurance and the corresponding market (health) insurance terms of exchange of income.

Figure 1 is an equilibrium for which a representative individual is faced with only two states of health: good health (g) with probability $1 - p$ and poor health (b) with probability p. Let us denote the person's income in state g by I^e; his loss function from poor health by $L(c)$, L being conditional on self-insurance expenditure in the amount of c "dollars"; the magnitude of market insurance purchased by s—the net income added to the insuree's income in state b via market insurance (the absolute amount of $L(c)$ covered through market insurance net of the premium paid); and the market health insurance implicit terms of exchange between net income in states b and g (defined in terms of state g's income) by π. The optimal combination of market and self-insurance occurs where [5]

(1)
$$\pi = - \frac{1}{L'(c) + 1}$$

In equilibrium, the market insurance line is tangent to the transformation curve of income between states g and b as determined by the productivity of self-insurance (point A in Figure 1). If there were no transaction costs associated with the provision of health insurance and if, as in Arrow's system, the amount collected in premiums exactly matched the expected amount of medical care expenditures covered by insurance, then the price of insurance would be actuarially fair, $\pi = p/(1 - p)$; the optimal coinsurance rate would be zero; and Equation (1) could be restated as $-pL'(c) = 1$, or by approximation

(2)
$$p \Delta L = \Delta c$$

where $p \Delta L$ denotes the expected absolute value of the marginal reduction in the financial costs of illness (its actual value for the representative individual)[6] and Δc is the marginal expenditure on self-insurance. Since in practice the transaction costs of market insurance may be nonnegligible, let $\pi = (1 + \lambda)p/(1 - p)$, where λ denotes the net loading factor (the proportion by which π exceeds the fair price of insurance). Then the optimal coinsurance rate would be greater than zero, and by similar analysis it can easily be shown that in this case

(3)
$$p \Delta L + \lambda p (\Delta L - \Delta c) = \Delta c$$

where, as before, $p \Delta L$ denotes the expected reduction in health-related losses and $\lambda p (\Delta L - \Delta c)$ represents the corresponding expected reduction in the transaction costs of insurance.[7] In a welfare-maximizing equilibrium position, the sum of these two terms must equal the marginal cost of self-insurance. Notice that for the representative individual, a decrease in the demand for self-insurance services and an increase in the demand for insured medical care services, for example, may involve a reduction in the price of self-insurance services and an increase in the price of medical care services if the relevant supply curves were upward sloping. Since a representative individual may be assumed to be both a producer and a user of health care and health insurance services, his expected utility would be affected only by real exchanges between self-insurance services and market-insured medical care. L, c, and s, the basic variables of the model, therefore will be defined throughout the following analysis in real rather than nominal terms.

Clearly, market health insurance, s, and self-insurance services, c, are substitutes in the sense that a decrease in the (real) price of one induces a greater demand for the other.[8] Moreover, any exogenous decrease in self-

FIGURE 1

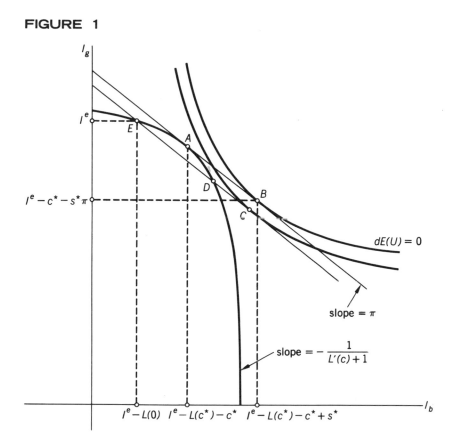

$$I_g$$

$$I^e$$

$$E$$

$$A$$

$$D$$

$$B$$

$$C$$

$$I^e - c^* - s^* \pi$$

$$dE(U) = 0$$

$$\text{slope} = \pi$$

$$\text{slope} = -\frac{1}{L'(c)+1}$$

$$I^e - L(0) \quad I^e - L(c^*) - c^* \quad I^e - L(c^*) - c^* + s^*$$

$$I_b$$

insurance would, by assumption, expand the potential losses from ill health and, hence, would increase the demand for coinsured medical care. Similarly, an exogenous decrease in health coinsurance rates, which necessarily implies an increase in s, unambiguously would lead to reduced resource expenditures on self-insurance, an increase in the actual losses in states of poor health, and an increase in the demand for medical care services (see Note 8). As long as the supply of market-insured medical services and self-insurance services are not perfectly inelastic, an exogenous change in health coinsurance rates is thus expected to generate allocative effects. However, the net effect on welfare depends on the overall change in the actual amount of resources allocated to medical care, market insurance, and self-insurance activities.

If the initial equilibrium position were optimal, then the welfare implications of changes in health coinsurance rates would be readily evident: any *exogenous* change in these rates would bring about an increase in the total amount of resources allocated to market- and self-insured health care services and a reduction in the market value of personal income (indicated by the height of the market insurance lines in Figure 1). The expected utility of a representative individual will fall. As Figure 1 illustrates, expected utility would decrease following any change in the market and self-insurance nexus away from points A and B, corresponding to the optimal values s^* and c^*. This is seen, for example, by a shift from the initial equilibrium to, say, points E and C following an exogenous decrease in self-insurance expenditure and a consequent decrease in the health coinsurance rate (and an increase in market insurance purchased). But precisely the same reduction in expected utility would be associated with an exogenous increase in self-insurance and a resulting decrease in market insurance and the health coinsurance rate relative to their optimal magnitudes (compare points D and C with A and B).The important implication of this analysis is that in comparing situations in which coinsurance rates are *suboptimal*, one cannot determine unambiguously whether a reduction in the coinsurance rate would increase or lessen the misallocation of resources. A reduction in health coinsurance rates could be corrective if, for example, initially self-insurance were less efficient than market insurance at the margin so that Equation (3) were an inequality such that

(4) $\quad p\,\Delta L + \lambda p\,(\Delta L - \Delta c) < \Delta c$

In this case more market insurance and medical care and less self-insurance services would be desirable.

Professor Arrow has focused attention on an important welfare issue associated with health coinsurance rates—namely, the potential resource misallocation arising from an increase in the wedge between buyers' and sellers' prices when the demand for health care services in each state of health is elastic with respect to its price. It has been argued in this comment, however, that in order to adequately analyze the direction of welfare effects resultings from (exogenous) changes in health coinsurance rates, one would wish to consider jointly the production of market-insured health services and alternative health insurance activities, including specific uninsured medical services. Since Arrow's general formula describing welfare effects does not account for resource shifts involving such alternatives to market-insured health services, empirical estimates of welfare effects relying solely on this formula would not appear to be complete.

NOTES

1. See Arrow (1973).
2. See Ehrlich and Becker (1972).
3. This assumption does not imply that the demand for insured medical care is unresponsive to changes in the coinsurance rate or the underlying price of insurance. As the following analysis demonstrates, a reduction in the coinsurance rate—an increase in the coverage ratio of ill-health-related losses—generally would enhance the demand for insured medical care because of a substitution away from self-insurance toward market insurance.
4. The analysis of the interaction between market health insurance and self-protection efforts designed to reduce the likelihood of states of ill health is more complicated than the analysis of

the interaction between market insurance and loss-reducing self-insurance, which is why the first analysis is ignored here. However, the basic implications developed in the following analysis concerning the welfare effects of changes in health coinsurance rates are general and would hold equally well when one's own efforts were expected to reduce the probabilities of poor states of health as well as the severity of illness and other related losses in such states.

5. The equilibrium condition is arrived at through maximization of the expected utility function

(1a) $E(U) = (1-p)U(I^e - c - s\pi) + pU[I^e - L(c) - c + s]$

with respect to c and s. Alternatively, let the coverage ratio (1 minus the coinsurance rate) be denoted by ∂ and let the loading factor be defined in terms of the gross amount paid in claims, $\lambda' \equiv (k-1)$. One then can proceed by maximizing the expected utility function

(1b) $E(U) = (1-p)U\left[I^e - c - kp\,\partial L(c)\right] + pU\left[I^e - c - \{1 - \partial(1-kp)\}L(c)\right]$

directly with respect to c and δ. The equilibrium condition then would be given by

(1c)
$$-\frac{1 + kp\,\partial L'(c)}{1 + [1 - \partial(1 - kp)]L'(c)} = \frac{kp}{1 - kp}$$

Notice that since self-insurance is assumed to be effective, the term $L'(c) + 1$ in Equation (1) is less than or equal to zero. The function $L(c)$ is also assumed to be continuously differentiable and convex.

6. Following Arrow's analysis, I assume that health risks are independently distributed among a large number of individuals, so that the expected change in resources devoted to market-insured medical care would be the same as the actual resources devoted to accomodate the representative individual.

7. Alternatively, using Equation (1c) in Note 5, the equilibrium condition can be restated more simply in terms of the gross loading factor as follows

(3a) $(1 + \lambda')p\Delta L = \Delta c$

8. Strictly speaking, this theorem holds unambiguously only insofar as the relation between $_c$ and $_s$, not the coverage ratio, ∂, is concerned. However, an *exogenous* increase in ∂, given L, implies an increase in the quantity of insurance, since quantity of insurance is defined by $s = \partial L(1 - kp)$. Furthermore, it can easily be shown through appropriate differentiations of Equation (1b) in Note 5 and utilization of the assumption that individuals are risk averse that an exogenous decrease in the coinsurance rate $r = 1 - \partial$ would necessarily reduce the optimal value of self-insurance expenditures, c. Such a decrease in r would thus raise L, hence the demand for (insured) medical care services, and the quantity of insurance purchased, s

REFERENCES

1. Arrow, Kenneth J., "The Theory of Discrimination," in Orly Ashenfelter and Albert Rees (editors), *Discrimination in Labor Markets* (Princeton: Princeton University Press, 1973).
2. Ehrlich, Isaac, and Gary Becker, "Market Insurance, Self-Insurance and Self-Protection," *Journal of Political Economy*, 80 (July–August 1972), pp. 623–648.

2

G. NORDQUIST
and
S. WU
University of Iowa

The Joint Demand for Health Insurance and Preventive Medicine

1. INTRODUCTION

In this paper we investigate the nature and properties of the joint demand for health insurance and preventive medicine. Our decision-maker is a globally risk-averse person whose welfare depends on his consumption and health. The decision horizon spans two periods, the present and the future. Present income and health are assumed to be given, but future income is uncertain because it depends on an uncertain future state of health. We suppose that the individual can manage this uncertainty in two

This paper represents an amalgamation of two earlier papers: "A Model of Demand for Preventive Medicine under Uncertainty," by Nordquist, and "The Consumer's Demand for Medical Goods and Services," by Wu. We wish to thank the conference participants, and especially R. Berg, M. Grossman, and S. Rosen, for many helpful comments. Notes 1, 4, and 7 have been added in partial response. We are indebted to our colleagues, M. Balch, J. Jeffers, and J. Heckman, for their help on earlier drafts. Of course, we alone assume responsibility for any shortcomings that may remain.

ways: (1) by purchasing an insurance policy that promises benefits (money payoffs) contingent on his future state of health, and (2) by choosing a bundle of medical goods and services called preventive medicine that promises to influence his future health prospect. Preventive medicine, unlike ordinary consumption, has little or no direct effect on utility; its value arises mostly from the beneficial changes it produces in the consumer's health prospect. We recognize, however, that many ordinary consumer goods play a dual role: They not only yield utility directly but also influence the health prospect. Although the main portion of this paper is devoted to what might be appropriately called "the pure aspects of insurance and prevention," the effect of including goods that play a dual role is examined in a separate section. Regardless of these variations, our basic premise is that the consumer will choose present outlays on health insurance and preventive medicine so as to maximize expected utility.[1]

Notice that insurance and prevention are alternative but fundamentally different approaches to planning for future health and welfare. Barring moral hazard of one kind or another, health insurance permits a person to alter the *payoffs* of a random experiment in which poor health is a possibility without affecting its probability. More specifically, the market insurance enables the consumer to *redistribute* his wealth from the present to the more hazardous, uncertain future. Prevention, on the other hand, alters the prospect for future health without changing the payoffs (except inasmuch as prevention may not be a free good).[2]

In an uncertain setting there are two ways to characterize the individual's preferences for present and future consumption. First, we might suppose that they are essentially unaffected by his state of health, in which case we characterize the individual's expected utility in the framework of von Neumann-Morgenstern. Symbolically,

$$Eu = \int_0^1 u(C_1, c_2) dF(h; \cdot)$$

where u is a von Neumann-Morgenstern utility index; C_1 and c_2, respectively, are the levels of present and future consumption; $h \epsilon$ (0,1) is the state of health; and F is the probability distribution function of h. Alternatively, we might insist that health has a conditional influence on consumer preferences—that the health state should really be an explicit argument in the utility function. In this case we describe the individual's expected utility in the framework of what some have characterized as conditional expected utility (Balch and Fishburn, 1974) and others, as the state-dependent approach to expected utility (Arrow, 1973). This expected utility is symbolically represented by

$$Eu^* = \int_0^1 u^*(C_1, c_2, h)dF(h; \cdot)$$

where u^* is a state-dependent utility index. Notice that in both of these expected utility formulations the probability distributions of h depend on various parameters. The analyses based on these alternative approaches are somewhat different and both require lengthy developments. Owing to limitation of space, we will restrict our analysis in this paper to the von Neumann-Morgenstern formulation.[3]

Now let us turn our attention to the constraints. First, define a health insurance policy by the pair $[I, x(h)I]$, where I is the stated premium, and $x(h)I$ is the total future payoff or benefit. Moreover, let ρI, $0 \leq \rho \leq 1$, be the private cost of insurance to the individual. The difference $(1 - \rho)I$ is the contribution of some third party such as employer or government. The consumer's present consumption, C_1, depends on his current income, Y_1, and current outlays for health insurance, ρI, preventive medicine, Z, and saving, S; i.e.,

$$C_1 = Y_1 - \rho I - Z - S$$

Future consumption, c_2, depends on future income, y_2; a schedule of health insurance payoffs, x; and the gross yield on savings, rS. Both y_2 and x are functions of the future random health state h and are therefore uncertain;[4] hence,

$$c_2(h) = y_2(h) + x(h)I + rS$$

Of course, the gross yield on savings may also be taken as random.

In the following development, we suppose that ordinary saving is identically equal to zero. Although the formal inclusion of saving presents little difficulty in either the specification or the solution of our problem, it does complicate the presentation. Furthermore, upon reflection one sees that saving and insurance are alike in that they both involve an intertemporal redistribution of income— insurance can be regarded as saving for specific future contingencies. The difference, of course, is that the yield on savings is not likely to be closely related to the state of health. In any case, we feel that the roles played by insurance and saving are sufficiently similar so that the exclusion of saving does not significantly weaken our solution.

Formally the consumer's choice problem now becomes

(1)   Maximize $Eu = \int_0^1 u(C_1, c_2)dF(h; \cdot)$
        I, Z

(2)   subject to $C_1 = Y_1 - \rho I - Z$

(3) $c_2 = y_2(h) + x(h)I$

where u is a von Neumann-Morgenstern utility index. We assume that the utility function possesses continuous first-, second-, and third-order derivatives.

We think that this model is of interest not only because of its bearing on the demand for health insurance and medical services but also because it represents a generalization of recent literature on the question of the optimal saving decision under uncertainty. Leland (1966) has analyzed precautionary saving when future income is uncertain. Sandmo (1969) has examined the case wherein the yield on saving is uncertain. In our model not only are both future income and the return on saving (or to be exact, the payoff from insurance) taken as random but we also permit the consumer to influence the distribution function of the random variable.[5]

This paper is divided into five sections. Section 2 introduces and defines three important concepts in our study. Section 3 develops the basic model in which the distribution of future health is assumed to depend on (1) the consumer's present outlay for prevention, and (2) an exogenous index of the future health environment. Section 4 extends the analysis to the case in which the distribution also depends on present consumption. Finally, in Section 5 we summarize our findings and suggest some policy implications. The proofs of various propositions have been placed in the Appendix to relieve the text of any cumbersomeness.

2. THREE RELEVANT CONCEPTS

In recent years there have been rather rapid advancements in theoretical concepts dealing with problems related to the economics of uncertainty. The concepts of stochastic dominance, risk aversion, and moral hazard play important roles in this paper. A brief specification of each of these concepts follows.

Stochastic Dominance

Stochastic dominance is a set of rules for ordering risky prospects (Hadar and Russell, 1971). Since we are dealing with a risk-averse consumer, it is appropriate to assume that prospects are ordered by second-degree stochastic dominance, denoted by $\mathcal{D}$.

Definition 1. Let $F(\theta)$ and $G(\theta)$ be two distinct probability distributions of the random variable θ, where $\theta \epsilon (0,1)$. Then $G \mathcal{D} F$ if and only if

$$\int_0^h G(\theta)d\theta \leq \int_0^h F(\theta)d\theta, \text{ for all } h \epsilon (0,1)$$

Now let $F(\theta,x)$ be the distribution function of the random variable θ, where x is a vector of shift parameters. ($F(\theta,x^0)$ is a given prospect of θ.) Assume that F_i and F_{ij} exist for all x_i and x_j and that they are continuous. Let h denote the health index, where $h \epsilon (0,1)$.

Definition 2. Let

$$R(h,x) = \int_0^h F(\theta,x)d\theta, \; h \epsilon (0,1)$$

$[1 - R(h,x)]$ is the measure of the stochastic size of a given health prospect.

Notice that definitions 1 and 2 imply that as F becomes larger, its size becomes smaller, and vice versa.

Definition 3. A factor (parameter) x_i is said to be beneficial (harmful) to the consumer's health prospect if

$$R_i = \int_0^h F_i d\theta < 0 \; (> 0)$$

If a factor x_i is beneficial to the consumer's health prospect, it is also plausible to assume that it exhibits diminishing returns. Likewise, if x_i is harmful to the consumer's health prospect, we assume that the harm will increase at an increasing rate. In both cases,[6]

$$R_{ii} > 0$$

Definition 4. The factors x_i and x_j are said to be biased toward benefit if $R_{ij} \leq 0$ and toward harmfulness if $R_{ij} \geq 0$.

Notice from our definitions that two factors may be biased toward benefit (harmfulness) regardless of the benefit or harm each one may produce on its own. For example, two factors could be benefit-biased even though each is classified as harmful, although it is difficult to think of good examples.

As previously indicated, we suppose that there are three factors that can directly affect the distribution function F, two of which are the consumer's present outlays for consumption and prevention, and the third being the general health environment that is beyond the consumer's influence. The inclusion of the choice variables Z and C_1 as parameters in F is not standard and warrants further elaboration. Since these effects turn out to be very similar, we restrict our discussion here to the effect of Z on F.

Suppose that the individual has access to a set of future health prospects wherein each prospect $F \epsilon \mathcal{F}$ is a probability distribution associated with an expenditure level Z. The mapping from Z to $\mathcal{F}$ is, however, not one-to-one. A person does not literally purchase a health prospect. Rather, he buys a particular bundle or mix of medical goods and services with a given sum of money. Since each expenditure level may purchase several, perhaps many, mixes of medical goods and services, there corresponds to each Z a whole set of health prospects $\mathcal{F}_Z$. Stochastic dominance permits us to confine our attention to the efficient set of prospects on the boundary of $\mathcal{F}_Z$. The concept asserts that for all risk-averse individuals a prospect G is preferred to a prospect F if and only if G is larger than F, as specified in Definition 1. Hence, we can assume that for a given Z our consumer will always choose a mix of medical goods and services that yields a dominant prospect as ordered by the relation $\mathcal{D}$.

Let $F^e(h,Z')$ be the dominant (i.e., the largest) probability distribution corresponding to the expenditure level Z'. As shown in Figure 1, $F^e(h,Z') \mathcal{D} F(h,Z')$ if in the closed interval $(0,h)$ the area under the distribution function $F^e(h,Z')$ is no greater than the area under any other distribution function $F(h,Z')$. The connection between R and Z is shown in Figure 2. For the expenditure level $Z', R(h,Z')$ is inversely related to the size of the distribution $F(h,Z')$. The region has an upper bound equal to 1, which reflects the worst possible health state regardless of the amount of money spent to

FIGURE 1

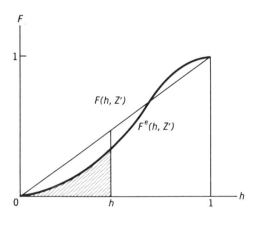

FIGURE 2

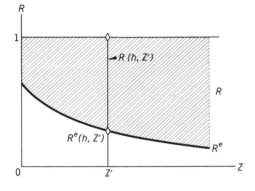

prevent it. The lower bound $R^e \epsilon \mathcal{R}$ is the locus of points representing the size of the dominant distribution for each and every conceivable outlay on preventive medicine. It is reasonable to assume that the efficiency frontier R^e decreases monotonically and is convex, reflecting both the general benefits to future health derived from larger outlays on preventive medicine and the diminishing marginal effectiveness of such activity.

Risk Aversion

When an individual's utility function is represented by a von Neumann-Morgenstern utility index $\phi(W)$ with $\phi'(W) > 0$, where W denotes his wealth, the individual is said to be globally risk averse if $\phi''(W) < 0$ for all W. To measure the *degree* of risk averseness, Arrow (1971, Ch. 3) and Pratt (1964) have defined a coefficient of absolute risk aversion

$$R_A(W) = - \frac{\phi''(W)}{\phi'(W)}$$

where, for small risks, R_A is a function of the maximum sum, or insurance premium, that the individual is willing to pay in order to avoid a given risk. It is generally supposed that an increase in the individual's wealth will reduce the maximum premium that he is willing to pay; i.e.,

$$\frac{dR_A}{dW} < 0$$

This proposition is widely known as the hypothesis of decreasing absolute risk aversion.

In the temporal framework postulated in this paper, the individual's utility function is represented by a von Neumann-Morgenstern utility index $u(C_1,c_2)$, where C_1 and c_2 denote present and future consumption, respectively, with C_1 certain and c_2 uncertain. With respect to future consumption, the individual is said to be risk averse if $u_{22}(C_1,c_2) < 0$. To measure the individual's aversion to risk, Sandmo (1969) has suggested the temporal risk-aversion coefficient

$$A(C_1,c_2) = - \frac{u_{22}(C_1,c_2)}{u_2(C_1,c_2)}$$

where $A(C_1,c_2)$ is also a function of the maximum premium that the individual is willing to pay when faced with a given risk. Analogous to the Arrow-Pratt hypothesis of decreasing absolute risk aversion, Sandmo proposed the following for the two-period case:

Definition 5. The individual's preferences are said to exhibit decreasing temporal risk aversion if

$$\frac{\partial A(C_1,c_2)}{\partial C_1} > 0 \text{ and } \frac{\partial A(C_1,c_2)}{\partial c_2} < 0$$

According to the principle of decreasing temporal risk aversion, (1) the higher the individual's present consumption, the greater the risk premium he is willing to pay in order to avoid a given gamble on future consumption, and (2) the higher his future consumption, the lower will be the risk premium. Notice that

$$\frac{\partial A(C_1,c_2)}{\partial C_1} > 0 \text{ implies that } u_{122}(C_1,c_2) < 0$$

and

$$\frac{\partial A(C_1,c_2)}{\partial c_2} < 0 \text{ implies that } u_{222}(C_1,c_2) > 0$$

Moral Hazard

In order to take advantage of the law of large numbers, suppliers of insurance must maintain safeguards so that the underlying stochastic law is not undermined as a consequence of providing the service. More specifically, the insurer must be certain that the act and the manner of insuring persons against a hazardous event or misfortune does not increase the frequency of its occurrence or amount of the claim. Often, the insured has the power to increase the probability of a hazardous event—either through deceptive or fraudulent behavior or through legitimate means.[7]

Definition 6. Moral hazard refers to the phenomenon whereby the method of insurance and the form of the insurance policy affect the behavior of the insured and, therefore, the probabilities on which the insurance company has relied (Arrow, 1971, Chs. 8 and 9; Pauly, 1968).

The presence of moral hazard is a real cost in the production of insurance protection and, hence, a genuine limit to its supply. Completely apart from the opportunities for fraudulent behavior, moral hazard arises in our problem because the consumer of health insurance can affect his future health prospect by changing his present pattern of consumption. If a change in the terms of the policy $(\rho I, x(h)I)$ causes the individual to purchase more insurance and less prevention, we have a clear instance of "moral" hazard.

Preliminary inspection of the constraints in our model also suggests several possible sources of moral hazard. It seems reasonable to suppose that pre-insurance income is a monotone increasing concave function of the health state reflecting diminishing returns; i.e., $y_2'(h) > 0$ and $y_2''(h) < 0$. Of course, post-insurance income can take many forms, depending on the payoffs $x(h)I$. Obviously, the insurance company would try to avoid the sale of contracts that (1) would make post-insurance income in better health states smaller than in worse health states, and (2) would make any payments in the state of perfect health. In order to avoid these pitfalls, the insurance company must offer a payoff schedule satisfying

Condition 1. $y_2(h) + x'(h)I > 0$ $\qquad$ for all $h \epsilon (0,1)$

and

Condition 2. $x(h)I$ $\begin{cases} = 0 & \text{for } h = 1 \\ < y_2(1) - y_2(h) & \text{for } h = 0 \end{cases}$

These conditions imply a monotonic decreasing payoff schedule.

Furthermore, in order to increase the size of a policy without inducing moral hazard, the insurance company will never choose a concave payoff schedule. Abstracting from the use of deductibles, we show that, given any concave schedule, there always exists a non-concave schedule that will yield a greater revenue for the insurance company. Let $x(h)$ in Figure 3 be a concave payoff

FIGURE 3

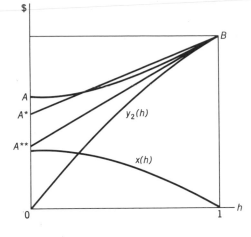

schedule and let $(I^0, x(h)I^0)$ be the largest insurance policy an individual can buy without violating conditions 1 and 2. In order to facilitate our analysis, let us construct a new curve, BA, where $BA = y_2(1) - x(h)I^0$. If $[I^0, x(h)I^0]$ is the maximum insurance policy given $x(h)$, then BA is tangent to OB at the point B. Now let $[I^*, x^*(h)I^*]$ be a policy with a linear payoff schedule $x^*(h)$, which is actuarially equivalent to $[I^0, x(h)I^0]$, and let $BA^* = y_2(I) - x^*(h)I^*$. Then it is evident that $[I^*, x^*(h)I^*]$ is not the largest policy that can be sold under the restriction of conditions 1 and 2. The largest linear policy is $[I^{**}, x^*(h)I^{**}]$, where $I^{**} > I^*$, with $BA^{**} = y_2(1) - x^*(h)I^{**}$. Following the same reasoning, a payoff schedule convex to the origin may improve the insurance company's revenue still further. In order to avoid violating conditions 1 and 2, however, the payoff schedule cannot be excessively convex. In fact, the limiting BA curve for convex schedules is OB itself. This result leads to a further restriction on the payoff schedule.

Condition 3. $x''(h) \geq 0$ and $y_2''(h) + x''(h)I < 0$

From these conditions we see that insurance companies must steer a fine course between "the rock" of moral hazard and the "whirlpool" of unattractive and unsalable policies. Ideally, coverage should be carefully tailored to the requirement of every client, but the heterogeneity of the population and the cost of information place definite limitations on this approach. Various devices such as coinsurance and deductibles are used, and though some work better than others, it is readily apparent that none is perfect.

3. THE BASIC MODEL

In this section we present the model in which it is assumed that the consumer maximizes a von Neumann-Morgenstern expected utility with the probability distribution of the health index dependent only on preventive medicine and the general health environment. From equations (1)–(3) we see that the consumer's problem is to choose I and Z so as to maximize[8]

(4) $$U(I,Z) = \int_0^1 u[Y_1 - \rho I - Z, y_2(h,\alpha) + x(h,\beta)I]dF(h;Z,\gamma)$$

where Y_1, α, ρ, β, and γ are parameters. The following assumptions are imposed both to generate stability of equilibrium and to produce some meaningful predictions concerning various equilibrium displacements.

Assumption 1. The consumer's utility function is strictly concave, and present and future consumption are noncompetitive; i.e.,

$$u_{11}, u_{22} < 0 \text{ and } u_{12} \geq 0$$

Assumption 2. The consumer exhibits decreasing temporal risk aversion; i.e.,

$$\frac{\partial A}{\partial C_1} > 0 \text{ and } \frac{\partial A}{\partial c_2} < 0$$

Assumption 3. Both pre-insurance and post-insurance future income are increasing concave functions of the future health state; i.e.,

$y_2'(h) > 0$ and $y_2''(h) < 0$, and $y_2'(h) + x'(h)I > 0$ and $y_2''(h) + x''(h)I < 0$, for $h \in (0,1)$

Assumption 4. The insurance payoff schedule is a decreasing convex function of the future health state; i.e.,

$$x'(h) < 0 \text{ and } x''(h) \geq 0, \text{ for } h \in (0,1)$$

From Assumption 3, we also have

$$x''(h) < -\frac{1}{I}y_2''(h)$$

Assumption 5. Expenditure for preventive medicine is beneficial to future health, subject to diminishing returns; i.e., $R_Z < 0$ and $R_{ZZ} > 0$. An increase in the riskiness of the general health environment reduces the size of the prospect; i.e., $R_Y > 0$, where γ is a risk-shift parameter.

Assumption 6. Preventive medicine and risk are biased toward benefit; i.e.,

$$R_{ZY} \leq 0.$$

Equilibrium Conditions

Suppose that an interior solution to the problem exists. Then the first-order equilibrium conditions are

(5.1) $$\int_0^1 u_1 dF = \frac{1}{\rho} \int_0^1 xu_2 dF$$

and

(5.2) $$\int_0^1 u_1 dF = \int_0^1 u dF_Z$$

Equations (5.1) and (5.2), respectively, supply the requirements for the optimal outlay on insurance and preventive medicine. The optimal outlay on insurance equates the expected marginal utility of present consumption with the expected marginal utility of future consumption, the latter weighted by the insurance payoff schedule and discounted by ρ. The optimal outlay on preventive medicine equates the expected marginal utility of present consumption with the gain in expected utility caused by an increment in spending on preventive medicine. Notice that the consumer must believe that money spent for preventive medicine will have a positive influence on his health prospect, no matter how small, otherwise he will spend nothing on it.

The implication of these first-order conditions can best be appreciated by comparing them with their counterparts in a single-period decision model. In the context of a single period, the optimal insurance equalizes income in all states as long as the insurance is actuarially fair. Moreover, in the special case in which prevention does not raise expected income, and barring moral hazard, a corollary proposition is that demand for prevention will be zero because full insurance eliminates the pecuniary advantage otherwise present in shifting the probabilities of particular events. These results do not obtain in the multiperiod model, however, for the simple reason that both insurance and prevention have positive opportunity costs in terms of present consumption. Thus, in general, the optimal outlay for prevention will be positive and the optimal insurance will be less than full coverage.

The equilibrium derived from Equation (5) is stable if

$$D = \begin{bmatrix} U_{II} & U_{IZ} \\ U_{ZI} & U_{ZZ} \end{bmatrix}$$

is negative definite, where

$$U_{II} = \int_0^1 (\rho^2 u_{11} - 2\rho x u_{12} + x^2 u_{22})dF$$

$$U_{ZI} = U_{IZ} = \int_0^1 (\rho u_{11} - x u_{12})dF = \int_0^1 (\rho u_1 - x u_2)dF_Z$$

$$U_{ZZ} = \int_0^1 u_{11}dF - 2\int_0^1 u_1 dF_Z + \int_0^1 u dF_{ZZ}$$

Negative definiteness of D requires that U_{II}, $U_{ZZ} < 0$ and $U_{II}U_{ZZ} > U_{IZ}^2$. $U_{II} < 0$ is guaranteed by Assumption 1. $U_{ZZ} < 0$ is guaranteed by assumptions 1–6 (see propositions 2 and 3 in the Appendix). In general, there is no *a priori* reason for signing U_{IZ}; however, in this case, the conditions that guarantee U_{II} and U_{ZZ} negative also make U_{IZ} negative.

Equilibrium Displacements

From (5), I and Z can be expressed as functions of the parameters Y_1, α, ρ, β, and γ. A shift in any one of them will change the optimal values of I and Z. In this subsection we examine and interpret these comparative static results. Notice that assumptions 1–6 not only guarantee that D is negative definite and U_{IZ} is negative,[9] but they also aid us in determining the signs of terms in the comparative statics.

1. A Change in Present Income

The optimal changes in I and Z following a change in Y_1 are

(6.1)
$$\frac{\partial I}{\partial Y_1} = \frac{\left[\int_0^1 (\rho u_{11} - x u_{12})dF \right] U_{ZZ}}{|D|} + \frac{\left(-\int_0^1 u_{11}dF + \int_0^1 u_1 dF_Z \right) U_{IZ}}{|D|}$$

(6.2)
$$\frac{\partial Z}{\partial Y_1} = \frac{\left(\int_0^1 u_{11}dF - \int_0^1 u_1 dF_Z \right) U_{II}}{|D|} + \frac{\left[-\int_0^1 (\rho u_{11} - x u_{12})dF \right] U_{ZI}}{|D|}$$

It is convenient to interpret the first term on the right-hand side of (6.1) and (6.2) as the *direct* income effect; it would measure the impact of a change in present income on the amount of insurance and preventive medicine purchased in the event that insurance and preventive medicine were independent alternatives; i.e., if $U_{IZ} = U_{ZI} = 0$. The second term on the right-hand side of (6.1) and (6.2) can then be called the *indirect* income effect; it measures the influence of any interdependence. Given assumptions 1–6, Proposition 2, and the stability requirement, the direct income effect on both I and Z is positive and the indirect income effect is negative. Of course, the total effect in each case is ambiguous, which is not unusual for pure income effects. The important implication is that since insurance and preventive medicine are competitive options, either one (perhaps both) could turn out to be *inferior* with respect to a change in present income.

2. A Change in Future Income

It is convenient to assume that the shift parameter for future income is nonstochastic and takes the form $\dfrac{\partial y_2(h, \alpha)}{\partial \alpha} = a$, where $a > 0$. Then the partial derivatives of I and Z with respect to α are:

(7.1)
$$\frac{\partial I}{\partial \alpha} = a \left\{ \frac{\left[\int_0^1 (\rho u_{12} - x u_{22}) dF \right] U_{ZZ}}{|D|} + \frac{\left(-\int_0^1 u_{12} dF + \int_0^1 u_2 dF_Z \right) U_{IZ}}{|D|} \right\}$$

(7.2)
$$\frac{\partial Z}{\partial \alpha} = a \left\{ \frac{\left(\int_0^1 u_{12} dF - \int_0^1 u_2 dF_Z \right) U_{II}}{|D|} + \frac{\left[-\int_0^1 (\rho u_{12} - x u_{22}) dF \right] U_{ZI}}{|D|} \right\}$$

As in the first case, the effect of a change in future income is separable into two parts with definite but opposite signs. However, the signs are now reversed. The first term on the right-hand side of (7.1) and (7.2) is negative and the second is positive. The direct income effect is now negative because, ignoring any cross effects, an increase in future income makes the purchase of insurance and preventive medicine less urgent. But the competitive nature of the two services produces an offsetting positive response so that we cannot definitely sign the total effect. In this case, if the direct effect on insurance (preventive medicine) outweighs the indirect effect, then insurance (preventive medicine) is inferior with respect to a change in future income. Notice also, since insurance and prevention are substitutes, the demand for either one (perhaps both) could increase with a rise in future income.

3. A Change in the Price of Insurance

From the individual's point of view, a variation in the price of insurance can take two forms: (1) a change in the private per unit cost ρ, and (2) a change in the payoff schedule $x(h)$. These price effects, however, are not symmetrical.

The displacement in the optimal values of I and Z with respect to a change in ρ can be divided into two parts, a present income effect and an intertemporal substitution effect:

$$(8.1) \qquad \frac{\partial I}{\partial \rho} = -I \frac{\partial I}{\partial Y_1} + \frac{\left(\int_0^1 u_1 dF \right) U_{zz}}{|D|}$$

$$(8.2) \qquad \frac{\partial Z}{\partial \rho} = -I \frac{\partial Z}{\partial Y_1} + \frac{-\left(\int_0^1 u_1 dF \right) U_{zI}}{|D|}$$

As we have seen in 3.1 (p. 47), the signing of the income effect depends on the relative magnitude of the direct and indirect terms. The sign of the substitution effect, however, is definite: It is negative in (8.1) and positive in (8.2). If insurance and prevention are both "normal goods" with respect to present income—which we feel is a very plausible assumption—then $\partial I/\partial \rho < 0$; i.e., a fall in the private cost of insurance will lead to an increase in demand for it. However, the sign of $\partial Z/\partial \rho$ is ambiguous. If it is positive, then a fall in the private cost of insurance will promote moral hazard.

Now assume that there is a change in the insurance payoff schedule $x(h)$. For simplicity, we suppose that the change is proportional to the original schedule; i.e.,

$$\frac{\partial x(h, \beta)}{\partial \beta} = bx(h, \beta^0)$$

where $b > 0$. Then the displacements of I and Z with respect to a change in β are:

$$(9.1) \qquad \frac{\partial I}{\partial \beta} = bI \left\{ \frac{\left[\int_0^1 x(\rho u_{12} - xu_{22}) dF \right] U_{zz}}{|D|} \right.$$

$$\left. + \frac{\left(-\int_0^1 xu_{12} dF + \int_0^1 xu_2 dF_z \right) U_{Iz}}{|D|} \right\} - \frac{b \left(\int_0^1 xu_2 dF \right) U_{zz}}{|D|}$$

$$
(9.2) \quad \frac{\partial Z}{\partial \beta} = bI \left\{ \frac{\left(\int_0^1 xu_{12}dF - \int_0^1 xu_2 dF_Z \right) U_{II}}{|D|} \right.
$$

$$
\left. + \frac{\left[\int_0^1 x(-\rho u_{12} + xu_{22})dF \right] U_{ZI}}{|D|} \right\} + \frac{b \left(\int_0^1 xu_2 dF \right) U_{ZI}}{|D|}
$$

We see immediately that the first two terms are future income effects. However, the expressions in the brackets are different from those in 3.2 in that the utility terms are weighted by the insurance payoffs. This difference does not change the signs of the direct and indirect income effects, but it may change the sign of the combined effect. The remaining term in (9.1) and (9.2) is again the intertemporal substitution effect; it is positive for insurance and negative for prevention. What can be said of the total effects? Assuming that the direct income effect dominates in (8.1) and (8.2), then insurance and prevention are both "inferior goods." Since in the case of insurance the substitution effect is positive, a proportional change in future insurance payoffs produces an ambiguous effect on the demand for insurance; $\partial I/\partial \beta > 0$ only if the substitution effect outweighs the combined income effect. Since in the case of prevention the income and substitution effects are both negative, the proportional change in payoff produces a definite negative effect on the demand for preventive medicine.

We emphasize in passing that although a change in ρ and a proportional change in $x(h)$ both produce income and substitution effects, in general they are not the same. The difference stems from the fact that a change in ρ produces a combined present income effect and a substitution effect involving present marginal utility, whereas the change in $x(h)$ produces a combined future income effect and a substitution effect involving future marginal utility.

4. A Change in Risk

Suppose that there is an exogenous change in the riskiness of the general health environment. Let a change in the parameter γ generate a mean-preserving change in the spread of all health prospects $F \epsilon \mathcal{F}$; i.e., $R_\gamma(h, \cdot) \geq 0$, with the equality holding for $h = 1$. Then the effects of a change in γ on the optimal levels of I and Z are:

$$
(10.1) \quad \frac{\partial I}{\partial \gamma} = \frac{\left[\int_0^1 (\rho u_1 - x u_2)dF_\gamma \right] U_{ZZ}}{|D|} + \frac{\left(-\int_0^1 u_1 dF_\gamma + \int_0^1 u\, dF_{Z\gamma} \right) U_{IZ}}{|D|}
$$

$$
(10.2) \quad \frac{\partial Z}{\partial \gamma} = \frac{\left(\int_0^1 u_1 dF_\gamma - \int_0^1 u\, dF_{Z\gamma} \right) U_{II}}{|D|} + \frac{\left[-\int_0^1 (\rho u_1 - x u_2)dF_\gamma \right] U_{ZI}}{|D|}
$$

Notice that as in the case of income effects, it is possible to divide the change in the optimal values of I and Z into two parts. We call the first and the second terms of (10.1) and (10.2), respectively, the direct and indirect risk effects. In order to sign these separate terms, we only need to sign the coefficients

$$
\int_0^1 (\rho u_1 - x u_2)dF_\gamma
$$

and

$$
\left(\int_0^1 u_1 dF_\gamma - \int_0^1 u\, dF_{Z\gamma} \right)
$$

By propositions 1 and 3 in the appendix, both coefficients are negative. Thus, the direct effects for both insurance and preventive medicine are positive and the indirect effects are negative. The combined effects will, of course, depend on the relative magnitudes of the separate terms.

Previous studies by Leland (1966) and Sandmo (1970) have shown that decreasing temporal risk aversion is sufficient to guarantee that an increase in risk will cause an increase in the optimal amount of saving (in our case, insurance). But we see from our model that the condition is more complex. First, by recognizing prevention as an alternative hedge against uncertainty, our model shows the existence of an indirect risk effect. Second, we find that the sufficient condition for a positive risk effect involves restrictions on the class of payoff functions as well as on the class of utility functions. An important implication of this latter finding is that the insurance company has in its choice of payoff schedule a significant weapon to combat moral hazard.

4. MODEL WITH CONSUMPTION AFFECTING HEALTH PROSPECT

As we mentioned in the introduction, preventive medicine is not the only factor that can influence the consumer's health prospect.

We need not go so far as to say "you are what you consume," but it is hardly controversial to admit that many nonmedical goods and services—food, housing, drink, tobacco—can and often do have an important bearing on future health, either positive or negative. In this section we examine the consumer's optimal outlay on insurance and prevention when present consumption, C_1, is a parameter of F as well as a variable in u. In order to analyze what we believe to be the most interesting case, we make two additional assumptions:

Assumption 7. Changes in present consumption involve goods that are harmful to health, subject to increasing negative returns; i.e.,

$$R_{C_1} > 0, R_{C_1 C_1} > 0$$

Assumption 8. Preventive medicine and present consumption are biased toward benefit, and risk and present consumption are biased toward harm; i.e.,

$$R_{Z C_1} \leq 0 \text{ and } R_{\gamma C_1} \geq 0$$

The consumer's expected utility can now be written as

$$V = \int_0^1 u(C_1, c_2) dF(h; Z, C_1, \gamma)$$

where u is again a von Neumann-Morgenstern utility index with continuous derivatives of the first, second, and third order. As in the preceding section the consumer will choose I and Z so as to maximize V subject to the constraints,

$$C_1 = Y_1 - \rho I - Z$$
$$c_2(h) = y_2(h) + x(h)I$$

The first-order maximization conditions become

(12.1) $$\int_0^1 u_1 dF = \frac{1}{\rho} \int_0^1 x u_2 dF - \int_0^1 u dF_{C_1}$$

(12.2) $$\int_0^1 u_1 dF = \int_0^1 u (dF_z - dF_{C_1})$$

and the second-order condition is that the matrix

$$A = \begin{bmatrix} V_{II} & V_{IZ} \\ V_{ZI} & V_{ZZ} \end{bmatrix}$$

is negative definite, where

$$V_{II} = \int_0^1 (\rho^2 u_{11} - 2\rho x u_{12} + x^2 u_{22})dF + 2\rho \int_0^1 (\rho u_1 - x u_2)dF_{C_1} + \rho^2 \int_0^1 u dF_{C_1 C_1}$$

(13)
$$V_{ZZ} = \int_0^1 u_{11}dF + 2\int_0^1 u_1(dF_{C_1} - dF_Z) + \int_0^1 u(dF_{C_1 C_1} - 2dF_{ZC_1} + dF_{ZZ})$$

$$V_{IZ} = V_{ZI} = \int_0^1 (\rho u_{11} - x u_{21})dF + \int_0^1 (\rho u_1 - x u_2)(dF_{C_1} - dF_Z)$$

$$+ \rho \int_0^1 u_1 dF_{C_1} + \rho \int_0^1 u(dF_{C_1 C_1} - dF_{ZC_1})$$

The first-order maximization conditions state that when current consumption affects the future health prospect, then (1) the consumer will choose an optimal insurance outlay by equating the expected marginal utility of present consumption with the expected marginal utility of future consumption discounted by ρ, net of the change in the expected utility from a shift in the probability distribution caused by a change in C_1; and (2) he will choose an optimal expenditure on preventive medicine by equating the expected marginal utility of present consumption with the net change in the utility of the health prospect stemming from changes in both Z and C_1. The implications of these first-order conditions can best be seen by comparing the equilibrium values of I and Z with those derived in the preceding section. Given Assumption 7 and according to Proposition 4 in the appendix, we find

$$\int_0^1 u dF_{C_1} < 0$$

Our interpretation is that the optimal present consumption will decrease if it has a harmful effect on the health prospect.[10] Consequently, the optimal outlays I and Z as determined by Equation (12) should be larger than those determined by Equation (5) in Section 3, where C_1 is assumed to have no effect whatsoever on the health prospect.

The second-order maximization conditions specify that V_{II}, $V_{ZZ} < 0$ and $V_{II}V_{ZZ} > V_{IZ}^2$. We will show that assumptions 1–8 are sufficient to make I and Z competitive. Notice first that by Assumption 1,

$$\int_0^1 (\rho u_{11} - x u_{21})dF < 0$$

Next, by propositions 2–5 in the appendix, we find that the terms

$$\int_0^1 x u_2 dF_{C_1} \text{ and } \int_0^1 u_1 dF_Z$$

are positive, and the terms

$$\int_0^1 u_1 dF_{c_1}, \int_0^1 xu_2 dF_z \text{ and } \int_0^1 u(dF_{c_1 c_1} - dF_{zc_1})$$

are negative. Then it follows from (13) that

$$V_{IZ} = V_{ZI} < 0$$

Having examined the maximization conditions, let us now turn to the comparative statics. As before, the equilibrium values of I and Z are determined by the parameters Y_1, α, ρ, β, and γ. The consumer's optimal expenditure on insurance and preventive medicine will change whenever there is an exogenous change in any of these parameters. Let the equilibrium values of I and Z be denoted by I^* and Z^*, and let $F^0 = F(h; C_1^0, \cdot)$. Symbolically, the comparative static results are:

$$(14) \quad \frac{\partial I^*}{\partial Y_1} = \left. \frac{\partial I^*}{\partial Y_1} \right|_{F=F^0} + \begin{cases} + \dfrac{\left[\int_0^1 (2\rho u_1 - xu_2) dF_{c_1} + \rho \int_0^1 u dF_{c_1 c_1} \right] V_{ZZ}}{|A|} \\[4ex] + \dfrac{ - \left[2 \int_0^1 u_1 dF_{c_1} + \int_0^1 u(dF_{c_1 c_1} - dF_{c_1 z}) \right] V_{IZ}}{|A|} \end{cases}$$

$$\frac{\partial Z^*}{\partial Y_1} = \left. \frac{\partial Z^*}{\partial Y_1} \right|_{F=F^0} + \begin{cases} + \dfrac{\left[2 \int_0^1 u_1 dF_{c_1} + \int_0^1 u(dF_{c_1 c_1} - dF_{c_1 z}) \right] V_{II}}{|A|} \\[4ex] + \dfrac{ - \left[\int_0^1 (2\rho u_1 - xu_2) dF_{c_1} + \rho \int_0^1 u dF_{c_1 c_1} \right] V_{ZI}}{|A|} \end{cases}$$

$$(15) \quad \frac{\partial I^*}{\partial \alpha} = \left. \frac{\partial I^*}{\partial \alpha} \right|_{F=F^0} + a \frac{\int_0^1 u_2 dF_{c_1} (\rho V_{ZZ} - V_{IZ})}{|A|}$$

$$\frac{\partial Z^*}{\partial \alpha} = a \left. \frac{\partial Z^*}{\partial \alpha} \right|_{F=F^0} + a \frac{\int_0^1 u_2 dF_{c_1} (V_{II} - \rho V_{ZI})}{|A|}$$

$$(16) \quad \frac{\partial I^*}{\partial \rho} = \left. \frac{\partial I^*}{\partial \rho} \right|_{F=F^0} - I \left\{ \frac{\partial I^*}{\partial Y_1} - \left. \frac{\partial I^*}{\partial Y_1} \right|_{F=F^0} \right\} + \frac{\left(\int_0^1 u dF_{c_1} \right) V_{ZZ}}{|A|}$$

$$\frac{\partial Z^*}{\partial \rho} = \frac{\partial Z^*}{\partial \rho}\bigg|_{F=F^0} - I \left\{ \frac{\partial Z^*}{\partial Y_1} - \frac{\partial Z^*}{\partial Y_1}\bigg|_{F=F^0} \right\} + \frac{-\left(\int_0^1 u\,dF_{C_1}\right)V_{IZ}}{|A|}$$

(17)
$$\frac{\partial I^*}{\partial \beta} = b\,\frac{\partial I^*}{\partial \beta}\bigg|_{F=F^0} + bI\,\frac{\int_0^1 xu_2\,dF_{C_1}(\rho V_{ZZ} - V_{IZ})}{|A|}$$

$$\frac{\partial Z^*}{\partial \beta} = b\,\frac{\partial Z^*}{\partial \beta}\bigg|_{F=F^0} + bI\,\frac{\int_0^1 xu_2\,dF_{C_1}(V_{II} - \rho V_{ZI})}{|A|}$$

(18)
$$\frac{\partial I^*}{\partial \gamma} = \frac{\partial I^*}{\partial \gamma}\bigg|_{F=F^0} + \frac{\int_0^1 u\,dF_{\gamma C_1}(\rho V_{ZZ} - V_{IZ})}{|A|}$$

$$\frac{\partial Z^*}{\partial \gamma} = \frac{\partial Z^*}{\partial \gamma}\bigg|_{F=F^0} + \frac{\int_0^1 u\,dF_{\gamma C_1}(V_{II} - \rho V_{ZI})}{|A|}$$

To simplify our notation, let

$t = (Y_1, \alpha, \rho, \beta, \gamma)$

In equations (14)–(18), the terms

$$\frac{\partial I^*}{\partial t}\bigg|_{F=F^0} \text{ and } \frac{\partial Z^*}{\partial t}\bigg|_{F=F^0}$$

have the same general form as the terms

$$\frac{\partial I}{\partial t} \text{ and } \frac{\partial Z}{\partial t}$$

in equations (6)–(10) of the basic model. The difference is that V_{II}, V_{IZ}, V_{ZZ} and $|A|$ are substituted for U_{II}, U_{IZ}, U_{ZZ} and $|D|$. Since U_{ij} and $V_{ij}, i,j = IZ$ are all negative, it is evident that the individual terms in

$$\frac{\partial I^*}{\partial t}\bigg|_{F=F^0} \text{ and } \frac{\partial Z^*}{\partial t}\bigg|_{F=F^0}$$

must have the same signs as the corresponding terms in

$$\frac{\partial I}{\partial t} \text{ and } \frac{\partial Z}{\partial t}$$

But because the magnitudes vary, the corresponding total effects may be different.

The remaining terms in equations (14)–(18) are new. They measure the effects of consumption-induced shifts in the health prospect on the optimal outlays for health insurance and preventive medicine. Observe that each coefficient shown contains a first- or second-order differential of F caused by the displacement of present consumption, C_1. Notice also that most of the additional terms can be properly classified as supplementary income or risk effects. The exception is Equation (16), in which there is also a supplementary substitution effect. It may seem odd at first glance that β does not generate an additional substitution term, but the explanation is to be found in the fact that size of marginal loss caused by consumption-induced harm to the future health prospect is proportional only to ρ, the private unit cost of insurance.

The predictions on the additional terms are exactly parallel to those in the preceding section. The income and risk effects can be divided into separate direct and indirect terms of definite and corresponding signs. Given assumptions 1–8, we find that

$$\int_0^1 u_1 dF_{C_1}, \int_0^1 u dF_{C_1 C_1} \text{ and } \int_0^1 u dF_{\gamma C_1}$$

are negative and

$$\int_0^1 u dF_{C_1} \text{ and } \int_0^1 u dF_{z C_1}$$

are positive. Hence the separate supplemental terms are all signed, but the combined effects are ambiguous. Again, the outcome in each case depends on the relative magnitudes of the opposing direct and indirect effects. The supplementary substitution terms in Equation (16) are definitely signed, but they are opposite from those in the basic model. However, the equilibrium conditions require

$$\int_0^1 u_1 dF + \int_0^1 u dF_{C_1} > 0$$

where

$$\int_0^1 u_1 dF$$

is a term in

$$\frac{\partial I^*}{\partial \rho}\bigg|_{F = F^0}$$

so that the signs of the combined substitution effects in the extended model are the same as in the basic model.

To summarize, the presence of consumption as a harmful influence on future health will increase the optimal outlay on insurance and prevention over what it would be otherwise. But given assumptions 7–8, the qualitative nature of the comparative static results derived in the basic model remains unchanged, although the magnitudes are likely to be different.

5. SUMMARY AND CONCLUSIONS

The problem studied in this paper is the optimal choice of health insurance and preventive medicine for an individual faced with uncertain future health. Insurance and prevention are fundamentally different approaches to health planning in that the former transfers income from the present to hazardous states in the future whereas the latter alters present consumption to benefit future health prospects. Our analysis is limited to the case in which the principal effect of the state of health is on net income (current earnings less necessary medical expenses), but we freely acknowledge the potential importance of health as a direct influence on consumer preferences.

In the basic model, we assume that current consumption can be partitioned into three mutually exclusive categories: insurance, pure prevention, and other consumption outlays. In this instance, preventive activity is assumed to have no direct influence on utility, and consumption is assumed free of any effects on future health prospects. In the extended model, we include a category of consumption in which the influence is mixed.

As is well known, the expected utility model is very general in the sense of admitting a wide range of risk attitudes and a broad set of probability distributions. In the context of optimal insurance and prevention, it is plausible to suppose that we are dealing with a generally risk-averse population and a set of prospects ordered by stochastic dominance. A few additional and, we hope, quite reasonable assumptions enable us to guarantee stability of equilibrium and to derive several meaningful results.

An important finding is that insurance and prevention are strictly competitive (net substitutes). This result has immediate implications for equilibrium displacements caused by changes in wealth, the amount of uncertainty in the environment, and the price of insurance. Total income effects turn out to be ambiguous, but we can definitely sign separate direct and indirect effects. If, as is likely, the direct effects outweigh the indirect effects, the combined effects are also signed: The demand for insurance and prevention will vary directly with present income and inversely with future income. Likewise, there are separate direct and indirect risk effects; again, if the direct effect is dominant, we predict that the demand for insurance and prevention will vary directly with the greater riskiness of the health environment. In addition to income effects, changes in the price of insurance yield definite substitution effects: A fall in the price of insurance (in the form of either a decline in the premium or a rise in benefits) will increase the amount of insurance and decrease the outlay on prevention. If the sign relationship between the combined income effect and the substitution effect produces a fall in the price of insurance and causes the individual to increase the optimal outlay on insurance and to decrease the optimal outlay on prevention, then we have a clear case of moral hazard.

There are further implications in this study concerning the phenomenon of moral hazard. The insurance company has within its control a device—the selection of a payoff schedule (together with deductibles and coinsurance)—to prevent moral hazard. The desired schedule must avoid any coverage that will cause post-insurance income to rise with greater misfortune or to increase at an increasing rate with an improved health state. A schedule with these characteristics can produce a bias toward insurance and against prevention and, hence, promote moral hazard.

The competitive character of insurance and prevention poses a problem in designing an efficient national health insurance program. Our analysis suggests that efforts to extend the coverage of health insurance through public subsidy should be weighed against the cost arising from possible reductions in the demand for prevention. Although we know of no way to avoid this opportunity cost altogether, it can and undoubtedly should be minimized. We see here that the terms of insurance potentially provide an important instrument of control. For example, if the price of insurance is reduced by a public subsidy to stimulate demand, there may be important differences in the way people respond, depending on whether the subsidy (1) reduces the current expenditure or (2) increases the future payoffs. In case (1), we would predict an increase in the volume of insurance because both the income and the substitution effects are likely to be negative. Moral hazard is indicated if the negative income effect on preventive expenditure is not outweighed by the positive cross-substitution effect. In other words, our model demonstrates that the income effect generated by a decline in the proportion of the premium paid by the beneficiary acts as a check on the tendency to substitute insurance protection for prevention. Of course, the importance of this restraint on moral hazard depends on the relative size of the income and substitution effects. As medical expenses and related costs of health care typically claim a significant share of budgets of middle- and low-income receivers, income effects are also likely to be significant.[11] In case (2), when the price reduction takes the form of a subsidy to future payoffs, the situation is reversed. The problem of moral hazard is now inescapable since both the income and substitution effects are negative. Any such implications, of course, must be qualified by possible limitations in the nature and the scope of the model. In particular, we recognize that the assumption of a state-independent utility function does bias our result toward insurance and against prevention, which tends to exaggerate the problem of moral hazard.

APPENDIX

Proposition 1. Let the shift in γ be a mean preserving increase in the spread of F. Given assumptions 1–4, then

$$\int_0^1 (u_1 - xu_2)dF_\gamma < 0$$

Furthermore,

$$\int_0^1 u_1 dF_\gamma < 0 \text{ and } \int_0^1 xu_2 dF_\gamma > 0$$

Proof. Integrating by parts twice, we obtain

$$\int_0^1 (u_1 - xu_2)dF_\gamma = -[(u_{12} - xu_{22})(y_2 + x'I) - x'u_2]R_\gamma(h,z,\gamma)\,|_0^1$$

$$+ \int_0^1 [(u_{122} - xu_{222})(y_2' + x'I)^2 + (u_{12} - xu_{22})(y_2'' + x''I)$$

$$- 2u_{22}x'(y_2' + x'I) - u_2x'']R_\gamma(h,z,\gamma)dh$$

(i) $-(\cdot)R_\gamma(h,z,\gamma)\,|_0^1 = 0$

follows from the assumption that the shift in γ represents a mean preserving increase in spread.

(ii) $(u_{122} - xu_{222})(y_2' + x'I)^2 < 0$

follows from A.2.

(iii) $(u_{12} - xu_{22})(y_2'' + x''I) < 0$

follows from A.1 and A.3.

(iv) $2u_{22}x'(y_2' + x'I) > 0$ and $u_2x'' \geqslant 0$

follow from A.3 and A.4. Therefore,

$$\int_0^1 (u_1 - xu_2)dF_\gamma < 0$$

Following the same reasoning,

$$\int_0^1 u_1 dF = \int_0^1 [u_{122}(y_2' + x'I)^2 + u_{12}(y_2'' + x''I)]R_\gamma(h,z,\gamma)dh < 0$$

and

$$\int_0^1 u_2 x dF_\gamma = \int_0^1 [u_{222}x(y_2' + x'I)^2 + 2u_{22}x'(y_2' + x'I)$$

$$+ u_{22}x(y_2'' + x''I) + u_2x'']\,R_\gamma dh > 0$$

Proposition 2.   Let the factor Z be beneficial to the consumer's health prospect. Given assumptions 1–4, then

$$\int_0^1 (u_1 - xu_2)dF_Z > 0$$

Furthermore,

$$\int_0^1 u_1 dF_Z > 0, \int_0^1 xu_2 dF_Z < 0, \text{ and } \int_0^1 u_2 dF_Z < 0$$

Proof.   Integrating by parts twice, we obtain

$$\int_0^1 (u_1 - xu_2)dF_Z = - [(u_{12} - xu_{22})(y_2' + x'I) - x'u_2]R_Z(h,Z,\gamma) \,|_0^1$$

$$+ \int_0^1 [(u_{122} - xu_{222})(y_2' + x'I)^2 + (u_{12} - xu_{22})(y_2'' + x''I)$$

$$- 2u_{22}x'(y_2' + x'I) - u_2x'']R_Z(h,Z,\gamma)dh$$

(i) $- [(u_{12} - xu_{22})(y_2' + x'I) - x'u_2]R_Z(h,Z,\gamma)\,|_0^1$

$$= - [(u_{12} - xu_{22})(y_2' + x'I) - x'u_2]R_Z(1,Z,\gamma)$$

follows from the fact that $R_Z(0,Z,\gamma) = 0$.

(ii) $R_Z(1,Z,\gamma) < 0$ follows from the assumption that Z is beneficial to the consumer's health prospect. $(u_{12} - xu_{22})(y_2' + x'I) > 0$ follows from A.1 and A.3, and $x'u_2 < 0$ follows from A.4. Therefore, $-(\cdot)R_z(1,Z,\gamma) > 0$.

(iii) $\quad \int_0^1 (u_1 - xu_2)dF_Z > 0, \int_0^1 u_1 dF_Z > 0,$ and $\int_0^1 xu_2 dF_Z < 0$

can be shown with the same reasons given in Proposition 1.

(iv) Similarly, it can be shown that

$$\int_0^1 u_2 dF_Z < 0$$

Proposition 3. Given assumptions 1–6: (a)

$$\int_0^1 u dF_{ZZ} < 0$$

and (b)

$$\int_0^1 u dF_{YZ} \geq 0$$

Proof.

(a) Integrating by parts twice, we obtain

$$\int_0^1 u dF_{ZZ} = uF_{ZZ}(h,Z,\gamma)\,|_0^1 - u_2(y_2' + x'I)R_{ZZ}(h,Z,\gamma)\,|_0^1$$
$$+ \int_0^1 [u_{22}(y_2' + x'I)^2 + u_2(y_2'' + x'I)]R_{ZZ}(h,Z,\gamma)dh$$

(i) $\quad F_{ZZ}(h,Z,\gamma)dh \equiv 0$ for $h = 0,1$. Therefore,

$\quad uF_{ZZ}(h,Z,\gamma)\,|_0^1 = 0$

(ii) $\quad -u_2(y_2' + x'I)R_{ZZ}(h,Z,\gamma)\,|_0^1 = -u_2(y_2' + x'I)R_{ZZ}(1,Z,\gamma) < 0$

follows from A.3 and A.5.

(iii) $\quad \int_0^1 [u_{22}(y_2' + x'I)^2 + u_2(y_2'' + x'I)]R_{ZZ}(h,Z,\gamma)dh < 0$

follows from A.1, A.4, and A.5.

(b) Integrating by parts twice, we obtain

$$\int_0^1 u dF_{YZ} = uF_{YZ}(h,Z,\gamma)\,|_0^1 - u_2(y_2' + x'I)R_{YZ}(h,Z,\gamma)\,|_0^1$$
$$+ \int_0^1 [u_{22}(y_2' + x'I)^2 + u_2(y_2'' + x'I)]R_{YZ}(h,Z,\gamma)dh$$

Again, we see that

$F_{YZ}(h,Z,\gamma)\,|_0^1 = 0$

regardless of the changes in γ and Z. By assumption 6, $R_{YZ} \leq 0$. The hypothesis of the proposition thus guarantees

$$\int_0^1 u dF_{YZ} \geq 0$$

which is what we wish to prove.

Proposition 4. Given assumptions 1–4 and 7, (a)

$$\int_0^1 u_1 dF_{C_1} < 0$$

(b)

$$\int_0^1 x u_2 dF_{C_1} > 0$$

and (c)

$$\int_0^1 u dF_{C_1} < 0$$

Proof.

(a) Integrating by parts twice,

$$\int_0^1 u_1 dF_{C_1} = -u_{12}(y_2' + x'I)R_{C_1}(h,Z,C_1,\gamma)\big|_0^1$$

$$+ \int_0^1 \left[u_{12}(y_2'' + x''I) + u_{122}(y_2' + x'I)^2 \right] R_{C_1}(h,Z,C_1,\gamma)dh$$

(i) $R_{C_1}(0,Z,C_1,\gamma) = 0$, and by A.7 $R_{C_1}(1,Z,C_1,\gamma) > 0$. Following A.1 and A.3, therefore,

$$-u_{12}(y_2' + x'I)R_{C_1}(h,Z,C_1,\gamma)\big|_0^1 > 0$$

(ii) A.1–4 and A.7 also imply that

$$\int_0^1 \left[u_{12}(y_2'' + x''I) + u_{122}(y_2' + x'I) \right] R_{C_1} dh < 0$$

Therefore,

$$\int_0^1 u_1 dF_{C_1} < 0$$

(b) Following a similar reasoning, we obtain (b) and (c).

Proposition 5. Given assumptions 1, 3, 4, and 8, (a)

$$\int_0^1 u dF_{\gamma C_1} < 0$$

(b)

$$\int_0^1 u dF_{C_1 C_1} < 0$$

and (c)

$$\int_0^1 u dF_{Z C_1} > 0$$

Proof.

(a) Integrating by parts twice, we obtain

$$\int_0^1 u \, dF_{\gamma C_1} = -u_2(y_2' + x'I) R_{\gamma C_1}(h, Z, C_1, \gamma) \Big|_0^1$$

$$+ \int_0^1 [u_{22}(y_2' + x'I)^2 + u_2(y_2'' + x''I)] R_{\gamma C_1} dh$$

(i) Again, $R_{\gamma C_1}(0, Z, C_1, \gamma) = 0$, and by assumption 8, $R_\gamma C_1(1, Z, C_1, \gamma) > 0$. A.3 therefore guarantees the result

$$-u_2(y_2' + x'I) R_{\gamma C_1}(h, Z, C_1, \gamma) \Big|_0^1 < 0$$

(ii) In addition, A.1, A.4, and A.8 guarantee

$$\int_0^1 [u_{22}(y_2' + x'I)^2 + u_2(y_2'' + x''I)] R_{\gamma C_1} dh < 0$$

Therefore,

$$\int_0^1 u \, dF_{\gamma C_1} < 0$$

(b) The same hypotheses also guarantee

$$\int_0^1 u \, dF_{C_1 C_1} < 0$$

and

$$\int_0^1 u \, dF_{zc_1} > 0$$

except that A.8 refers to $R_{C_1 C_1} > 0$ and $R_{ZC_1} < 0$, respectively.

NOTES

1. Considerable doubt, however, exists in the medical profession regarding the effectiveness of preventive medicine, especially that part concerned with the early detection and treatment of diseases. If preventive medicine is of doubtful value, then why would a rational person purchase any of it? We have no particular ax to grind on this issue except to point out that preventive medicine need not be so narrowly conceived: it might just as well include any consumption activity, medical or otherwise, having a potential benefit on future health. Moreover, the crucial consideration in our model is the individual's *subjective* view of the effectiveness of prevention, the opinions of medical experts to the contrary notwithstanding.

2. Prevention is sometimes characterized as an activity that reduces the probabilities of hazardous states of health. Although this description is correct, it is not the whole story because it is silent on what happens to the probabilities of less hazardous states, including those that are totally free of hazard. As the hypothesis of risk avoidance strongly suggests, prevention is not confined to activities that uniformly "roll up" probabilities toward less hazardous states; it also includes those that reduce the frequencies of both the most and the least

hazardous states but leave the average state of health unaffected. To cite an example: A drug or operation that reduces the chances of a person's becoming very ill may also involve side effects that lower the chances of one's being extremely well. A risk-averse person might favor such a prospect even though it does not offer much hope of raising his health expectation.

3. For analyses based on conditional expected utility, see Arrow (1973), Nordquist (1970), and Parkin and Wu (1972).

4. Future income, y_2, is assumed to be net of (a) anticipated future medical expenses, and (b) reductions in earning power caused by illness. We assume that the individual can purchase insurance to compensate for both sources of loss to future consumption opportunities.

5. In their seminal paper, Ehrlich and Becker (1972) provide a similar analysis in a setting of a single period and two states.

6. We recognize that some factors may be beneficial in some range of consumption and harmful in others.

7. The principal objective of this paper is to develop a rigorous formulation of the joint demand for insurance and prevention. Thus, we adhere to the conventional atomistic specification of consumer choice and decline to make the market price of insurance depend directly on any of the individual's choice variables, as is done in the article by Ehrlich and Becker (1972, p. 640). Although it is quite likely that a *mohopolistic supplier* of insurance would perceive and be concerned about the presence of moral hazard, we argue that the same will not be true of the *small and independent purchaser*.

8. Properly specified, the problem should include the further restriction $I \leq I^0$, where I^0 is the premium of the largest insurance policy (with payoff $x(h)I$) that the consumer is allowed to purchase. For simplicity, we assume that this inequality constraint is never binding.

9. We should add the reminder that the conditions cited here are sufficient but not necessary to sign the separate income terms.

10. If a change in present consumption involves goods that are beneficial to health, these results will be reversed.

11. For other possible checks to moral hazard, see Arrow (1971, Ch. 8) and Ehrlich and Becker (1972, pp. 641–642).

REFERENCES

1. Arrow, K.J., *Theory of Risk Bearing* (Chicago: Markham Publishing Co., 1971).

2. _____., "Optimal Insurance and Generalized Deductibles," The Rand Corporation, February 1973.

3. Balch, M., and P.C. Fishburn, "Subjective Expected Utility for Conditional Primitives," in M. Balch, D. McFadden, and S. Wu (editors), *Essays on Economic Behavior under Uncertainty* (Amsterdam: North-Holland, 1974).

4. Dreze, J.H., and F. Modigliani, "Consumption Decisions under Uncertainty," *Journal of Economic Theory*, 4 (December 1972), pp. 308–335.

5. Ehrlich, Isaac, and G.S. Becker, "Market Insurance, Self-Insurance, and Self-Protection," *Journal of Political Economy*, 80 (July–August 1972), pp. 623–649.

6. Feldstein, Martin S., "The Welfare Loss of Excess Health Insurance," *Journal of Political Economy*, 81 (March–April 1973), pp. 251–280.

7. Frech, H.E., III, and Paul B. Ginsburg, "Imposed Health Insurance in Monopolistic Markets," mimeo. (November 1971).

8. Grossman, Michael, *The Demand for Health: A Theoretical and Empirical Investigation*, Ph.D. dissertation, Columbia University, 1970.

9. _____., "The Economics of Joint Production in Households," Center for Mathematical Studies, University of Chicago, September 1971.

10. _____., "On the Concept of Health Capital and the Demand for Health," *Journal of Political Economy*, 80 (March–April 1972), pp. 223–255.

11. Hadar, J., and W. Russell, "Stochastic Dominance and Diversification," *Journal of Economic Theory*, 3 (September 1971), pp. 288–305.

12. Hirshleifer, J., "Investment Decision Under Uncertainty: Application of the State Preference Approach," *Quarterly Journal of Economics*, 80 (May 1966), pp. 252–277.

13. Leland, Hayne, "Saving and Uncertainty: The Precautionary Demand for Saving," *Quarterly Journal of Economics*, 82 (August 1966), pp. 465–473.

14. Luce, D., and D.H. Krantz, "Conditional Expected Utility," *Econometrica*, 39 (March 1971), pp. 253–271.

15. Mossin, J., "Aspects of Rational Insurance Purchasing," *Journal of Political Economy*, 76 (July–August 1968), pp. 553–568.

16. Nordquist, G., "A Model of the Demand for Preventive Medicine under Uncertainty," Working Paper No. 70–6, College of Business Administration, The University of Iowa, August 1970.

17. Parkin, J.M., and S.Y. Wu, "Choice Involving Unwanted Risky Events and Optimal Insurances," *American Economic Review*, 62 (December 1972), pp. 982–987.

18. Pauly, Mark, "The Economics of Moral Hazard: Comment," *American Economic Review*, 58 (June 1968), pp. 531–537.

19. _____., "Efficiency, Incentive, and Reimbursement for Health Care," mimeo. (August 1969).

20. _____., *National Health Insurance: An Analysis*, American Enterprise Institute, August 1971

21. Pratt, J.W., "Risk Aversion in the Small and in the Large," *Econometrica*, 32 (January 1964), pp. 122–136.

22. Rosett, Richard N., and Lein-fu Huang, "The Effect of Health Insurance on the Demand for Medical Care," *Journal of Political Economy*, 81 (March–April 1973), pp. 281–305.

23. Sandmo, Agnar, "Capital Risk, Consumption and Portfolio Choice," *Econometrica*, 37 (October 1969), pp. 586–599.

24. _____., "The Effect of Uncertainty on Savings Decisions," *Review of Economic Studies*, 37 (July 1970), pp. 353–360.

25. Zeckhauser, R., "Medical Insurance: A Case Study of the Tradeoff between Risk Spreading and Appropriate Incentives," *Journal of Economic Theory*, 2 (March 1970), pp. 10–26.

2 COMMENTS

Robert L. Berg, M.D.
University of Rochester

The influence that variable insurance coverage has on the purchase of preventive services represents a particularly thorny issue in the health care field. In general, we can expect that the consumer will choose such a mix as to maximize his expected utilities. In an open-market situation, in which the individual chooses his expenditures, then there is a real possibility that he might underspend on prevention; that is, he might underspend if preventive services represent a separate good such that the purchase of curative services does not entail the purchase of preventive services. With perfect information he should be expected to choose an optimal mix of insurance and prevention to maximize utility. However, information is imperfect, especially in the health field. Prevention has been oversold as an idea in many areas, except that only some consumers overbuy, such as in purchasing annual physical exams. Prevention makes a big difference if it leads more people to wear seat belts or stop smoking cigarettes, but behavioral modification has been the least successful approach to prevention. Much must be done in educating the public in any system of health care, but the transmission of information alone does not insure compliance with the optimal program.

There is also a considerable problem of moral hazard. It is not so much that the consumer will run great health risks because health care costs are going to be paid with full entitlement or increased entitlement and thus would tend to avoid obtaining necessary preventive services, but that full entitlement will lead to unnecessary hospitalization and unnecessarily long hospitalization with overly expensive work-ups.

Another feature is unnecessary office visits. But who is to define unnecessary office visits? When initiated by a patient, an office visit represents de facto demand.

Although all this is true from the point of view of the consumer, the program must face tradeoffs between curative and preventive medicine. Fees will presumably be replaced by capitation payments. In this circumstance, who should determine the contents of the preventive package when the public is so poorly informed? Somebody must accept the responsibility for maximizing societal utilities, and this is difficult to do without knowledge of the value society attaches to the outcomes of medical care. Much additional research is needed on health status indexes and the societal values placed on the conditions of life to provide a basis for such judgments.

Whatever the decision, it may be difficult to keep preventive services within reasonable bounds. With a few crucial exceptions (e.g., the control of hypertension to prevent strokes, and immunizations to prevent certain infectious diseases), prevention is of little use at the present time, regrettably, and we tend to overdo it. On net, the consumer will have little to say about the mix of preventive and curative services, and even when preventive services become more effective, he may well resist diverting money to preventive services if it means longer queues and personal inconvenience.

Sherwin Rosen

University of Rochester

This is a very careful and competent investigation of the economics of self-protection. The authors consider a two-period model in which individuals with known health states in the first period reduce second-period medical risk by self-protection and market insurance. Self-protection (i.e., preventive medicine) shifts the actual distribution of risky outcomes. Market insurance doesn't change the distribution, but transfers the risks to others, at a price. As long as preventive expenditures shift the cumulative probability density function of poor health states, they are productive; and individuals extend expenditures in both directions up to the appropriate margins. Of course, the practical importance of self-protection for the allocation of health resources depends on the extent to which it does in fact shift medical risks, a point on which there is little evidence one way or the other.

Nordquist and Wu specialize their argument to a case wherein health states affect only income and not the capacity to consume: They ignore "pain and suffering," which otherwise introduces asymmetry between self-protection and market insurance. Market insurance reduces financial risks but not pain and sufferings, whereas self-protection affects both. Inclusion of health-utility effects involves conceptually straightforward extensions of their methods and perhaps that is sufficient justification for ignoring them at this stage.

Another maintained assumption strikes me as having less justification. Nordquist and Wu assume that the price of market insurance is independent of preventive expenditures. That is, they assume that insurance premiums per dollar of coverage are independent of medical risks individuals choose to run. This could be a valid assumption at the individual level if transactions costs are sufficiently high, for then insurance companies do not find it worthwhile to classify individuals according to risk. But even those factors must be a matter of degree, and the empirical validity of the assumption surely depends on the productivity of preventive expenditures. The observation that insurance companies do not vary premiums across individuals in different risk classes is evidence that policing and information costs are large relative to preventive expenditure productivity on health.

But whatever is the true assumption for any person at random, it surely cannot be true for the market as a whole or for the "representative" individual, as the authors implicitly recognize in discussing moral hazard. Suppose that some exogenous event, such as those considered in the paper, induces all individuals to change self-protection expenditures and thereby to change the average health state among all persons. Insurance companies now experience unanticipated changes in profit, and price competition and new entry must alter premium rates. This sets off another chain, with feedbacks to optimal self-protection expenditures, and so on. All these secondary and higher-order effects are ignored in the paper and how they affect the conclusions is not very obvious. For example, the process depicted above may not be stable. But assuming that it was, some information on the long-run, steady-state response could be obtained if the authors had considered the other polar extreme in which insurance premiums and health state probabilities are perceived to be related to each other rather than completely unrelated.

Some other limitations of the specification should be mentioned.

1. Nordquist and Wu use an index, h, as a health state indicator. What is the operational content of h and precisely what does it measure? Even if health states could be ranked according to an objective univariate index, it still must be an ordinal index. The authors arbitrarily normalize the index to lie between zero and 1, but any monotonic transformation would do just as well. If so, what sense does it make to talk about the convexity of the insurance payoff schedule?

2. As pointed out above, the authors focus only on financial risks of illness. Income (in period two) is what it would have been in the absence of illness minus the cost of medical treatment. Income received from the insurance company in the event of illness, xl, covers some fraction of the medical bill. Thus they assume that illness does not affect earning capacity and, more important, each illness is associated with a unique exogenously determined remedy available to all at a fixed fee. All the much discussed effects of insurance and payments by third parties on the type and quality of care are ignored. Moreover, the quality of care and self-protection may be good substitutes.

Turn now to the theorems established by the authors. For ease of interpretation and exposition, their argument will be simplified by considering a one-period problem and collapsing the continuous distribution of possible health states into a familiar binomial process. Although these simplifications ignore some of the elegant technical sophistication of their model, they retain its spirit and, I believe, help pinpoint the intuitive economic content of the analysis.

Consider a one-period problem in which the individual chooses preventive expenditures Z and insurance l to maximize

(1) $$Eu = (1 - p)u(Y_0 - \rho l - Z) + pu(Y_1 + xl)$$

In this formulation $u(\cdot)$ is the utility function (assuming risk aversion), p is the probability of a "standard" illness, Y_0 is income if illness doesn't occur, Y_1 is net income if illness does occur [$(Y_0 - Y_1)$ is the medical bill], ρ is the price of insurance, and xl is the amount of medical bills paid by the insurance company. Assume that p is a function of preventive expenditure, $p(Z)$, with

$dp/dz = p' < 0$ so that preventive medicine is productive. The marginal conditions for a maximum of (1) subject to $p(Z)$ are

(2) $\quad \partial Eu/\partial I = -(1-p)pu'_0 + xpu'_1 = 0$

(3) $\quad \partial Eu/\partial p = -p'(u_0 - u_1) - (1-p)u'_0 = 0$

where u'_0 is shorthand for marginal utility evaluated at the appropriate value of non-illness net income and u'_1 is marginal utility evaluated at the appropriate value of illness net income, and similarly for u_0 and u_1.

Just as in Nordquist and Wu's more sophisticated model, the content of this theory is obtained by differentiating the marginal conditions with respect to exogenous parameters and exploiting second-order conditions, as usual. A geometrical interpretation can be given in the present case by using the indirect utility function. We want to derive indifference curves between Z and p conditional on the individual's buying the optimum amount of insurance coverage at every value of p. Condition (2) above defines the optimum amount of insurance for all values of p. If the functional form of u were given, (2) could be solved for I in terms of p, Z, and the other variables and substituted into (1), resulting in a synthetic, indirect utility function relating Eu to p, Z, Y_0, Y_1, p, and x. Values of I are "optimized out" as it were. If a specific functional form is not given, the indirect utility function is defined only implicitly by equations (1) and (2). In other words, ignore (3) for the moment and treat (1) and (2) as two equations in which I and Z are considered to be dependent variables and p, Eu, x, p, Y_1 and Y_0 are considered to be independent variables. Then the function $Z(p, Eu, ...)$ implicitly defined by (1) and (2) yields a family of indifference curves between Z and p at alternative values of Eu.[1] In distinction to the usual case, the entire indifference map relating Z and p shifts when x, p, Y_1, and Y_0 change, because in each case the optimum amount of insurance changes.

The implicit function theorem applied to (1) and (2) establishes all the essential properties of $Z(p, Eu, ...)$. In particular it readily shows that $\partial Z/\partial Eu$, $\partial Z/\partial p$, and $\partial^2 Z/\partial p^2$ are all negative. Therefore, the indifference curves appear as E_0, E_1, and E_2 in Figure 1. Since Z and p are "bads," it should come as no surprise that the indifference curves are concave and expected utility rises as we move toward the origin. The constraint relating preventive medical expenditure and the probability of illness is shown in Figure 1 as the curve labeled $p(Z)$. Hence the optimum amount of self-protection and resulting probability of illness occur as usual at a point of tangency between an indifference curve and the constraint. Since $\partial Z/\partial p = -(u_0 - u_1)/(1-p)u'_0$ along an indifference curve, the geometry and Condition (3) are internally consistent.

Think of the slope of an indifference curve, $-\partial Z(p, Eu, ...)/\partial p$, as a reservation price. It is the (incremental) amount the individual is willing to pay to reduce medical risk by a small amount. The theory of utility maximization and risk aversion places no restrictions on how reservation prices vary with the level of welfare, Eu (i.e., the derivative $\partial^2 Z/\partial p \partial Eu$ is unsigned and could be either positive or negative). This is the fundamental reason why Nordquist and Wu get so few positive predictions from their theory. Income effects resulting from parameter changes can go in either direction, and even if substitution effects are unambiguous, the total, uncompensated effects are not. Thus, to get unambiguous predictions it is necessary to make a *priori* assumptions about the sign of income effects. To capture the essence of their crucial assumptions in the present simplified model, assume that the marginal reservation price of medical risk falls with real income. Then the slopes of the indifference curves in Figure 1 become steeper as we move up any vertical line. I find it difficult to say whether such an assumption is "reasonable" or not. Perhaps it is equally plausible to assume that the amount a person will pay to reduce medical risk increases with wealth instead of decreasing. Here would seem to be a case where ignoring pain and suffering might make a difference. Whatever, let us examine the implications of this kind of assumption.

Suppose that the price of insurance, p, decreases. Repeated application of the implicit function theorem to the definition of the indifference map (equations (1) and (2)) has two implications. First, the entire indifference map shifts up ($\partial Z (p, Eu, \ldots)/\partial p$ is negative) and the individual is unambiguously better off at the new equilibrium. Second, the new indifference curves are not so sharply inclined as the old ones were ($\partial^2 Z/\partial p\, \partial p$ is negative): The compensated marginal offer price-risk *schedule* for reductions in medical risk shifts downward. Now without some a *priori* specification of the income effect, the net outcome in the new situation could involve either more or less risk than the old one. However, if reservation prices fall with increases in Eu, the new equilibrium must be at a point on $p(Z)$ such as B. Preventive expenditure falls, real risks rise, and there is a clear case of moral hazard.

Consider next an increase in x, the share of medical remedy costs reimbursed by market insurance. Again the indifference curves shift upward and the individual must be better off at the new equilibrium. But in this case it turns out that the simple theory does not provide an unambiguous prediction about what happens to the reservation price (i.e., $\partial^2 Z/\partial p\, \partial x$ is unsigned). There is only a presumption that the indifference map tilts in the same way as it did for the above case of a decrease in p. If it does, we get the same kind of outcome; a move to the new equilibrium at a point such as B, a decrease in Z, and an increase in p and moral hazard.

This simple theory by itself is silent about both income and substitution effects for changes in x, whereas for changes in p it does make an unambiguous prediction about substitution effects, but of course not about income effects.[2] Nordquist and Wu get a similar result in their more sophisticated model, except that the substitution effect is definitely signed for changes in x but not for changes in p (see their equations (8.2) and (9.2)).

Finally, consider a change in the risk-expenditure constraint $p(Z)$. In fact, suppose that $p(Z)$ simply shifts to the left in Figure 1 without changing its slope, a pure income effect, owing, for example, to an increase in public health. In this case we get a very puzzling result if the same income effect assumption as above is maintained: As long as the new equilibrium is interior, preventive care falls and real risks rise. Of course, it is possible that the shift in $p(Z)$ is so large that the new equilibrium occurs along the p axis, in which case Z falls to zero and p definitely decreases. But for marginal changes, the above assumption about income effects implies that slight improvements in public health induce individuals to expose themselves to greater risks. There is more illness after the improvement than before! This outcome does not appear very "reasonable" to me at all, but then again it is only a product of the assumption and not necessarily an implication of the pure theory.[3]

In sum, the theory presented by Nordquist and Wu contains very few empirical predictions. Given the technical sophistication of their model, it seems doubtful whether further theorizing will result in a more authoritative theory. Clearly, here is a case in which careful empirical study is the next order of business. This theory is useful for organizing the structural relations to be estimated from data and for clarifying thought. But it does not give much guidance in advance about what these relationships should look like.

NOTES

1. Alternatively, p and I can be treated as "dependent" and Z, Eu, x, ρ, Y_1, and Y_2 as "independent" variables, yielding a function $p(Z, Eu, \ldots)$. Of course, $p(Z; \ldots)$ is simply the inverse of $Z(p; \ldots)$ and contains the same information about the indifference map.
2. To keep within the spirit of Nordquist and Wu's model, notice that Z is not subtracted from $Y_1 + xI$ in Equation (1). In the context of a straight one-period model, it makes some sense for Z to be subtracted from income in both states. The conceptual basis of the diagrammatic exposition in Figure 1 is unchanged in that case, but my cursory examination of it shows analysis is much more difficult: It is not even clear that the indifference curves can be shown to be concave. If so, then not even many of the pure substitution effects can be signed.
3. Improvements in public health must change insurance premiums and affect the result. I have ignored these general equilibrium repercussions because Nordquist and Wu ignored them.

3

G. S. GOLDSTEIN and M. V. PAULY
Northwestern University

Group Health Insurance as a Local Public Good

1. INTRODUCTION

Group health insurance is an important topic for at least two reasons. First, its quantitative importance is large and growing. Second, the management, level, and form of group insurance are increasingly a matter of concern for public policy, as are other benefits often provided as fringe benefits. For example, the Nixon administration proposed to use health insurance as a fringe benefit as the main vehicle of its national health policy, and employee pensions have recently been the subject of congressional investigation and legislation.

In one of the few papers that deal with fringe benefits (Lester, 1967), the author concludes

> We lack a theory of the collective purchase of insurance-type benefits for employees, either unilaterally by management or through union-management negotiations. Without such a theory one is unable to give an adequate explanation of . . . changes . . . in the wage benefit mix in the American economy. . . .

In this paper, we shall attempt to outline such a theory and provide some empirical tests of parts of it. Data deficiencies prevent a complete test of all implications of the theory. The critical element in this theory is that group insurance has institutional characteristics similar to those of local public goods. There are two important similarities:

1. The level of insurance coverage must, over broad categories of employees, be equal for all, just as the level of the textbook local public good must be shared equally by all.
2. Persons not in the employee group receive no benefits, and benefits can be lost or acquired by "migration" among groups, just as for many local public goods.

These similarities make it possible to use some parts of the theory of local public goods to draw conclusions about group insurance. But they also mean that a theory of fringe benefits will fall prey to the many unsettled theoretical problems of local public goods.

There are differences as well, and they are equally instructive for the light they shed on the question of how analysis of the provision of local public goods might be affected under similar arrangements. For example, one model we shall develop assumes that the employer determines the level of group insurance, without group choice by employees, but with a view toward minimizing his labor costs. The analogous model for the theory of public goods might be a developer of a "new town" choosing the level of local public services so as to maximize his profits from sales or rentals.

2. WHY FRINGE BENEFITS?

The first question to be answered is the most basic one—why fringe benefits exist. Why doesn't the employer pay the equivalent cash wage? Why should either the employer or employees, organized as a union, choose to receive some income in kind as health insurance? There are two elements in any answer. First, group health insurance as a fringe benefit may be cheaper than individual purchases on the market. Second, the configuration of employee preferences may be such as to permit group purchasing of health insurance to be relatively efficient.

Only the first rationale appears to be emphasized in the literature on this subject. Rice, for example (1966), emphasized economies of group purchasing and tax advantages as the major rationales for variations in fringe benefits in general, though he found that group life and health insurance did not seem strongly related to the empirical variables he could find to serve as proxies for these notions. A similar explanation, with particular emphasis on the advantages of group purchases, was given by Phelps (1973). Although their purpose is descriptive rather than analytical, Feldstein and Allison (1974) also emphasize tax advantages, whereas Feldstein (1973) cites, in addition to group purchasing and tax reductions, the supposed desire of unions and employers to provide visible benefits.

The tax laws do impose some restrictions on group insurance. Only certain kinds of insurance benefits qualify for tax exemption. The level of those benefits must, ostensibly at least, be chosen by the employer or through collective bargaining, rather than be subject to the choice of each individual employee.

But it is obviously not true that all employee groups take maximum possible insurance benefits. Even at a net price lowered by tax considerations or the economies of group purchase, a net price that on average may, according to Feldstein and Allison, be below the actuarially fair price, group demand is not infinite, or even as large as the tax laws permit.

The reason for this may be that employees do not necessarily all have the same preferences. Both tax and technological considerations require that group health insurance be uniform over groups of employees, if not over all employees. If employees did have identical preferences, a single level of benefits would be optimal for all. This paper suggests that the dispersion of preferences may help to explain the level of coverage actually chosen by or for a group.

The rudiments of a theory of fringe benefits must include consideration of the problem of combining diverse preferences. In what follows a series of simple models will be developed to illustrate these points.

3. FORMAL MODELS

Model 1: A Tiebout-Type Model

The first model is intended to be analogous to Tiebout's (1956) classic model of providing local public goods. We assume that employees are perfectly mobile, that firms are all at least as large as that size at which the marginal advantage for group purchasing approaches zero,[1] and that workers are perfectly homogeneous with respect to the kind of labor they supply and to their expected medical expenses, but differ in their attitudes toward risk. We shall also assume that the incidence of the cost of fringe benefits falls wholly on the employees of the firm offering those benefits. Finally, we assume (1) that the number of firms is sufficiently "large" that a level of insurance corresponding to any level of employee preferences can be provided, (2) that the number of employees with any set of preferences is at least twice the number needed to exhaust group-purchase economies, and (3) that employees have perfect information.

Employee Equilibrium

We assume a competitive market for labor. Thus, given any method of determining the level of group insurance premiums, it must be true that, in every firm:

(1) $$MRP_L = Y = Y_w + \pi(k)$$

where MRP_L is the marginal revenue product of labor, Y is labor cost per employee, Y_w is the money wage, and π is the premium for whatever level of insurance coverage k is chosen. In effect, Equation (1) defines a supply curve of group insurance to the employee. From the set of all existing insurance-wage combinations satisfying (1), the employee will locate at one that maximizes his utility function.

Here, as in the remainder of the paper, we will consider two possible methods of determining the level of group insurance benefits. Fringe benefits are sometimes determined collectively, by the set of present employees, usually through union bargaining. We call this method "union choice." Sometimes, however, fringe benefits are determined by the employer, with a view toward minimizing his labor cost. We first consider employer choice.

Employer-Choice Equilibrium

Given a distribution of employee preferences and assuming that optimally sized groups can always be created, employers may find it worthwhile to adjust the quantity of insurance they provide. Equilibrium therefore requires that no employer be able to create an excess supply of labor to his firm by altering his wage-fringe benefit package. A sufficient condition for this is that there exists no wage-fringe benefit package that could be offered by any firm that is preferred by any worker to the package he is now receiving.

Suppose, for example, that a subset of all employers is initially providing a subset of employees with a mix of wages and benefits that is not the employees' optimal mix. All other employees are receiving their optimal package from their employers. The employees for whom the level of coverage is not optimal will require a higher money wage to work in those firms than they would for firms offering their optimal quantity. Employers will be able to reduce labor costs by providing a package that is optimal to their employees.

Equilibrium therefore requires that every employee be in a firm that provides a utility-maximizing bundle of the public good. For if this were not so, some employer could reduce his labor cost by offering such a bundle. Thus, in equilibrium all groups will offer the package of insurance that maximizes that utility of all of their employees, and all employees in any group will have identical preferences with respect to insurance.

Union Choice

We assume that union groups are at least as large as the firm (though they can be larger). We first show that the employer equilibrium described above is also a union equilibrium. Union equilibrium is assumed to require that each group (firm) choose a level of coverage equal to the optimum of the median individual. One equilibrium would clearly involve the distribution of employees into groups with homogeneous preferences for insurance. For such homogeneous groups, the optimum of the worker with the median preference is also the optimum of all other group members, so that no worker will be motivated to move. And we have just shown that employer equilibrium occurs when employees are distributed into homogeneous groups. Hence, employer equilibrium is a union equilibrium.

There may be other union equilibria. Some differ from employer equilibrium in that they involve different alternative configurations into homogeneous groups, because a union group can exceed an employer-formed group in size. There also are equilibria in which groups are not homogeneous. But any equilibrium in which any group is not homogeneous is unstable. Suppose that there are two kinds of employees and the optimal number of groups is two, but the types of employees are evenly divided between the groups. The median preferences in both groups will be the same, and so will the levels of coverage. If one group should provide a slightly higher level of coverage than the other group, it will attract one type of employee and repel the other. Equilibrium will be reestablished when groups are homogeneous.

Group-Size Variable

We now relax the assumption that employee group size must be optimal. This seems reasonable. For some industries, premiums appear to fall with group size up to sizes well in excess of the work forces of some firms. One possible solution would be for employee groups to combine for insurance purposes. Practical difficulties may prevent employers from sanctioning this procedure, though we might expect unions to do so. But if there is no combination, it follows that wage costs per employee will initially have to be higher in small firms than in large ones, and that, moreover, the difference will have to be still greater at high levels of coverage than at low levels of coverage. As a consequence, we would not expect to find high levels of coverage as common among small firms as among large firms, under employer or union choice. Conversely, we should expect those employees with strong demands for insurance to be more likely to work for large firms. Prices of the outputs of industries characterized by small firms would rise relative to those of industries characterized by large firms until labor costs and marginal products are equalized.[2]

Adverse Selection

Assume now that not all workers have the same expected medical expenses. Expected expenses can differ either because the incidence of illness differs or because the quantity of care (medical loss) consumed for any given illness differs.[3] It is clear that in such a situation bad risks may find it worthwhile to join groups of good risks. Consequently, exclusionary devices may come into play. Such devices may take the form of medical examinations, or the characteristics of the job itself may be sufficient to exclude bad risks. If adverse selection still remains, one might expect some individuals to be driven out of the group-purchase market altogether, whereas others will pay a "weighted average" rate. The relationship between quantity of insurance and level of risk is likely to be positive.

It is also possible that equilibrium may not exist.[4] For example, suppose that because of an influx of bad risks the price of insurance rises so high that good risks no longer wish to buy insurance. They will gather in a firm or group providing no insurance. But such a group could provide insurance advantageously to its members. Yet if it begins to do so, it will attract bad risks again and all the good risks will again drop out. It may also be worthwhile for the employer to provide less than the amount of insurance that would minimize labor costs, since large quantities of insurance may attract bad risks. Likewise, if the median worker is a good risk, limiting insurance quantities may be worthwhile and may be stable.

Empirical Implications

The purpose of this paper is to estimate a demand-for-insurance equation of the form

$$k = k(x) + e$$

where k is the fraction of expenses covered by insurance, x is a set of independent variables, and e is a random error term. If the conditions above hold, under either method of choice the employees of a firm will be homogeneous with respect to their insurance preferences; their characteristics, part of the set x, will differ only because of the random error e. Hence, it will be appropriate to use mean values of x in the empirical specification.

Another implication of this model is that the method of choice will not affect the quantity of insurance chosen. We will test for this both by including the extent of unionization as an independent variable in a regression using all observations and dividing the observations into predominantly union and nonunion sets, and by testing to see if the estimated coefficients on other independent variables differ.

Model 2: Imperfect Mobility

A model in which the variety of options is sufficiently large to permit homogeneous groups of employees may not be descriptive of the world. Workers in a single group may have heterogeneous preferences for insurance for two reasons. First, efficient production may require the hiring of labor forces that are heterogeneous with respect to characteristics (e.g., education, sex), which might affect the demand for insurance. Although separate groups might be created for some kinds of employees (e.g., separate plans for executives and production workers), it may be too costly or too cumbersome to maintain separate plans for each worker type. Second, the number of groups available to a set of employees may not be large enough to permit the formation of homogeneous groups of sufficient size to capture economies of scale or inhibit adverse selection.[5] Whatever the reason, the result will be the formation of insurance groups in some of which it will be impossible for the quantity provided to be the optimum for all group members.

Heterogeneous Labor

In what follows we analyze both cases. We show that, if groups are heterogeneous for the first reason, employer equilibrium generally will exist but will differ from union equilibrium. In the second case, we show that employer equilibrium is unlikely to exist. We begin with the first case.

Suppose that there are two kinds of workers, A and B. Each kind of worker provides a qualitatively different type of labor input; each type has a quantitatively different identical-within-type demand for health insurance. Both types of workers are useful in producing output, and there is no perfect substitutability between types. Hence, most firms will end up hiring some of each type of labor. Because of supply and production considerations, we assume that most firms hire more type-A than type-B employees when labor costs per employee equal their relative marginal revenue products. We also assume that different levels of insurance cannot be provided to different types of employees.

Now suppose that the employer can provide health insurance. For each employer, labor supply of each type of employee will be a function of the money wage and the level of fringe benefits offered. Assume that the incidence of fringe benefit payments falls wholly on employees. Then, if their respective demand curves for insurance are like D_A and D_B in Figure 1, A-type workers will optimally want k^*_A units of insurance, and B-type workers, k^*_B units.[6] Each of the optimal quantities is the quantity that would minimize labor cost for that type of employee. At any other level of coverage, a firm could offer a quantity close to k^*, permit the employee to capture some of the utility gain, and recoup the remainder in the form of lower wages.

But the optimal level of coverage for a firm consisting of both types of employees requires a tradeoff between the optimums of both groups. Suppose that firm i's employment of each labor type, L_{A_i} and L_{B_i}, is given. Its wage bill is therefore:

$$W^i = C_A L_{A_i} + C_B L_{B_i}$$

FIGURE 1

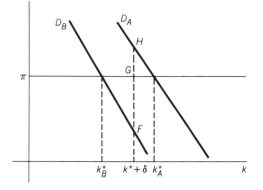

where C_A is the labor cost per type-A employee and C_B, the labor cost per type-B employee.

Assume that the wage package available to type-J employees at other firms is (w^{Jo}, k^o). Hours of work are fixed. Workers have utility functions of the form:

(2) $\quad U = U(w, k)$

For every type-J employee for firm i, equilibrium requires that $U^J(w^{Ji}, k^i) \geq U^J(w^{Jo}, k^o)$. If firm i wishes to minimize its labor costs, it will set the wage rate of type-J workers, for a given $k^i = \bar{k}^i$, so that:

(3) $\quad U^J(w^{Ji}, \bar{k}^i) = U^J(w^{Jo}, k^o)$

Suppose that the firm is considering offering an increment in k that has a premium cost π. The change in the money wage that permits (3) to continue to hold is given by that decrease in money wages that holds utility constant at the level indicated in (3), or:[7]

(4) $\quad \dfrac{dw^{Ji}}{dk^i} = \dfrac{u_k^J}{u_{wJ}^J}$

Hence, the change in total labor cost per employee is:

(5) $\quad \dfrac{dC_j^i}{dk^i} = \dfrac{u_k^J}{u_{wJ}^J} - \pi$

since the firm must pay the premium, π. Minimizing total labor cost for all classes of employees implies:

(6a) $\quad \dfrac{dW^i}{dk^i} = \dfrac{dC_A^i}{dk^i} L_{A_i} + \dfrac{dC_B^i}{dk^i} L_{B_i} = 0$

or

(6b)
$$- L_{A_i} \left[\frac{U_k^A}{U_{w \cdot A}^A} - \pi \right] = L_{B_i} \left[\frac{U_k^B}{U_{w \cdot B}^B} - \pi \right]$$

Thus cost-minimizing equilibrium requires equalizing weighted-average marginal labor cost per employee of each type. Changes in k^i beyond the optimum of type-B workers require an increase in their wages, but this increase may be more than offset by the decrease in the wages of type-A workers. In terms of Figure 1, increments in coverage beyond k_B^* require an increase in type-B employees' wages equal to the difference between D_B and π; e.g., measured by distance GF at quantity $k^* + \delta$. If, for example, $L_B GF < L_A GH$, then k should be increased further, whereas if $L_B GF = L_A GH$, $k^* + \delta$ is the cost-minimizing level of the fringe benefit.

Union equilibrium, on the other hand, simply requires that the quantity chosen equal the optimum of the individual with median preferences. Since the median worker is a type-A employee, union equilibrium requires equating type-A marginal rates of substitution with the premium to be charged per unit of insurance. The employer has an incentive to consider all workers' preferences in a way that the union does not. If type-A (union-dominant) workers generally prefer more insurance than type-B workers, unions will prefer different quantities of insurance than nonunionized firms. Moreover, the greater the number of type-B employees, as long as it is less than half of the total number of workers, the greater will be the difference between employer and union choice.

In particular, suppose that type-A employees demand larger quantities of insurance than do type-B employees. Unions will cater to the demands of type-A employees. Those firms that provide larger quantities of insurance will tend to be unionized. The exceptions would be (1) those firms containing only one type of employee and (2) those firms with more type-B than type-A employees. With more kinds of employees, it becomes more difficult to predict the direction of the union effect. In general, union choice will differ to the extent that the marginal rate of substitution of the median worker differs from a weighted average of the marginal rates of substitution of all marginal workers.

It is worth mentioning that employer equilibrium is also Pareto optimal, whereas union equilibrium is not. For if we rearrange terms in (6b), we get:

$$(6c) \qquad L_{A_i} \frac{u_k^A}{u_{w_A}^A} + L_{B_i} \frac{u_k^B}{u_{w_B}^B} = (L_{A_i} + L_{B_i})\,\pi$$

Since the cost of a unit of the "public good" insurance provided equally to all is given by the term on the right, Equation (6c) is equivalent to the Samuelson optimality condition, equating summed marginal rates of substitution with marginal cost.[8]

The preceding model shows that union and employer choice may differ, and that those differences depend on a comparison of the marginal benefit of health insurance to the median voter with the average marginal benefit of all marginal workers. Unions will systematically provide more insurance, *ceteris paribus*, if the former is consistently greater than the latter. If we assume that all employees are equally likely to be marginal, one reason why unions might be expected to provide more insurance is that the median union voter will typically have a higher marginal benefit than the average worker's marginal benefit.

This may occur for two reasons. First, even in unionized firms, not all workers are union members, and yet reasons of administrative economy may well require them to share the insurance package bargained by the union. Those nonmembers tend to be women and low-income and young male workers, all of whom will have low demands for insurance. In addition, it is likely that those workers with low marginal benefits who are union members are less likely to vote in union elections. The constituency of voters to which union leaders respond will therefore be one with a high demand for insurance, whereas the employer, if he chooses the level of coverage, will have an incentive to consider the effect of his choice on the wages he must pay all workers.

Homogeneous Labor

We now turn to the second case, in which labor is homogeneous but in which there are not "enough" groups. Workers are homogeneous with respect to the amount and type of labor they supply and have different preferences with respect to the level of insurance they prefer. These differences might result both from differences in demands at equal prices and from the different prices that tax considerations pose for different income groups. The number of employment opportunities is not sufficiently large to permit formation of homogeneous groups for every employee preference. The supply of labor to any firm, therefore, becomes a function of both its money wage rate and the level of insurance it offers.

In order for equilibrium to exist in this market, the quantity of insurance being provided to the members of a group must be an equilibrium under the choice rule being used for that set of individuals. In addition, given the quantity of insurance chosen, each firm or group must be an equilibrium location for the members of the group; employee equilibrium must prevail.

In employee equilibrium, no employee may confront a wage-fringe benefit package in some other firm that he prefers to the one he is now receiving. The characteristics of this equilibrium depend on whether or not the employer can adjust the money wage of each employee individually. If he cannot, but must (for practical or institutional reasons) pay the same money wage to each employee, employee equilibrium would require that the employee at the margin be indifferent between the wage-insurance package of this employer and that of his next best alternative.

Call $w_{ij}|k = \bar{k}$ worker i's reservation wage for working at firm j. This is the minimum money wage at which, given the level of insurance coverage, worker i would be willing to work for firm j. Call $\bar{w}_j|k = \bar{k}$ the actual money wage being paid by firm j. For simplicity, the level of insurance coverage will be suppressed in what follows. Obviously, if $w_{ij} < \bar{w}_j$, the worker will work for firm j, and vice versa. Obviously, too, w_{ij} depends on worker i's alternative opportunities. Thus, employee equilibrium is characterized by:

(7) $\qquad w_{ij} \leq \bar{w}_j | k_j = \bar{k}_j$

for all workers who work at any firm j.

Equilibrium with respect to the employer's insurance decision requires two conditions to apply. First, no firm can alter its labor cost per employee by slight changes in its level of coverage. Assume that each firm believes that other firms' levels of coverage will not change in response to changes in its level of coverage. Let π be the cost per unit of insurance k. If a unit change in coverage is made, a worker who formerly did not do so will choose to work for firm j if, and only if:

(8a) $\qquad \dfrac{u_k^i}{u_{w}^i} - \pi > w_{ij} - \bar{w}_j$

Conversely, a worker who works for firm j will leave if, and only if:

(8b) $\qquad \dfrac{u_k^i}{u_{w}^i} - \pi < w_{ij} - \bar{w}_j$

Equilibrium requires that the number of workers for which (8a) holds equal exactly the number of workers for which (8b) holds.

The second employer equilibrium condition is that no firm be able to make a nonmarginal change in coverage such that it can hire the same number of employees at a lower labor cost. If this number is $\bar{L}$, this means that the number of workers for which (9a) and (9b) hold must be less than $\bar{L}$ for all j:

(9a) $\quad U(\bar{w}_j, \bar{k}_j) \leqq U(w, k)$

and

(9b) $\quad w\bar{L} + \pi k\bar{L} < \bar{w}_j\bar{L} + \pi\bar{k}_j\bar{L}$

Conditions 9 require that there be no set of $\bar{L}$ workers who can obtain as much as or more utility from hypothetical package (w, k) than they are now getting, if the hypothetical package has a lower labor cost than the package they are presently receiving. The actual number of workers $\bar{L}$ to be hired would then be determined in the usual way by equating marginal factor cost to marginal revenue product of labor.

To show that the two conditions (8) and (9) are unlikely to be satisfied simultaneously, let us begin with the case in which the supply of labor to the market as a whole is perfectly inelastic with respect to the real wage. The only function of the level of fringe benefits is then to determine for which employer a worker will work. At the margin, given any set of levels of insurance k being offered by a given number of firms, $\bar{w}_j = w_{ij}$. A slight alteration in k will bring the level of coverage closer to the optimums of the employees at one margin and move it further away from the optimums of the employees at the other margin. Suppose that we have a frequency distribution of the optimums of workers in the labor market. Call $f(m_1)$ the frequency of optimums of employees who are at the one margin and $f(m_2)$ the frequency of employees at the other margin. To make (8a) = (8b) therefore requires that $f(m_1) = f(m_2)$. This can happen only if the distribution contains a mode between m_1 and m_2, or if it is rectangular over the interval m_1 to m_2. For unimodal distributions, the only level of coverage satisfying marginal equilibrium occurs at a mode.

However, if all firms offer the level of coverage at the mode, persons whose optimums are not close to the mode will be willing to work at lower wages for firms that offer levels of coverage nearer their optimums. Hence, conditions (9) may well not hold. If the only points that satisfy (8) do not satisfy (9), no equilibrium exists.

This problem is formally similar to Hotelling's locational problem, and a brief geometric exposition may help to explain the foregoing discussion and to make the similarity clear. It is assumed that, marginal labor cost held constant, workers will choose to work for the firm whose level of k is closest to their optimum. If five firms offered the levels of coverage k_1 through k_5, respectively, the margins would be at the point indicated by the dashed lines in Figure 2. For simplicity, these positions have been chosen so that each firm has the same number of employees (i.e., the integrals between the margins are the same). It is apparent that these firms are not in marginal equilibrium; movements toward the mode gain more workers than they lose for all firms except firm 3. But if all firms locate at the mode, dividing the total labor supply into five parts, it is obvious that a firm that took up, say, position k_2 could attract an excess supply of labor, since it would lure all the workers from the left tail up to the margin m. Hence, marginal and global equilibrium cannot coexist.

Although it will not be proved here, it can be shown that if the labor supply is not perfectly inelastic with respect to the real wage, equilibrium by chance may occur even in situations with "large" unimodal distributions. But such occurrences would not be particularly likely.

It is worth pointing out that these conclusions about the nonexistence of equilibrium can be generalized to the local public goods case as well. Questions are raised about the existence of equilibrium if property owners are thought of as choosing the level of local public goods to maximize rents. For the purpose of characterizing reality, the foregoing model is somewhat unsatisfactory.

Union equilibrium obviously requires that the employees be in equilibrium and that the employer be in equilibrium with respect to the number of employees he hires, given the level of insurance

FIGURE 2

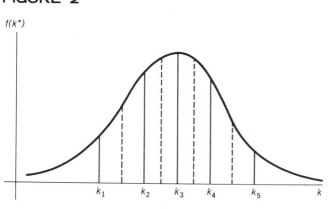

coverage and the supply of labor function. The level of insurance coverage, however, is set at the level of the optimum of the individual with median preferences in the present group of workers.

Two observations are relevant here. First, it is clear that there can be multiple equilibria. It may be, for example, that *every* employee-employer equilibrium is also the optimum of the individual with median preferences. But second, it is also clearly possible that no equilibrium exists. Suppose that every individual's utility depends in a linear way on the difference between his optimum and the level of coverage chosen for the group. Suppose that the distribution of individual optimums is as in Figure 3. Finally, suppose that there are three firms.

The conditions for equilibrium are the following, where $f(x)$ is the distribution of optimum quantities and it is assumed that the wage costs per worker are the same in all firms:

(10)   Employee equilibrium $m_1 d_1 = d_1 m_2$
$$m_2 d_2 = d_2 m_3$$

(11)   Union-choice equilibrium $\int_0^{m_1} f(x)dx = \int_{m_1}^{d_1} f(x)dx$

$$\int_{d_1}^{m_2} f(x)dx = \int_{m_2}^{d_2} f(x)dx$$

$$\int_{d_2}^{m_3} f(x)dx = \int_{m_3}^{\infty} f(x)dx$$

FIGURE 3

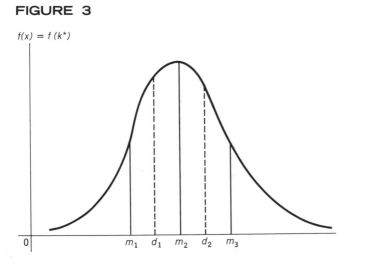

$f(x) = f(k^*)$

m_1 d_1 m_2 d_2 m_3

The positions of d and m in Figure 3 are drawn to satisfy these conditions. However, it is also clear from that figure that the number of employees in each firm is not equal. But at equal wage cost per employee, each firm will want to hire the same number of employees. Hence, no equilibrium exists. If the marginal wage cost per employee differs across firms (because elasticities of supply differ), firms may not all want to have the same size labor forces. But whatever pattern they choose, it need not correspond with the numbers that satisfy (10) and (11).[9]

Empirical Implications

Without a robust characterization of equilibrium, it is difficult to specify *a priori* what one would expect to find from empirical data. What we can say is that under either equilibrium notion presented above, the level of coverage an employer would choose will tend to be related more to the characteristics of all employees in a given labor market than to the characteristics of those particular employees he hires, whereas union choice will tend to be related only to characteristics of the median person. Insofar as the employer is in marginal equilibrium, what will be relevant are the characteristics of his marginal employees. Union choice, on the other hand, should still be related to the individual with median preferences.

Contributory Plans

Up to this point, the only choice available to union or employers is to decide how much tax-free fringe benefit to offer. But many firms have so-called contributory plans, in which the employer does not "pay" the entire health insurance premium. The employees pay all or part of the premium as an explicit and voluntary payroll deduction. The critical differences are that those employees who choose not to participate in the plan can retain their share of the premium and that the employee's share is taxed as ordinary income.

We first show, in the context of the two-employee-types model, how a contributory plan can be preferred by an employer to a noncontributory plan. We also show that a union will in general *not* choose a contributory plan. Then we indicate how the employer chooses the optimal share-coverage combination. For simplicity, we consider a model in which the same contributory share applies to all units of coverage.

Why Contributory Plans?

Suppose that a firm has exactly twice as many type-A employees as type-B employees and that their demand curves are as shown in Figure 4, where π is the unit premium for group insurance. The noncontributory equilibrium package is at k_n^*, where $GH = 2HF$. The total welfare loss suffered by a type-B person is given by area JHG.

The line π' represents the cost to type-B employees for individual insurance. Type-B employees will be better off dropping out of the group plan if the effects of extra premium costs for an individual plan, or area $J\pi\pi'M$, are less than the welfare loss from group insurance.

When is an employer more likely to offer a contributory plan? Such a plan is more likely to materialize if the costs imposed on type-A persons are low, i.e., if their marginal income tax rate is relatively low. It is also more likely to be advantageous if the welfare loss of type-B persons under a noncontributory plan is relatively high, which tends to occur if the optimums of both groups are widely separated.

Optimal Employee Share

In the two-type model, a contributory plan will make all employees who take the maximum amount of insurance worse off, relative to a noncontributory plan, because it subjects a part of the

FIGURE 4

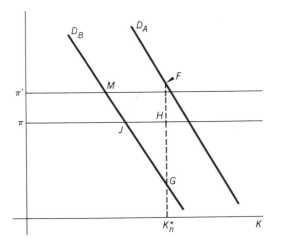

premium to income taxation. Hence, a noncontributory plan can benefit type-B workers only if they are induced to opt out of the group insurance plan. Then they save the employer the total amount of the premium that would have been paid for them. Suppose that a contributory plan is introduced, with a given employer share s. There are two equilibria possible. On the one hand, if type-B employees do not drop out, the optimal k is analyzed as in the noncontributory case. On the other hand, if type-B employees do drop out, k is set at the optimum of type-A individuals, and the money wages of type-B workers are increased to make up for the loss of insurance. If they are worse off with insurance than without it, the employer would want to set w^B at such a level that $U^B(w^B, 0) = U^B(w^{Bo}, k^o)$ and set w^A such that $U^A\{[w^A - t(1 - s)k_A^* \ \pi], k_A^* \} = U^A(w^{Ao}, k^o)$. Notice that $k_A^{*\prime}$ will differ from k_A^*, since the increase in the fraction of premium that is taxable income raises the net price of insurance to type-A employees. Clearly, w^A is minimized if s is as large as possible, and w^B does not vary with s once type-B employees have dropped out. Hence, the optimal s would appear to be the largest s at which opting out is legal.

But this assumes that type-B workers will indeed opt out. From the viewpoint of any individual worker, his money wage will not depend on whether he chooses insurance or not (for if it did, the employer payment would not be tax free). He will not be likely to opt out at a high s, since his *perceived* benefit from doing so is $(1 - s)k\pi$, whereas his perceived cost is the loss of the entire insurance package k. The employer may need to lower s much below 1 to induce type-B employees to opt out. The cost of providing this inducement is the extra tax on the income of type-A workers.

The type-B worker's *perceived* utility level, if he opts out, is $U^B [w^B + (1 - s)k_n\pi, 0]$, and he compares it to $U^B (w_i^B, k_n^*)$, where k_n^* is the optimal mixed equilibrium. (We assume here that the firm does not "force" him out by providing, say, k_A^* units, although the analysis would be roughly similar.) The firm's problem is to choose the largest s such that opting out occurs. The lower the evaluation the worker puts on the k_n units of insurance (i.e., the greater the welfare loss he bears at k_n), the higher this s can be, as long as s is less than 1.

There is a fundamental difference in the effect of worker characteristics on premiums. For noncontributory insurance, the lower B's demand relative to A's demand, the lower k_n, and hence the lower the premium. For contributory plans, the lower B's demand, the *higher* will be optimal s. If the B's do not participate, k_n can be higher. Premiums can increase, decrease, or be unaffected by changes in variables related to B's demand.

Unions and Contributory Plans

It would appear that a union should never choose a contributory plan, for the optimum of the median worker always involves a noncontributory (fully tax free) plan providing his optimal level of coverage. Of course, if the employer has some influence in the decision, or if vote-trading or consideration of the effect of worker group characteristics induces the union to consider the preferences of other employees, unions may be associated with contributory plans. But in general we should expect unions to be less likely to have contributory plans.

General Equilibrium

The world that we will be analyzing empirically is one in which group insurance is provided in many firms and the quantity is sometimes chosen by unions and sometimes by employers. The supply curve of labor to a particular firm depends both on the wage-insurance package of that firm and also on that of all other firms. But, assuming that a general equilibrium exists, the partial equilibrium conditions outlined above must be satisfied for every firm, the particular set of conditions depending on whether the employer or the employee chooses the quantity. In addition, it requires that wage cost per employee be equated across firms. This means that those firms which are prevented from offering the labor-cost minimizing insurance package will sustain losses and will go out of business. If they are concentrated in particular industries, and if new nonunionized firms cannot be formed, average firm size must shrink until marginal products are equalized.

Empirical Specification

The empirical models of union choice that we test are similar to studies of the demand for local public goods by Borcherding and Deacon (1972) and by Bergstrom and Goodman (1973). Both of these studies rely on the proposition that, in a majority rule model, the group choice is identical with the optimum of the individual with median preferences. Coupled with the assumption (implicit in Borcherding and Deacon and explicit in Bergstrom and Goodman) that the median quantity is demanded by the citizen with the median income, they provide an empirical estimate of the price and income elasticities of demand as well as an estimate of a "crowding" or "(dis)economy of scale" parameter.

There are three major empirical variables in both of these studies. Both use median income. In addition, quantity of the public good is regressed on a measure of the price of the public good and the number of persons in the sharing group.

We have mentioned above that for group insurance, the loading is likely to vary inversely with group size up to some limit. The extent to which it does so would correspond to the "crowding" notion. Unfortunately, it does not appear that we will be able to use an independent measure of price. Insurance is produced in a national market, so there seems to be no reason to expect prices for a given group size to differ across areas or industries. And it seems reasonable to assume that all employees pay equal shares of the total cost, so "tax shares" will not differ. One could argue that differential concentrations of bad risks might affect the price paid by a representative median individual, but to get a measure of the actual price variation we need to know by how much, e.g., a larger proportion of high-risk blacks raises the premium per individual for a given level of coverage.

Thus we are limited to estimating the effects on quantity of insurance demanded of income and group size alone. Data limitations will require us to work with average pay, rather than median income. A further difficulty is that we do not have a measure of k, the fraction covered by insurance. Instead, we get a measure of total premiums. This means that, since we do not know price, we are estimating an expenditure equation rather than a demand equation. And since total premiums depend on expected losses as well as on the fraction of those losses covered by insurance, we either need to find a way of removing influences on losses in order to determine what affects choice of coverage for a given loss or need to interpret our coefficients as including both effects. After the empirical results are presented, some illustrative calculations directed at removing these effects will be presented.

4. DIFFERENCES BETWEEN UNION CHOICE AND EMPLOYER CHOICE

We will be able to estimate separate demand relationships for industries in which the choice method is primarily by unions and industries in which it seems reasonable to think of the employer as choosing insurance. The hypothesis that employers choose differently from unions for a given set of employee characteristics might be extended to include the premise that employers are likely to respond differently from unions to *differences* in the set of employee characteristics. In particular, since the employer responds to characteristics of the marginal worker, we would expect the mean income to have less of an effect on employer-chosen insurance than it does on union-chosen insurance. For mean and median incomes are likely to be highly correlated, whereas the relationship between mean income and the income and other characteristics of the marginal worker is likely to be relatively weaker.

In addition, the finding that union choice leads to larger total premiums is consistent with the notion that the union's choice is more likely to ignore the strong preferences of those who would want less insurance. Finally, to the extent that those union members whose preferences are relevant tend to be higher risks than employees in general (because they tend to be older and have larger families or higher incomes), we would also expect to find unions choosing higher levels of health insurance. No recourse to a "union leader" or "visibility" argument is necessary.

5. THE DATA

The Bureau of Labor statistics periodically conducts a survey of employer expenditures for supplementary compensation.[10] The data used in this study are drawn from a 1971 survey of 3,772 establishments across the United States. The questionnaire distinguishes between the records of office and nonoffice employees and asks whether union-management agreements covered a majority of either group of workers. The questions concerning fringe benefit plans distinguish among health, life, and accident insurance. Specifically, the questionnaire asks whether or not an establishment had a health, life, or accident insurance plan, and if so whether the plan (or plans) was (were) noncontributory or contributory. Unfortunately, the question about employer expenditures for these private welfare plans asked only for the total expenditure on all plans together. Other information drawn from the survey for this study includes gross annual payroll, total employment, the SIC code, the region in which the establishment was located, and a further geographical code distinguishing metropolitan from nonmetropolitan locations.[11] For purposes of this study, annual employer expenditures per worker for health, life, and accident insurance and total payroll per worker were calculated separately for the office and nonoffice divisions of establishments.

6. THE EMPIRICAL WORK

We are unable to directly examine all the distinctions suggested by the theory between employer-choice and union-choice models. Ideally, we would need data on the characteristics of workers in each establishment. We would then attempt to show that premiums in the employer-choice model respond to selected measures of dispersion of the various employee characteristics, whereas in the union-choice model premiums would be expected to be related only to selected characteristics of the median worker.

The data restrict us considerably since there is no information on the distribution of characteristics of the workers. So the model to be estimated is basically of the following form:

$$\text{Premium} = a + b \text{ pay} + c(\text{size of group}) + d(\text{size of group})^2 + \sum_{i=1}^{7} g_i$$

(seven binary variables representing the types of plans) $+ \sum_{i=1}^{32} f_i$

(thirty-two binary variables representing SIC codes) $+ s$(binary variable for the South) $+ t$(binary variable for unionization) $+ V$(binary variable for office worker group).

The variables will be discussed individually. The "pay" variable is simply the annual wage and salary payment per worker. The "size" variable is used as a proxy variable for the price of the plan. The price per unit of group insurance is expected to decline with the size of the group. The quadratic term, "(size)^2," is used to pick up any nonlinearity between size and price per unit of group insurance.

As mentioned, the survey asks about health, life, and accident insurance plans. Since the size of the premium is related to the combination of plans offered, we must control for this variation. There are twenty-six possible combinations of plans. It was felt that the accident insurance component of fringe benefit payments was likely to be insignificant, and as a result this component was ignored in the empirical work. The eight possible combinations of plans are presented in Table 1 of Appendix 1.

The binary variables for the SIC codes are presented in Table 2 of Appendix 1. These are designed to capture the industry-specific characteristics that might affect the size of the premium. They will be discussed further below.

The binary variable for location in the South is entered to control for the lower costs of medical services in the South, and a negative sign for the coefficient of this variable is expected.

The union variable takes the value of 1 if the group is covered by a collective bargaining agreement, and premiums are expected to be positively related to this variable for reasons discussed above.

Finally, there is the binary variable that takes the value of 1 if the group is made up of office workers. This is a control variable to account for possible different attitudes toward these fringe benefits, *ceteris paribus*, on the part of office workers.

There are several possible samples that can be used to calculate the regression above. The decision unit could be all office and nonoffice groups in the sample considered individually. This would be reasonable if office and nonoffice groups were always covered by their own separate plans. If the two groups were sometimes covered by the same plan, then using simply the pay of one group in an establishment to explain the premium for that group alone would be misleading. The pay figure that would be relevant would be some combination of the pay of this group and the pay of the other group in the establishment. A similar argument applies to the union variable. As for the size variable, clearly the size of the entire insurance group is the desired variable. The sample that will be used therefore includes only those firms for which the office and nonoffice groups have different plans, and for which it is legitimate to conclude that employee groups were not pooled. The decision units are the office and nonoffice groups of these firms.[12]

In Appendix 2, Table 1, we summarize the results of the initial regression, with union and nonunion observations pooled. As expected, premiums are positively related to pay, with the income elasticity of demand at the mean being 0.64. Premiums are positively related to the size of the group, but negatively related to the quadratic term for size as hypothesized. If the establishment is located in the South, the premium per worker is $28 less, *ceteris paribus*, than outside the South. The sets of binary variables for types of plans and industry classification are often statistically significant, whereas the binary variable for office workers is not.[13] Finally, the union variable is positively related to premiums as hypothesized. The presence of a union-management agreement adds $81 to the premium per worker, *ceteris paribus*.

We have demonstrated thus far that unions do indeed make a difference in the premium and coverage per worker. The theoretical discussion above, however, suggested that unionized groups act differently from nonunionized groups in making a decision on premiums. The sample was subdivided into unionized and nonunionized groups, and the same model was tested on each subgroup (with the exclusion, now, of the union variable, of course). An *F* test rejected the hypothesis of equality between the sets of coefficients in the two regressions at the 1 per cent level of significance.

In Appendix 2, Tables 2 and 3, we present the regression results for unionized groups and for nonunionized groups, respectively. The most important difference between the two groups is in the income elasticity of demand for premiums. For the unionized groups, the elasticity is now 0.87, whereas for the nonunionized group it is 0.45. Of significance also is the fact that the coefficient of size is statistically insignificant in the nonunion results, whereas the coefficient of the quadratic term is insignificant in both cases.[14] Furthermore, in the nonunion results, the binary variable for office workers is now significant and positive. Being in an office group, *ceteris paribus*, adds $86 to the premium.

The sample can be further subdivided on the basis of type of plan. In Appendix 3, Tables 1 through 4, we present the results of regressions calculated for unionized establishments with noncontributory plans, unionized establishments with contributory plans, nonunionized establishments with noncontributory plans, and nonunionized establishments with contributory plans.[15] For unionized establishments with noncontributory plans, the income elasticity of demand for premiums is 0.90; for nonunionized establishments with noncontributory plans, only 0.17. For unionized establishments with contributory plans, the income elasticity of demand for premiums is 0.67; for nonunionized establishments with contributory plans, the figure is 0.70. To discuss these results further, it is useful to briefly present some other results on choice of plan.

In Appendix 4, results are presented for a regression using only groups with plans in which the dependent variable is a binary variable that takes the value of 1 if the establishment has a noncontributory welfare plan, and 0 if the plan was contributory.[16] *Ceteris paribus*, unionized establishments are 28 per cent more likely to have a noncontributory welfare plan than nonunionized establishments, following the argument presented in the theoretical section.

It is difficult to find a rationale for the lower income elasticity of contributory as compared to noncontributory plans among unionized groups, since the theory does not predict that unionized groups will have contributory plans. A somewhat plausible argument can be suggested for the nonunionized group. In this case the income elasticity of demand for premiums in the contributory subsample is larger than in the noncontributory subsample. In nonunionized establishments the employer must respond to varying preferences, not just to the median individual. If a noncontributory plan is chosen, then the employer must be careful not to provide too much in the way of benefits relative to pay, because no one can opt out. In the contributory case, however, the employer has much more freedom to vary benefits since individuals may opt out. The level of benefits will be more responsive to income in the contributory case than in the noncontributory case.

7. ILLUSTRATIVE CALCULATIONS OF PRICE AND INCOME ELASTICITIES OF DEMAND FOR INSURANCE

The elasticity estimates of the preceding section are only estimates of the response of gross premiums to income and group size. To estimate the parameters of the demand for insurance, we need to introduce some additional information.

Assume that insurance is sold at a constant price Φ per unit of coverage. Then the elasticity of premiums with respect to the size of the group, s, can be defined as:

(12) $\eta_{\pi s} = (\eta_{k\Phi} + 1)\eta_{\Phi s}$

where $\eta_{k\Phi}$ is the price elasticity of demand and $\eta_{\Phi s}$ is the elasticity of price with respect to the size of the group (i.e., a measure of the rate at which changes in group size reduce the premium). Clearly, to estimate $\eta_{k\Phi}$, one needs to know $\eta_{\Phi s}$.

Similarly, the net (of tax advantages) premium $\tilde{\pi}$ can be defined as:

(13) $\tilde{\pi} = (1 - t)\lambda(s)kE(x)$

where t is the marginal income tax rate, λ is the loading (a function of group size), and $E(x)$ is expected medical expenses. The elasticity of gross premiums with respect to income is therefore:

$$(14) \qquad \eta_{\pi y} = \eta_{k\Phi}\eta_{ty} + \eta_{E(x)y} + \eta_{ky}$$

where η_{ty} is the income elasticity of marginal tax rates and $\eta_{E(x)y}$ is the income elasticity of demand for medical care. To estimate η_{ky}, one must have estimates of the other elasticities. This formulation ignores the effect that increased losses arising from increased income might have on the level of coverage chosen.

We use some estimates of the missing elasticities that, although not precise, should give some idea of the magnitudes involved. A schedule of group health premium discounts with size, presented in Dickerson (1968), has an elasticity of loading with respect to firm size of approximately −0.031. If the elasticity of premiums with respect to size is 0.03, the price elasticity is approximately −2.0. If the average loading is about 0.2, this yields an estimate of the elasticity with respect to *loading* of approximately −0.33.

The income elasticity of marginal income tax rates, at the average income in our sample, is approximately 0.07. Feldstein (1973) has estimated the income-elasticity of demand for medical care to be 0.54. Using a price elasticity estimate of 2.0 and our income elasticity estimate of 0.64, and ignoring the payroll tax, one obtains an income elasticity of demand for insurance of −0.04. This very low estimate is consistent with Feldstein's finding, in cross-sectional state-aggregated data, of no pure effect of income on the demand for health insurance. However, there is a positive income elasticity of demand for unionized groups, whereas the elasticity for nonunionized groups is negative, although small.

8. CONCLUSION

The theory developed in this paper has some important implications for empirical work, although the possibility of the nonexistence of equilibrium raises difficulties. The data available did not permit direct testing of all of these implications. What tests we were able to perform confirm the predictions of the theory, in that they show that unions and employers behave differently in their choice of group insurance levels. Data on the distribution of firm characteristics will be necessary for more direct empirical testing.

APPENDIX 1

TABLE 1   Fringe Benefit Plan Binary Variables

HOLC	no health plan, contributory life insurance plan
HOLN	no health plan, noncontributory life insurance plan
HCLO	contributory health plan, no life insurance plan
HCLC	contributory health plan, contributory life insurance plan
HCLN	contributory health plan, noncontributory life insurance plan
HNLO	noncontributory health plan, no life insurance plan
HNLC	noncontributory health plan, contributory life insurance plan
Reference group: HNLN	noncontributory health plan, noncontributory life insurance plan

TABLE 2   SIC Code Binary Variables

Reference group:		
	1	Construction, special trade contractors
	2	Agricultural services, forestry, fishing
	3	Mining
	4	General building construction, other construction
	5	Ordnance
	6	Food
	7	Tobacco, textiles, apparel
	8	Lumber
	9	Furniture
	10	Paper
	11	Printing and publishing
	12	Chemicals
	13	Petroleum refining, rubber
	14	Leather
	15	Stone
	16	Primary metal
	17	Fabricated metal
	18	Machinery except electrical
	19	Electrical machinery
	20	Transportation equipment
	21	Instruments
	22	Miscellaneous
	23	Railroads

TABLE 2 (concluded)

Reference group:	24	Local and interurban transportation, other transportation
	25	Motor freight
	26	Electric, gas, and sanitary services
	27	Wholesale trade
	28	Retail building, retail general merchandise apparel, furniture
	29	Retail food
	30	Automobile dealers and service stations
	31	Eating and drinking establishments
	32	Finance
	33	Services

APPENDIX 2

TABLE 1

Variable	Coefficient	Standard Error
Pay[a]	$.2360 \times 10^{-1}$	$.1902 \times 10^{-2}$
Employ[b]	$.3117 \times 10^{-1}$	$.1708 \times 10^{-1}$
(Employ)^{2}[c]	$-.2270 \times 10^{-5}$	$.1704 \times 10^{-5}$
South[b]	-28.0705	16.6032
Union[a]	81.5864	20.5623
Office	14.8572	22.2622
HCLO	-113.2745	37.4564
HCLC	-86.5932	17.4216
HCLN	-59.3872	31.7672
HNLO	-32.0808	28.4242
HNLC	-9.1734	32.2892
IND. 3	262.7475	30.4385
IND. 4	-4.0026	37.6809
IND. 5	85.1385	123.3323
IND. 6	51.8220	30.0988
IND. 7	-11.7399	37.0554
IND. 8	102.7528	60.0224
IND. 9	35.1830	71.6291
IND. 10	47.2370	46.2737
IND. 11	-72.5394	71.8307
IND. 12	-124.9947	69.0594
IND. 13	163.4320	61.0997

TABLE 1 (concluded)

Variable	Coefficient	Standard Error
IND. 14	−89.7814	150.8334
IND. 15	71.6416	43.1703
IND. 16	187.7605	27.0916
IND. 17	165.4972	42.8687
IND. 18	138.7482	33.6760
IND. 19	31.6347	53.3250
IND. 20	70.4452	47.0344
IND. 21	46.2840	124.2524
IND. 22	102.5244	55.1915
IND. 24	−11.1003	67.7551
IND. 25	48.1036	43.5189
IND. 26	−76.6522	149.8810
IND. 27	16.8561	41.5541
IND. 28	−40.1884	48.3839
IND. 29	11.7315	56.8736
IND. 30	27.9368	66.1347
IND. 31	−7.7350	42.9379
IND. 32	−17.0243	49.1655
IND. 33	6.9831	30.4050
Constant	50.0110	25.5113

$N = 1139$
$R^2 = 0.3378$
$F = 13.6479$
[a] Significant at the 1 per cent level of significance using a one-tailed test.
[b] Significant at the 5 per cent level of significance using a one-tailed test.
[c] Significant at the 10 per cent level of significance using a one-tailed test.

TABLE 2 Unionized Groups

Variable	Coefficient	Standard Error
Pay[a]	$.3841 \times 10^{-1}$	$.3232 \times 10^{-2}$
Employ[c]	$.3247 \times 10^{-1}$	$.2085 \times 10^{-1}$
(Employ)^{2}[b]	$-.2211 \times 10^{-5}$	$.1993 \times 10^{-5}$
South	−44.6729	26.2218
Office	−76.9843	66.0872
HCLO	−62.9760	78.4928
HCLC	−103.4328	34.4361
HCLN	−95.7251	62.2356
HNLO	.8046	47.7489

TABLE 2 (concluded)

Variable	Coefficient	Standard Error
HNLC	−110.5753	79.0453
IND. 3	370.4995	42.4451
IND. 4	−18.9182	53.0407
IND. 5	116.5961	225.7463
IND. 6	36.4339	42.4022
IND. 7	−15.4366	59.8475
IND. 8	61.0942	84.5065
IND. 9	8.4334	109.7024
IND. 10	94.5771	68.5686
IND. 11	−172.1880	114.5963
IND. 12	−133.8114	112.2699
IND. 13	197.8371	92.1663
IND. 14	39.9854	162.0159
IND. 15	95.8523	73.1455
IND. 16	192.3440	38.0959
IND. 17	209.6347	67.2601
IND. 18	176.8147	51.5436
IND. 19	38.8871	91.1344
IND. 20	74.0772	67.7042
IND. 21	30.1787	157.2047
IND. 22	−40.2380	92.3222
IND. 24	36.1261	92.1104
IND. 25	6.8042	64.3555
IND. 27	49.8022	74.0300
IND. 28	−123.5410	100.0552
IND. 29	71.5459	78.4637
IND. 30	115.7510	217.5840
IND. 31	−34.0095	126.8290
IND. 32	−14.0974	127.1777
IND. 33	−8.3702	63.1849
Constant	9.8736	32.0272

$N = 572$
$R^2 = .3950$
$F = 8.9078$
[a] Significant at the 1 per cent level of significance using a one-tailed test.
[b] Significant at the 5 per cent level of significance using a one-tailed test.
[c] Significant at the 10 per cent level of significance using a one-tailed test.

TABLE 3 Nonunionized Groups

Variable	Coefficient	Standard Error
Pay[a]	$.1325 \times 10^{-1}$	$.2288 \times 10^{-2}$
Employ	$.1129 \times 10^{-1}$	$.3553 \times 10^{-1}$
(Employ)^2	$-.1523 \times 10^{-5}$	$.4096 \times 10^{-5}$
South	-20.5244	20.4538
Office[a]	85.7691	23.2286
HCLO	-108.0411	40.6329
HCLC	-37.9779	20.6210
HCLN	-21.7960	36.0258
HNLO	-17.6038	34.8915
IND. 3	104.8398	42.3542
IND. 4	71.2975	51.8767
IND. 5	45.9567	139.0909
IND. 6	62.1844	41.6817
IND. 7	-13.7153	45.0955
IND. 8	170.9656	81.8337
IND. 9	59.9171	89.2962
IND. 10	15.8361	61.2696
IND. 11	17.7774	88.8277
IND. 12	-121.4522	83.0313
IND. 13	131.0928	77.6114
IND. 15	53.1949	50.8759
IND. 16	170.0372	36.9433
IND. 17	127.7391	53.0766
IND. 18	120.1987	43.2132
IND. 19	32.2442	62.0061
IND. 20	107.2002	63.8566
IND. 21	58.2886	198.6398
IND. 22	190.8957	65.0109
IND. 24	40.3944	99.1579
IND. 25	83.4148	58.9521
IND. 26	-48.3575	138.1063
IND. 27	-14.2430	47.7058
IND. 28	-31.4968	52.1833
IND. 29	-35.0852	81.2892
IND. 30	11.5089	65.1347
IND. 31	-8.3230	43.7159
IND. 32	-48.0040	50.9116
IND. 33	-4.5165	34.1299
Constant	73.9285	29.8791

$N = 567$
$R^2 = .3350$
$F = 6.8078$
[a] Significant at the 1 per cent level of significance using a one-tailed test.

APPENDIX 3

TABLE 1 Noncontributory Union

Variable	Coefficient	Standard Error
Pay	$.4152 \times 10^{-1}$	$.3879 \times 10^{-2}$
Employ	$.1635 \times 10^{-1}$	$.1604 \times 10^{-1}$
South	-42.3737	30.6757
Office	.8947	150.9988
IND. 3	379.0296	45.1782
IND. 4	-16.2282	59.8149
IND. 6	32.8301	54.5310
IND. 7	77.9837	80.2042
IND. 8	98.8492	105.3201
IND. 9	67.3969	134.2085
IND. 10	150.3697	96.8831
IND. 11	-165.6497	231.1611
IND. 12	-147.7895	163.9522
IND. 13	215.7386	119.4212
IND. 15	153.5582	90.7415
IND. 16	203.6861	44.0708
IND. 17	261.0186	83.3650
IND. 18	220.3621	62.9921
IND. 19	53.9260	117.5788
IND. 20	61.9820	94.4213
IND. 21	101.2534	231.3503
IND. 22	-50.5028	134.2346
IND. 24	-100.4000	231.9547
IND. 25	-53.2847	98.7247
IND. 27	27.1488	88.5110
IND. 28	-114.9369	134.3569
IND. 29	135.5957	104.5338
IND. 30	123.6867	232.5082
IND. 31	-49.0194	165.0196
IND. 32	-21.7028	164.7800
IND. 33	-9.8884	91.6538
Constant	-21.1256	37.9593

$N = 454$
$R^2 = 0.3827$
$F = 8.4402$

TABLE 2 Contributory Union

Variable	Coefficient	Standard Error
Pay	$.2216 \times 10^{-1}$	$.8539 \times 10^{-2}$
Employ	$-.3030 \times 10^{-2}$	$.1593 \times 10^{-1}$
South	124.6589	72.7539
Office	−111.9219	91.8847
IND. 4	−225.0749	154.0686
IND. 6	114.3624	91.7063
IND. 7	−284.3558	123.0155
IND. 8	−4.1756	128.9841
IND. 10	−.5782	115.0574
IND. 11	−93.1873	182.7301
IND. 12	−69.6146	128.0180
IND. 13	156.6614	112.7175
IND. 14	−137.3590	156.2430
IND. 16	154.5355	72.6874
IND. 17	94.8389	115.2763
IND. 18	103.7329	168.0169
IND. 19	−62.9834	157.3418
IND. 20	189.6651	169.7042
IND. 21	.1941	163.0831
IND. 24	−50.9480	95.0793
IND. 25	204.7270	175.5142
IND. 29	−107.7528	175.4910
IND. 31	−88.8023	156.8024
IND. 33	−165.6519	154.0572
Constant	99.8306	73.9427

$N = 56$
$R^2 = 0.5580$
$F = 1.6304$

TABLE 3 Noncontributory Nonunion

Variable	Coefficient	Standard Error
Pay	$.5338 \times 10^{-2}$	$.3752 \times 10^{-2}$
Employ	$-.3001 \times 10^{-2}$	$.4095 \times 10^{-1}$
South	−84.2868	38.8259
Office	146.9658	42.2269
IND. 3	93.2499	199.8618
IND. 4	−31.7060	96.4642
IND. 6	87.9809	118.3455

TABLE 3 (concluded)

Variable	Coefficient	Standard Error
IND. 7	−82.9149	75.8292
IND. 8	188.9954	102.2741
IND. 10	−46.1270	93.2270
IND. 11	66.9251	119.3414
IND. 12	−347.3340	203.8687
IND. 13	65.4376	200.8328
IND. 15	−97.0990	142.1633
IND. 16	70.2285	77.6841
IND. 17	−3.5564	119.2246
IND. 18	41.3707	77.7683
IND. 19	132.8449	199.4682
IND. 20	64.7879	114.7006
IND. 22	1597.8103	200.6054
IND. 24	51.7718	119.4195
IND. 25	40.7810	87.2553
IND. 26	−98.4091	199.3910
IND. 27	−45.4775	103.8643
IND. 28	−64.9899	102.8961
IND. 29	−130.4693	117.9913
IND. 30	−33.9875	142.8651
IND. 31	−110.3982	80.3047
IND. 32	−181.0119	79.9211
IND. 33	−58.6157	58.2030
Constant	159.1605	47.7670

$N = 165$
$R^2 = 0.5200$
$F = 4.8388$

TABLE 4 Contributory Nonunion

Variable	Coefficient	Standard Error
Pay	$.1966 \times 10^{-1}$	$.3923 \times 10^{-2}$
Employ	$.7432 \times 10^{-1}$	$.6341 \times 10^{-1}$
(Employ)^2	$-.7667 \times 10^{-5}$	$.6409 \times 10^{-5}$
South	23.4893	30.2928
Office	48.6150	36.6571
IND. 3	109.5375	45.8571
IND. 4	13.9091	108.7873

TABLE 4 (concluded)

Variable	Coefficient	Standard Error
IND. 5	232.1925	185.4734
IND. 6	125.2553	57.5479
IND. 7	29.3740	74.1326
IND. 9	182.3184	132.2361
IND. 10	55.4584	110.8921
IND. 11	−316.7350	193.4660
IND. 12	76.3260	133.3111
IND. 13	251.2017	117.8779
IND. 15	133.0822	70.4645
IND. 16	184.0137	45.2669
IND. 17	131.1661	79.0090
IND. 18	211.3406	77.8495
IND. 19	1.3106	96.0196
IND. 20	160.8269	96.1539
IND. 22	63.2844	95.0369
IND. 25	95.7776	94.9226
IND. 26	−36.3840	186.9200
IND. 27	−37.3047	86.6681
IND. 28	−34.7703	77.3517
IND. 29	67.2898	132.4986
IND. 30	24.7555	96.1113
IND. 31	82.3387	68.8227
IND. 32	−6.4284	89.3205
IND. 33	34.8311	57.9816
Constant	−39.2046	47.1898

$N = 240$
$R^2 = 0.3676$
$F = 3.900$

APPENDIX 4

TABLE 1

Variable	Coefficient	Standard Error
Employ	-2.4995×10^{-5}	1.6441×10^{-5}
Union	.2835	3.8577×10^{-2}
Office	−.1679	3.9066×10^{-2}
IND. 3	-9.8381×10^{-2}	5.9778×10^{-2}
IND. 4	7.2523×10^{-2}	7.5004×10^{-2}

TABLE 1 (concluded)

Variable	Coefficient	Standard Error
IND. 5	$-.3149$	$.2460$
IND. 6	-9.8988×10^{-2}	5.8525×10^{-2}
IND. 7	-7.2216×10^{-2}	7.2542×10^{-2}
IND. 8	$.1385$	$.1198$
IND. 9	$.1098$	$.1431$
IND. 10	$-.1328$	9.1344×10^{-2}
IND. 11	-8.3941×10^{-2}	$.1435$
IND. 12	-2.2569×10^{-2}	$.1371$
IND. 13	-4.7230×10^{-2}	$.1206$
IND. 14	$-.3088$	$.3014$
IND. 15	$-.2239$	8.5211×10^{-2}
IND. 16	-8.8429×10^{-2}	5.3201×10^{-2}
IND. 17	-1.7157×10^{-2}	8.4889×10^{-2}
IND. 18	6.6508×10^{-2}	6.4383×10^{-2}
IND. 19	$-.1595$	$.1056$
IND. 20	-8.1747×10^{-2}	9.3898×10^{-2}
IND. 21	-4.4670×10^{-2}	$.2471$
IND. 22	$-.2000$	$.1085$
IND. 24	$-.1204$	$.1359$
IND. 25	-2.2485×10^{-4}	8.6189×10^{-2}
IND. 26	$-.1184$	$.3022$
IND. 27	9.9731×10^{-2}	8.2196×10^{-2}
IND. 28	$-.1388$	9.6017×10^{-2}
IND. 29	-4.0330×10^{-2}	$.1128$
IND. 30	$-.2500$	$.1316$
IND. 31	$-.1293$	8.4508×10^{-2}
IND. 32	8.2696×10^{-2}	9.6228×10^{-2}
IND. 33	1.0251×10^{-2}	5.8155×10^{-2}

Dependent Variable: Occurrence of a noncontributory welfare plan.
$N = 1139$
$R^2 = 0.22$
$F = 9.6910$
Constant is 0.6188.

NOTES

1. An illustrative schedule of the variation in premiums with group size is presented in O. D. Dickerson, *Health Insurance*, 3rd ed. (Homewood, Illinois: Richard D. Irwin, 1968), p. 592. This schedule indicates that group size economies would be exhausted at a group size of about 500 employees, assuming a monthly premium per employee family of $50.

2. This assumes that small firms are more efficient in the production of outputs in particular industries.

3. Moral hazard is obviously ignored here.

4. In a more general context, Rothschild and Stiglitz have shown that no equilibrium may exist in cases of adverse selection. See M. Rothschild and J. Stiglitz, "Equilibrium in Insurance Markets: The Economics of Imperfect Information," unpublished manuscript, Yale University, 1973.

5. In equilibrium, the number of firms will be such that no firm will have a work force homogeneous with respect to health insurance preferences or risk of illness. In other words, the distribution of preferences and/or risk over the labor force is such that the frequency of workers at any preference or risk level is insufficient to permit a firm to operate profitably with only these workers. There is then some minimal size needed to operate profitably, and this requires attracting more workers than there are at any given preference or risk level.

6. These demand curves make quantity of insurance a function of gross (of tax savings) price. In part, the differences in demands at a given gross price could be caused by differential tax advantages that cause net prices to differ.

7. Here again, marginal utilities depend in part on tax savings. Thus, u_k^j is not equal to $\partial U^j / \partial k$, but also includes a utility valuation of the reduction in taxes which occurs when k increases and taxable (money) income declines.

8. The critical assumption is that an employer can separate workers of different types. He can then pay each group a different money wage to ensure that, given the level of health insurance, each group is at the margin (Equation (4)). If it is too costly to separate all types of workers, then it is certainly possible that some workers will not be at the margin, and yet will still be better off in their job than in alternatives currently available for a range of values of health insurance benefits. The employer will not need to take their preferences into account in choosing the level of health insurance. Consequently, there is no presumption that such a situation will be Pareto optimal.

9. The earlier assumption about the incidence of fringe benefits falling wholly on employees is actually a consequence of the free entry and mobility assumptions. With free entry of firms, if one employer tries to shift more than the cost of the fringe benefits onto his workers, some potential employer can offer a slightly higher wage, attracting all the employees of the former and still being able to operate profitably.

10. For a description of this data, see *Employee Compensation in the Private Nonfarm Economy, 1970*, Washington, D.C., 1973.

11. The four-digit SIC code for each establishment is given. The regional code takes on four values, for Northeast, South, North Central, and West.

12. This procedure obviously sacrifices some observations. There will be firms in which the office and nonoffice workers have the same type of plan, but in which the plans are separate. Our procedure is a conservative one that cuts the sample from almost 7,000 observations to just over 1,600 observations. Moreover, if union-wide contracts cover more than one firm, again we will have imprecise measurement of group characteristics. Use of the SIC code may help to control this. Our procedure also eliminates all groups providing no insurance whereas a more reasonable procedure would involve using a Tobit form of analysis on all observations.

13. *F*-tests indicated that both the plan classification and the industry classifications added significantly to the explanation of premiums at the 1 per cent level.

14. The elasticity of premiums with respect to the size of the group in Table 1 is 0.02, whereas the elasticity in Table 2 is 0.03. In the unionized subsample, 3

per cent of the workers are office workers; in the nonunionized subsample, 71 per cent are office workers.

15. The sets of coefficients calculated using the nonunion subsample are statistically significantly different from each other at the 1 per cent level. In the union case, the two sets are not significantly different at the 10 per cent level.

16. Use of a binary dependent variable makes the assumption of homoscedasticity untenable. The OLS estimator is unbiased, but the estimates of the standard errors of the regression coefficients are biased and inconsistent.

REFERENCES

1. Bergstrom, Theodore, and Robert Goodman, "Private Demands for Public Goods," *American Economic Review*, 63 (June 1973), pp. 280–296.

2. Borcherding, Thomas A., and Robert Deacon, "The Demand for the Services of Non-Federal Governments," *American Economic Review*, 62 (December 1972), pp. 891–901.

3. Feldstein, Martin, "The Welfare Loss of Excess Health Insurance," *Journal of Political Economy*, 81 (March–April 1973), pp. 251–280.

4. _____ , and Elizabeth Allison, "Tax Subsidies of Private Health Insurance." In *The Economics of Federal Subsidy Programs*, A Compendium of Papers Submitted to the Subcommittee on Priorities and Economy of Government of the Joint Economic Committee, Part 8—Selected Subsidies, July 29, 1974 (Washington, D.C.: U.S. Government Printing Office, 1974).

5. Lester, R. A., "Benefits as a Preferred Form of Compensation," *Southern Economic Journal*, 34 (April 1967), pp. 488–495.

6. Phelps, Charles, "The Demand for Health Insurance," R–1054–OEO, The Rand Corporation, July, 1973.

7. Rice, Robert D., "Skill, Earnings, and the Growth of Wage Supplements," *American Economic Review, Papers and Proceedings*, 56 (May 1966), pp. 583-593.

3 ‖ COMMENTS

Donald Richter
University of Rochester

Professors Goldstein and Pauly should be complimented on their effort to construct a theory of the collective purchase of insurance-type benefits, and more important, on deriving some very interesting implications of their theory that are in principle subject to empirical test. Their paper is a refreshing change from much other empirical work in that they take some care in developing the theory that underlies their empirical hypotheses. My comments will be confined primarily to the theoretical part of their paper, in particular to the two general types of equilibria discussed—employer-choice equilibrium and union-choice equilibrium.

I will first discuss the concept of employer-choice equilibrium. In order to facilitate comparison with analogous equilibrium concepts in the theory of public goods, and because the precise requirements of employer-choice equilibrium were a bit obscure to me from reading the paper, I will restate its definition in the following terms. An employer-choice equilibrium is a set of employee groups, each with a wage-fringe benefit package, such that:

1. producers maxliniiæ profito;
2. no employee wishes to switch to another group;
3. there is no other conceivable set of groups and associated wage-fringe benefit packages that could make all employees better off.

Notice that the authors introduce condition (3) by saying that employers choose their wage-fringe benefit package so as to minimize their labor cost. This requirement implies that the equilibrium is Pareto optimal.

Let me compare this equilibrium concept with two equilibrium concepts relevant to the theory of value with public goods. The consumers of the economy are partitioned into a set of governmental jurisdictions, which provide public goods to their residents and collect taxes so as to balance their respective budgets. The consumers are assumed to maximize their utility over their private goods bundles, given the amounts of public goods provided by their jurisdictions and subject to their after-tax budget constraint. For simplicity, assume that each jurisdiction can levy a proportional wealth tax, whose rate varies across jurisdictions.

The partition of consumers into jurisdictions and the provisions of public and private goods, the tax rates, and private goods prices are endogenous and determined by the following equilibrium concepts. The first, which I will refer to as a "local mobility equilibrium," requires that the supply and demand for private goods be equated such that:

1'. producers maximize profits;
2'. no consumer wishes to move to another existing jurisdiction;
3'. for any of the existing jurisdictions, there is no alternative provision of public goods and taxes to pay for them which can make everyone better off.

The other equilibrium concept, which I will refer to as a "global mobility equilibrium," replaces (3') with the following condition (3"): there is no other set of jurisdictions and associated public goods provisions and taxes that will make everyone better off.

Condition (3') amounts to what Ellickson (1973) has referred to (in a somewhat different context) as Pareto optimality relative to a partition. It simply means that the equilibrium is Pareto optimal when compared to all other attainable allocations consistent with the endogenously determined partition. Condition (3″) is a much stronger condition, which implies (3′) but also requires that there be no Pareto superior allocation among the class of attainable allocations corresponding to all conceivable partitions of the consumers, not just the equilibrium one.

The global mobility equilibrium is the direct analogue of the Goldstein-Pauly employer-choice equilibrium. It is an extremely strong equilibrium that is unlikely to exist under general conditions. On the other hand, the local mobility equilibrium can, I think, be shown to exist under rather general conditions. It also seems like an interesting equilibrium concept in the public goods context. In particular, it seems reasonable that consumers will shop around among the various existing jurisdictions, comparing public goods-tax packages, but there does not seem to be a compelling decentralized mechanism that would lead to a global Pareto optimum. This suggests that perhaps the authors should use the analogue of the local mobility equilibrium in their arguments. The advantage is that their equilibrium is then likely to exist. The disadvantage is that one loses the interpretation that sees the employer as choosing the wage-fringe benefit package with an eye to minimizing labor cost.

The other equilibrium concept discussed in the paper—the union-choice equilibrium—would correspond in the public goods context to determining the amount of public goods in each jurisdiction according to the median voter's preferences. Again, existence is likely to be a problem. Models demonstrating the existence of a general economic equilibrium wherein public goods provisions are determined by some (highly simplified) type of political behavior are precious few.

Let me close by pointing out that it is very unfortunate that the empirical implications that really draw on the richness of the authors' model are precisely the ones that the authors have not been able to test because of data limitations. Future relaxation of these data limitations would be very interesting indeed.

REFERENCES

1. Ellickson, B., "A Generalization of the Pure Theory of Public Goods," *American Economic Review,* 63 (June 1973), pp. 417–432.

William Vickrey
Columbia University

I have only a few rather peripheral remarks to add to this paper. One is that the use of medical examinations as an exclusionary device is likely to be somewhat less important than might at first appear. One of the motives for group insurance is precisely the savings in underwriting costs, of which the medical examination is an important element. Underwriters of group plans generally expect to encounter a certain proportion of risks that would be selected out or subjected to higher premiums if insured on an individual basis. They protect themselves against an undue amount of adverse selection, in the case of contributory optional plans, by requiring the inclusion in the plan of a certain minimum proportion of the eligible risks before the plan will be put into effect. In the case of plans with compulsory participation, whether noncontributory or otherwise, the limited elasticity of substitution among jobs will ordinarily be sufficient to limit the inclusion of bad risks to a tolerable level. To be sure, employers often require a medical examination prior to employment, but it is not clear to what extent such examinations are a means of protecting insurance programs against bad risks and to what extent they are intended to protect the employer from workmen's compensation claims based on preexisting conditions, or to ensure that the employee will be physically capable of performing the required work, or to weed out employees likely to leave after too short a period to yield a return on their initial on-the-job training and recruitment costs.

Another point is that to treat a union as a mechanism for making decisions on the extent of insurance according to majority rule, with the decision according with the preferences of the median "voter," is, I think, a grossly unrealistic approach. At best the union leadership is elected on the basis of a large number of issues, the most salient of which is probably the degree of general militancy and skill evinced in dealing with employers; and the particular issue of how much insurance to include in the wage package would be considered only in conjunction with a large number of other matters. In the union's decision on the package to bargain for, there would be considerable scope for weighing intensity of individual preferences concerning the relative amounts of insurance against other elements of the package, so that the median voter rule would be inapplicable. In practice, rather than being an ideal democracy, the typical union has a leadership that is to a large extent self-perpetuating and subject to serious challenge only under very unusual circumstances. Such a leadership would tend to make decisions that are fairly strongly biased toward the preferences of the senior members with the longest tenure, which in turn is likely to be a preference for larger amounts of insurance, since the older members are likely to have the higher risk. This is to me a more persuasive explanation of the statistical findings that premiums are higher if unions exist.

Finally, it is perhaps worth mentioning that among the industry coefficients the only ones that appear to have substantial statistical significance levels are those for mining, primary metal, fabricated metal, and machinery, except electrical, all of which have positive coefficients with t ratios ranging from about 4 to 8. There may be some significance to the fact that only industries in this rather closely interconnected group show insurance levels above the general run.

4

CHARLES E. PHELPS
The Rand Corporation

Demand for Reimbursement Insurance

The theory of demand for insurance has been studied by Arrow (1963, 1973a,b), Mossin (1968), Smith (1968), Pratt (1964), Ehrlich and Becker (1973; hereafter EB), and others; and demand estimates have been published by Fuchs and Kramer (1972), Feldstein (1973), and Phelps (1973). These works have generally specified insurance contracts in which (1) the losses are not affected by the amount of insurance (EB is an exception), or (2) the amount of insurance in each period can be chosen directly. I will investigate here demand for insurance under two more restrictive conditions that normally apply to health insurance: (1) the insurance coverage rate must be equal in all insured states of the world (i.e., constant coinsurance in all insured states) and (2) states of the world are aggregated in some fashion before a loading fee is computed.

I assume that the consumer has a utility function in a composite good (x) and health (H), where health is produced by medical care (h) and own-time in fixed production coefficients, and where the stock of health H is subject to random losses ("illnesses") having a known distribution $f(l)$, where l is the illness amount. Hence, the final level of health is $H_0 - l + g(h)$, where H_0 is the endowed level

This research was supported by Grant Number HS 01029 from the National Center for Health Services Research and Development. The author is indebted to Bridger M. Mitchell and Joseph P. Newhouse for helpful comments, although residual errors are mine. Bryant Mori provided careful and prompt computational assistance.

of health. To capture the essence of the model I assume that the consumer may choose only some coinsurance rate C (the fraction of medical care bills paid by the consumer) and a maximum payment amount h^* (in units of care). The insurance is a subsidy for purchasing medical care, so calculating the optimal values of C and h^* must take into account that more h is purchased for lower values of C (Phelps, 1973; Phelps and Newhouse, 1974).

The consumer pays for his insurance with a premium, R, that reflects both the expected expenses for medical care and administrative costs of the insurance process. Several specifications of the insurance premium will be investigated to examine differential effects of different pricing systems on demand for insurance.

In addition, effects of income, and of income tax subsidy of insurance, will be investigated. It can be shown that estimates of the income elasticity of demand for insurance include (1) a "pure" income effect and (2) a substitution effect that depends on the progressiveness of income taxes. Estimated income elasticities of demand for insurance can be separated into these components.

Finally, I will investigate effects of changes in the price level of medical care. It has been asserted that rising prices for medical care induce additional demand for insurance (Feldstein, 1971). This model shows that that conclusion does not hold except under specific circumstances.

The model to be used assumes that consumers maximize expected utility over all possible states of illness. The distribution of illnesses $f(l)$ is assumed to be continuous and smooth in the range $0 \leq l < \infty$. Thus, expected utility can be written as

(1)
$$Z = s_0 U(x_0, H_0) + \int_0^{l^*} U\left[x, H_0 - l + g(h)\right] f(l) dl$$
$$+ \int_{l^*}^{\infty} U\left[x, H_0 - l + g(h)\right] f(l) dl$$

where l^* is the loss that induces the consumer to purchase h^* units of care,[1] and where

$$s_0 + \int_0^{\infty} f(l) dl = 1$$

For $l \leq l^*$, the budget constraint is:

(2)
$$I = x + Cp_h h + R$$

reflecting the insurance subsidy for medical care.

For the second integral, in which insurance no longer pays, the budget constraint is:

(3)
$$I = x + p_h h + R - (1 - C) p_h h^*$$

where $(1-C)p_n h^*$ is the maximum amount paid by the insurance plan. Optimal levels of C and h^* are derived by solving the first derivatives when set to zero. When Z is differentiated with respect to C and h^* and set to zero subject to the appropriate budget constraints (2) and (3), the results are:[2]

(4)
$$s_0(-R_c) \cdot \lambda(l_0) + \int_0^{l^*} \lambda(l)\left[-R_c - p_n h(l)\right]f(l)dl$$

$$+ \int_{l^*}^{\infty} \lambda(l)(-R_c - p_n h^*)f(l)dl = 0$$

and

(5)
$$s_0(-R_{h^*}) \cdot \lambda(l_0) + \int_0^{l^*} (-R_{h^*}) \cdot \lambda(l)f(l)dl$$

$$+ \int_{l^*}^{\infty} \left[-R_{h^*} + (1-C)p_n\right]\lambda(l)f(l)dl = 0$$

where R_c and R_{h^*} are the partial derivatives of R with respect to C and h^*, respectively, and $\lambda(l)$ is the marginal utility of income for the health loss l.

Expressions (4) and (5) are subject to an interpretation parallel to that used by EB. In (5), if h^* increases, the net income flow out of all states more favorable than h^* is $-R_{h^*}$, the derivative of the premium as h^* changes. For states less favorable than l^* (i.e., larger losses), the net income transfer rate is $-R_{h^*}$ (the premium still changes) plus $(1-C)p_n$, the last expression reflecting the additional rate of income flow into those states with illnesses greater than l^*. The real price of insurance, defined in the EB sense, is $R_{h^*}/[-R_{h^*} + (1-C)p_n]$, the negative of the ratio of income flow rates between states below and above h^*. Equation (5) can be solved for this price, showing

(6)
$$P_{h^*} = \frac{R_{h^*}}{(1-C)p_n - R_{h^*}} = \frac{\int_{l^*}^{\infty} \lambda(l)f(l)dl}{s_0\lambda(l_0) + \int_0^{l^*} \lambda(l)f(l)dl} = \frac{\overline{U}'}{\underline{U}'}$$

The optimal h^* is chosen so that the ratio of *expected* marginal utility of incomes above and below h^* is equal to the real price of insurance—the ratio of income transfers between less favorable and more favorable states. This is analogous to the two-state problem analyzed by EB, except that here the consumer divides all possible states of nature into two categories on the basis of his choice of h^*.

It is possible to show that some insurance is optimal with the loading fee sufficiently small. To prove this point, notice that where

$$R = \int_0^{l*} (1-C)p_h f(l)dl + \int_{l*}^{\infty} (1-C)p_h h*f(l)dl$$

is an actuarily fair premium (no load), then

$$\frac{\partial R}{\partial h*} = R_{h*} = (1-C)p_h \int_{l*}^{\infty} f(l)dl = (1-C)p_h Q(l*)$$

Then to show that some $h*>0$ is optimal, I evaluate (5) at $h* = 0$. At that point, (5) becomes

(7a)
$$-s_0 \lambda(l_0)(1-C)p_h Q(l*) + \int_0^{\infty} \lambda(l) \left[(1-C)p_h - (1-C)p_h Q(l*)\right] f(l)dl$$

$$= \left\{-s_0 \lambda(l_0) Q(l*) + (1-s_0)\bar{\lambda}[1-Q(l*)]\right\} (1-C)p_h$$

where $(1-s_0)\bar{\lambda} = \int_0^{\infty} \lambda(l)f(l)dl$ is expected marginal utility for all states of the world with losses. Notice that for $l = 0$, $Q(l) = 1-s_0$, so (7a) becomes

(7b)
$$\left[-\lambda(l_0)(s_0)(1-s_0) + \bar{\lambda}(1-s_0)(s_0)\right](1-C)p_h$$

$$= \left[\bar{\lambda} - \lambda(l_0)\right](1-C)p_h s_0(1-s_0) > 0$$

since $\lambda(l_0)$, the marginal utility of income with no loss, is less than $\lambda(l)$ for any larger l. (A loss, l, can be translated into an income loss, so that $\partial \lambda/\partial l > 0$.) Thus for "small" θ, *some* purchase of insurance is optimal.

It also follows that some loading fee of sufficient size exists to deter purchase. Let the premium function be $R = (1+\theta)E$(benefits), where θ is the load. Then $R_{h*} = (1+\theta)(1-C)p_h Q(l*)$, and $\partial E(U)/\partial h*$ at $h* = 0$ is:

(8)
$$- s_0 \lambda(l_0)(1+\theta)(1-C)p_h Q(l*) + \int_0^{\infty} \lambda(l)\left[(1-C)p_h\right.$$

$$-(1+\theta)(1-C)p_h Q(l*)f(l)dl \left.\right](1-C)p_h$$

$$\left\{- s_0 \lambda(l_0)(1+\theta)(1-s_0) + (1-s_0)\bar{\lambda}\left[1 - (1+\theta)(1-s_0)\right]\right\}$$

$$= (1-C)p_h(1-s_0)\left\{s_0(1+\theta)\left[\bar{\lambda}-\lambda(l_0)\right] -Q\bar{\lambda}\right\}$$

This expression is negative (i.e., $E(U)$ falls as $h*$ rises from $h* = 0$) if

(9)
$$\theta > \frac{s_0\left[(\bar{\lambda} - \lambda(l_0)\right]}{s_0\lambda(l_0) + (1-s_0)\bar{\lambda}} = \frac{s_0 \Delta\lambda}{E(\lambda)}$$

That is, if the loading fee at $h* = 0$ exceeds the difference between marginal utilities of income in the states with and without loss (relative to their expectation), times the probability of no loss, then no insurance will be purchased. Notice the similarity between the right-hand-side of (9) and the usual risk-aversion measure.

The problem with respect to choice of C is more complex and is in fact the major difference between choice of single-coverage reimbursement insurance and other forms of insurance. The consumer must select one level of coinsurance C that maximizes expected utility over all possible insured states.

As seen from Equation (10) below, R_c is negative. The income flow rate into any state with $l \leqslant l^*$ is $(p_h h + R_c)$. For small losses ("favorable states") the flow rate is negative. There is some loss l between 0 and l^* such that the net income flow is zero.[3] For larger losses, the net income flow is positive, including those for $l > l^*$, in which case the income flow rate is $(p_h h^* + R_c)$. The "real price" of insurance for state l" is $(-R_c)/[p_h h(l) + R_c)$, the ratio of income transfers from the least serious state $(h=0)$ to the more serious states. If this "price" is negative, the income flow is away from that state. Notice that the consumer does not choose some income transfer for each state, but rather only one value for C. Hence, he is really not directly allocating incomes according to the prices in each state; that allocation follows from the choice of C and from his choice of h given l. Only for the trivial case of $h = \bar{h}$ for all $l \leqslant l^*$ is a direct solution of (4) possible. Thus, it is difficult to speak of "the price of C" in the usual sense. I shall show below that where $P_l = -R_c/[p_h h(l) + R_c]$, the price of C for loss l, the comparative statics of demand for C will hinge crucially on how p_l changes with l. Since changes in income or medical prices change both R (and hence R_c) and $h(l)$, an income-generated own-price effect on demand for care may translate into a modified price effect of demand for insurance. I will show that if P_l increases with l (for whatever reason), then demand for C falls commensurately. It is by this method that comparative statics of demand for C may be analyzed. It can be shown also that some insurance is optimal (i.e., $C < 1$) for a sufficiently small loading fee and small s_0. For this proof, I make the simplifying assumption that $h^* = \infty$, because this simplifies the calculation of the premium change function R_c. In general, the premium function is

$$R = (1 + \theta)\left[\int_0^{l^*} (1-C)p_h h(l)f(l)dl + \int_{l^*}^{\infty} (1-C)p_h h^* f(l)dl\right]$$

so

(10) $\quad -R_c = (1 + \theta)\left\{\int_0^{l^*} \frac{p_h h(l)}{C}\left[C - (1-C)\eta_{hc}\right]f(l)dl + p_h h^* Q(l^*)\right\}$

Clearly, at $\theta = 0$ and at $C = 1$, this becomes $-R_c = p_h \bar{h} + p_h h^* Q(l^*)$. For $h^* = \infty$, $-R_c = p_h \bar{h}$, the average expense in states with positive illness, where h is a function of p_h, l, and C, but is evaluated at $C = 1$. Expression (4), showing how expected utility changes with C, can be evaluated at $C = 1$ to determine if $E(U)$ rises or falls with C—if it falls ($dZ/dC < 0$), then some insurance purchase is optimal. Expression (4), using the above substitution for $-R_c$, becomes

(11)
$$ s_0 \cdot \lambda(l_0) \cdot (p_h \bar{h}) - \int_0^\infty \lambda(l) \left[-p_h \bar{h} + p_h h(l) \right] f(l) dl $$
$$ = s_0 \cdot \lambda(l_0) \cdot (p_h \bar{h}) - p_h \int_0^\infty \lambda(l) \left[h(l) - \bar{h} \right] f(l) dl $$

The expression in the integral is positive; if $\lambda(l)$ were constant over all losses, then the integral would merely be the integral of deviations of $h(l)$ about its mean; but each value is weighted by $\lambda(l)$, which increases as l increases. Thus the larger terms in the integral (recall that $h(l)$ increases with l) carry a larger weight, and the integral itself is positive. Therefore, (11) is negative for a sufficiently small value of s_0, or if the marginal utility of income rises sufficiently between the state with no loss (l_0) and all other states, which means that $E(U)$ will rise if C is reduced from 1 to some smaller value—some insurance is purchased.

When selecting C less than 1, the model shows that the larger the coinsurance elasticity of demand for h, the larger will be the optimal coinsurance level. Optimal C is chosen so that for any smaller C, expected utility (Z) falls; in other words, dZ/dC becomes positive, which can happen only if $-R_c$ grows "large" relative to the average expense $p_h \bar{h}$. From (10), $-R_c$ obviously becomes large as either θ increases or as η_{hc} increases in absolute value. If η_{hc} is sufficiently large, the optimal C could be near 1.[4]

One prediction that might be made informally from this model is that the equilibrium coinsurance rate (*ceteris paribus*) will be larger (less insurance), the larger the own-price elasticity of demand for that service.

1. COMPARATIVE STATICS OF DEMAND FOR MAXIMUM COVERAGE

First, I will analyze effects of income, medical prices, and various insurance pricing strategies on the demand for h^*.

Income

The comparative statics are developed by fully differentiating the first-order conditions and solving the resultant equation for the appropriate derivative. Let ∂Z represent Equation (5) and X represent any independent variable of interest. Then the full derivative is

(12) $$dz = \frac{-\partial(\partial Z)}{\partial X}\, dX + \frac{\partial(\partial Z)}{\partial h^*}\, dh^*$$

which must be set at zero in order to maintain the optimality of (5). Hence

(13) $$dh^*/dX = \frac{-\partial(\partial Z)}{\partial X}\bigg/\frac{\partial(\partial Z)}{\partial h^*} = \frac{-\partial^2 Z}{\partial h^*\partial X}\bigg/\frac{\partial^2 Z}{\partial h^{*2}}$$

The denominator of this expression is simply the second-order condition for optimality with respect to h^*—it must be negative if expected utility is maximized.[5] Thus the sign of dC/dX is identical to the sign of the cross-partial derivative $\partial^2 Z/\partial C\, \partial X$; i.e., the derivative of (5) with respect to X. A similar result holds, of course, for the comparative statics with respect to C, where the derivative of (4) is taken. That is,

(14) $$\frac{dC}{dX} = \frac{-\partial^2 Z}{\partial C^*\partial X}\bigg/\frac{\partial^2 Z}{\partial C^2}$$

The basic income effect on h^* is found by establishing the sign of:[6]

(15) $$\frac{\partial^2 Z}{\partial h^*\partial l} \propto \int_0^{l^*} (-R_{h^*})\,\frac{\partial \lambda(l)}{\partial l}\,f(l)dl + \int_{l^*}^{\infty} \left[-R_{h^*} + (1-C)p_h\right]\frac{\partial \lambda(l)}{\partial l}\,f(l)dl$$

$$= \int_0^{l^*} (-R_{h^*})(-\lambda)(l)r(I,l) + \int_{l^*}^{\infty}\left[-R_{h^*} + (1-C)p_h\right](-\lambda)(l)r(I,l)f(l)dl$$

where $r(I,l)$ is the Arrow-Pratt risk-aversion measure, defined as $r(I,l) = -\partial^2 U/\partial I^2/\partial U/\partial I = -(\partial \lambda/\partial I)/\lambda$. Equation (15) is obviously just the negative of the first-order condition (5) weighted by the risk-aversion measure. If the person exhibits constant risk aversion over all illness levels (equivalent to constant risk aversion over all incomes), then this "income effect" on demand for maximum coverage is zero. If risk aversion increases with illnesses (decreases with income), then $r(I,l)$ acts as a weighting scheme making (15) negative, so that demand for h^* falls as income rises. If risk aversion is increasing in income (decreasing as illnesses increase), then (15) becomes positive and demand for h^* increases as income increases.

This "basic income effect" appears throughout the comparative statics of demand for reimbursement insurance. Invariably, expressions appear where an income effect is present, based on how the marginal utility of income ($\lambda(l)$) changes as some variable, X, changes. The income effect in these derivatives is always determined by how $\partial \lambda/\partial X$ changes over values of l. Hence, it is sufficient to determine the behavior of $\partial \lambda/\partial X$ over l in order to determine the "income component" of effects of any variable, X, on demand.

Medical Prices

In addition to the pure income effects, this model can show the effects of a change in p_h on demand for maximum coverage. The income effect of a change in p_h is determined by the behavior of $\partial \lambda/\partial p_h$ as l changes. That derivative is

(16)
$$\frac{\partial \lambda(l)}{\partial p_h} = \begin{cases} \left(-Ch - \dfrac{\partial R}{\partial p_h}\right) \cdot r(I) \cdot \lambda + C\lambda \dfrac{\partial h}{\partial I} \text{ for } h \leqslant h^* \\[2ex] \left[-(h - h^*) + Ch^* - \dfrac{\partial R}{\partial p_h}\right] r(I) \cdot \lambda + \lambda \dfrac{\partial h}{\partial I} \text{ for } h > h^* \end{cases}$$

which (in elasticity form) becomes the "weights" in the integral similar to how $r(I)$ acts as weights in (15). These weights are

(17)
$$\frac{p_h}{\lambda(l)} \cdot \frac{\partial \lambda(l)}{\partial p_h} = \begin{cases} -(\omega_h + \omega_R \eta_{Rp_h}) \cdot r^*(I) + \omega_h \eta_{hI} \text{ for } h \leqslant h^* \\[1ex] -(\omega_h + \omega_R \, \eta_{Rp_h}) \cdot r^*(I) + [\omega_h \eta_{hI} + (1-C)p_h h^*]\eta_{hI} \\ \text{for } h > h^* \end{cases}$$

where ω_h is the *out-of-pocket* budget share—i.e., $Cp_h h/I$ for $h \leqslant h^*$, and $[p_h(h - h^*) + Cp_h h^*]/I$ for $h > h^*$, η_{hI} is the income elasticity of demand for h, η_{Rp_h} is the total elasticity of the premium R with respect to p_h, and ω_R is the budget share of R itself.

Although this income effect appears complex, its sign is basically determined by whether $r^*(I)$—the income elasticity of the marginal utility of income—is larger or smaller than the income elasticity of demand for medical care.[7] The factors are offsetting—when medical prices rise, the income effect η_{hI} induces demand for higher coverage, but general purchasing power falls commensurately, tending to reduce demand for h^*. Empirical estimates of $r^*(I)$ are in the range of 1.5 to 2.5, whereas estimates of η_{hI} are in the range of 0.1 to 0.5, so the general income effect is likely to dominate the income effect of demand for h.

Several things are worth remembering about this phenomenon. First, if C is small (nearly zero coinsurance), then the budget share terms ω_h tend to vanish in (17), but ω_R will be larger. Thus at one extreme (low C, low η_{hI}), only the terms involving $r^*(I)\omega_R\eta_{Rph}$ would remain, which are negative. In this case, the income effect of a change in p_h would be negative—higher p_h would mean lower h^*. At another extreme, if η_{Rph} is near zero—as would occur if demand for medical care were nearly of unitary elasticity—and if C were near zero, then only the final term $(1-C)p_hh^*\eta_{hI}$ would remain in the last integral, which is positive. In this case, demand for h^* would rise as p_h increased, via this income effect. Thus it appears that there are interactions between demand for C and h^*, and even interactions between demand for h^* and demand for h. The resultant derivatives are, however, ambiguous.

There is no substitution effect on demand for h^* as p_h changes, because the price of medical care is simply a numeraire for that problem. This is most easily shown by noting that the "real price of insurance," defined as $P_{h*} = R_{h*}/[-R_{h*} + (1-C)p_h]$, does not change as p_h changes. This is true because $R_{h*} = (1+\theta)(1-C)p_hh^*f(l^*)$ and the partial derivative of that with respect to p_h is simply equivalent to dividing through by p_h. Since p_h is a common factor in all terms in P_{h*}, there is no change in P_{h*} as p_h changes.

If the maximum payment is described in physical units (such as h^*), then, except for the net income effects, there is no effect from a change in p_h. If the limit is in terms of dollars, then the effect is positive, and the measured elasticity should center around unity, not zero. Put differently, people shouldn't change their demand for maximum coverage as the price of care changes, except for effects introduced by income considerations.

Loading Fees

Finally, I would like to investigate how demand for h^* changes as the loading fee on insurance changes. To do this, I shall introduce several forms of an insurance premium, specifying different types of loading. One common specification is that the loading fee, θ_1, is applied uniformly to all expected benefits, so that

(18) $\qquad R_1 = (1+\theta_1)\left[\int_0^{l^*} (1-C)p_hh(l)f(l)dl + (1-C)p_hh^* \int_{l^*}^{\infty} f(l)dl\right]$

so

$\qquad R_{h*} = (1+\theta)(1-C)p_hQ(l^*)$

and

$\qquad \dfrac{\partial^2 R}{\partial h^* \partial \theta} = (1-C)p_hQ(l^*) > 0$

In this case, it can be shown that demand for maximum coverage behaves much as a usual good—there is a negative substitution effect (demand falls as θ_1 rises), and an income effect that depends on whether demand for h^* rises or falls with income (i.e., whether h^* is a superior or inferior good). If $\partial h^*/\partial I$ is positive, then the income effect (as in the usual case) is negative, and demand for h^* falls as θ_1 rises.

The substitution component of this derivative is simply

$$(19) \qquad \int_0^{l^*} [\lambda(l)] \left(\frac{\partial^2 R}{\partial h^* \partial \theta}\right) f(l)dl + \int_{l^*}^{\infty} [\lambda(l)] \left(\frac{\partial^2 R}{\partial h^* \partial \theta}\right) f(l)dl$$

i.e., the expected value of marginal utility of income times $-\partial^2 R/\partial h^* \partial \theta$, which is positive. Hence, the substitution effect is negative. I compute the income effect by making $\partial \lambda/\partial \theta = (\partial \lambda/\partial I) \cdot R\theta$, where R_θ is the first partial derivative of R with respect to θ (holding C and h^* constant) and is positive. Hence, the income effect of a change in θ is proportional to the pure income effect and therefore depends on whether risk aversion is increasing or decreasing. If $r(I)$ is increasing in income, so that $\partial h^*/\partial I$ is positive, then the entire derivative $\partial h^*/\partial \theta$ is negative, just as in a "standard" consumer demand problem.

Consider now a second possible formulation of the premium function

$$(20) \qquad R_2 = \theta_2 + \int_0^{l^*} (1-C)p_h h(l)f(l)dl + \int_{l^*}^{\infty} (1-C)p_h h^* f(l)dl$$

In this formulation, there is a fixed loading fee, (say, sales costs) but no administrative costs otherwise. Then $\partial R/\partial \theta_2 = 1$, and $\partial^2 R/\partial h^* \partial \theta_2 = 0$. In this case, an increase in θ_2 produces an income effect, but no substitution effect, and will be proportional to the income effect $\partial h^*/\partial I$.

A third possible premium function combines the first two—a fixed loading charge, θ_3, and a declining proportional addition, θ_4—so that

$$(21) \qquad R_3 = \theta_3 - \theta_4 \left[\int_0^{l^*} (1-C)p_h h(l)f(l)dl + \int_{l^*}^{\infty} (1-C)p_h h^* f(l)dl \right]$$

Under this pricing scheme, there would be a positive fixed charge and a declining marginal cost of coverage, as measured by expected benefits. There is a declining marginal cost of h^*, and such a pricing scheme can occur only if there are scale economies in coverage. Clearly, the greater the scale economies (i.e., the higher is θ_4 in absolute value), the more h^* would be demanded.

Now consider a premium with rising marginal costs of coverage:

$$\text{(21a)} \quad R_4 = \int_0^{l*} (1-C)p_h h(l)\left[\theta_5 h(l)\right]f(l)dl + \int_{l*}^{\infty} (1-C)p_h h^*(\theta_5 h^*)f(l)dl$$

so

$$\text{(21b)} \quad R_{h*} = (1-C)p_h\,(2\theta_5 h^*)\,Q(l^*) > 0$$

and

$$\text{(21c)} \quad \frac{\partial^2 R}{\partial h * \partial \theta_5} = 2(1-C)p_h Q(l^*) > 0$$

Notice that the EB "real price of insurance" can rise with h^*, unlike the other premium functions considered. The real price—the rates of income transfer rates between insured and uninsured states—is defined by

$$\text{(22a)} \quad P_{h*} = \frac{R_{h*}}{(1-C)p_h - R_{h*}}$$

For this premium function (21a),

$$\text{(22b)} \quad P_{h*} = \frac{(1-C)P_h(2\theta_5 h^*)Q(l^*)}{(1-C)P_h - (1-C)P_h(2\theta_5 h^*)Q(l^*)} = \frac{Z}{1-Z}$$

where $Z = 2\theta_5 h^* Q(l^*)$.
Thus, price changes with h^* according to

$$\text{(22c)} \quad \frac{\partial P_{h*}}{\partial h *} = \frac{\partial Z/\partial h *}{(1-Z)^2} = 2\theta_5\left[h^*\frac{\partial Q(l^*)}{\partial h *} + Q(l^*)\right]$$

$$= 2\theta_5 Q(l^*)\,(1+E)$$

where E is the elasticity of $Q(l^*)$ with respect to h^*. Thus, as long as $Q(l^*)$ is inelastic with respect to h^*, the real price of insurance (in the EB sense) rises with h^*. Hence, P_{h*} changes with the distribution of l, and can fall and then rise as l^* increases. Such a pricing function is consistent with observed finite maximum amounts of insurance coverage in health insurance policies. Notice that $E = -f(l) \cdot l/Q(l)$, since $\partial Q(l)/\partial l = -f(l)$. The ratio of $f(l)/Q(l)$ is known in statistics as the hazard function. Thus, P_{h*} increases with h^* for illness distributions in which the hazard function decreases faster than l increases, since in that case $(1+E) > 0$.

It is quite clear, since R_{h*} and $\partial^2 R/\partial h * \partial \theta$ are of appropriate sign, that the price effect computed for the premium function R_1 also holds for this premium function; namely, that increases in θ_5 will reduce demand for h^* as long as the income component of the price effect is normal.

2. COMPARATIVE STATICS OF DEMAND FOR COINSURANCE

Selecting the coinsurance level, C, is a more complicated analysis (at least for the analyst!), the complication arising primarily because coinsurance subsidizes purchase of a market good (medical care) rather than simply providing an income transfer. The second major complication arises because one and only one level of coinsurance C is selected, which must apply to all states of the world less than l^*. Because of the interdependence of the different states, comparative statics effects are complex. First, I identify the basic income effect, found here by establishing the sign of $\partial^2 Z/\partial C \, \partial I$.

$$(23) \quad \frac{\partial^2 Z}{\partial C \, \partial I} = \frac{\partial}{\partial I} \left[\int_0^{l^*} \lambda(l) \ [-R_c - p_h h(l)] \ f(l)dl + \int_{l^*}^{\infty} \lambda(l) \ (-R_c - p_h h^*) f(l)dl \right]$$

The "income-component" is

$$(24) \quad \int_0^{l^*} [-R_c - p_h h(l)] \ \frac{\partial \lambda(l)}{\partial I} f(l)dl + \int_{l^*}^{\infty} (-R_c - p_h h^*) \ \frac{\partial \lambda(l)}{\partial I} \ f(l)dl$$

$$= - \left[\int_0^{l^*} (-R_c - p_h h \,) r(I) \lambda(l) f(l)dl + \int_{l^*}^{\infty} (-R_c - p_h h^*) r(I) \lambda(l) f(l)dl \right]$$

which is the negative of the first-order condition weighted by the Arrow-Pratt risk-aversion measure. The expression $(-R_c - p_h h)$ becomes more negative as l increases, so increasing risk aversion in income (decreasing risk aversion in l) lends less weight to the more negative values, making the expression in brackets positive. Hence, $\partial C/\partial I$ becomes more negative through this component—demand for insurance rises (lower C) if risk aversion in income increases. The substitution component produced by a change in income is shown by

$$(25) \quad \int_0^{l^*} \lambda(l) \left[\frac{\partial(-R_c)}{\partial I} - p_h \frac{\partial h}{\partial I} \right] f(l)dl + \int_{l^*}^{\infty} \frac{\partial(-R_c)}{\partial I} \ f(l)dl$$

This is most easily understood by treating the case wherein $h^* = \infty$, so that (25) is simply

$$\int_0^{\infty} \lambda(l) \left[\frac{\partial(-R_c)}{\partial I} - p_h \frac{\partial h}{\partial I} \right] f(l)dl$$

Notice now that the way the premium derivative R_c changes with income is simply the average over all insured states of $(1 + \theta)$ times the average income effect—i.e.,

$$\frac{\partial(-R_c)}{\partial I} = (1+\theta) \int_0^\infty \left[p_h \frac{\partial h}{\partial I} - (1-C)p_h \frac{\partial^2 h}{\partial C\, \partial I} \right] f(l)dl = (1+\theta)p_h \frac{\partial h}{\partial I}$$

(assuming no income interaction with the price effect, $\partial h/\partial C$). Thus, the substitution effect produced by a change in income is

(26) $$\int_0^\infty \lambda(l) \left[(1+\theta)p_h \frac{\partial h}{\partial I} - p_h \frac{\partial h\,(l)}{\partial I} \right] f(l)dl$$

For this to be negative (i.e., making dC/dI negative, so that more insurance is demanded with income), the income effect, $\partial h/\partial I$, must be increasing with the level of illness; if $\partial h/\partial I$ is constant or decreasing as l increases, it is easy to see that (26) is positive, since $\lambda(l)$ increases with l. An important point is that since changes in income change the relative prices of insuring different states of the world, a substitution effect on demand for C is introduced when I changes. Thus one cannot infer anything about risk-aversion characteristics of the utility function from income elasticities of demand for coverage; the income elasticity is a composite effect of a "pure" income effect (dependent on the risk-aversion measure) and a substitution effect (dependent on how $\partial h/\partial I$ changes over losses).

One conclusion that may be drawn from statistical studies of demand relates to pricing policies of the health insurance industry. If rates are set independently of income, then $\partial(-R_c)\partial I = 0$, and the only subsidy effect is obviously to increase demand for coverage as I rises. Thus, unless possible decreasing risk aversion outweighs the substitution effect, "community-rated" insurance should lead to a positive income elasticity of demand for coverage. Since the Blue Cross and Blue Shield plans have been traditionally community-rated rather than experience-rated, enrollment shares of the Blues should be higher in high-income areas than in low-income areas, *ceteris paribus*, since the Blues also offer high-coverage insurance.[8]

Medical Prices

Changes in the price of medical care can also affect demand for C, although in complex ways, and the sign of the effect is indeterminate. As with demand for h^*, there is an income effect and a substitution effect. The income effect is determined by how the net change in income varies over different l. The income effect of a change in p_h is proportional to

$$(27) \quad \int_0^{l*} (-R_c - p_h h) \frac{\partial \lambda}{\partial p_h} f(l)dl + \int_{l*}^\infty (-R_c - p_h h*) \frac{\partial \lambda}{\partial p_h} f(l)dl$$

where $\partial \lambda/\partial p_h$ is given in (16) and restated in (17).

Similar conclusions can be drawn with respect to demand for C as are drawn for $h*$ when p_h changes. First, suppose that $\partial h/\partial I$ is zero, so that the income effect is entirely a function of $r(I)$, since $\partial \lambda/\partial p_h = -S \cdot r*(I) - \omega_h \eta_{hI}$. The income effect is then simply the first-order condition weighted by $r*(I)$ and by the expression $S = (\omega_h + \omega_R \eta_{Rph})$. The out-of-pocket budget share, S, must increase with l, so there are larger and larger weights applied to the more and more negative values in (27), and $\partial C/\partial p_h$ falls (demand for insurance increases as p_h rises). If risk aversion in income is increasing ($r(I)$ is falling with l), then that produces an offsetting effect, but the net must be to increase demand for insurance (reduce C) unless the risk-aversion measure falls faster than the out-of-pocket budget share rises. I view this as unlikely.

Finally, if the assumption that $\partial h/\partial I = 0$ is removed, then there is an offsetting income effect—there is lower demand for h at all levels of l because of the income effect, so that portion of the income effect reduces demand for coverage (increases C) as p_h rises.

The substitution effect as p_h changes is

$$(28) \quad \int_0^{l*} \lambda(l) \left[-\frac{\partial^2 R}{\partial C \partial p_h} - h(1 + \eta_{hh}) \right] f(l)dl + \int_{l*}^\infty \lambda(l) \left[-\frac{\partial^2 R}{\partial C \partial p_h} - h* \right] f(l)dl$$

where η_{hh} is the own-price elasticity for h at any given l and is a function of l. The components in brackets in (28) show how the "real price of coverage" changes as p_h changes, the change being a function of how the net income transfer ($p_h h + R_c$) changes. The premium slope ($-R_c$) changes with p_h, as does the expenditure $p_h h$, the latter as a function of the own-price elasticity for h. The premium slope $-R_c$ changes according to:[9]

$$(29) \quad \frac{-\partial^2 R}{\partial C \partial p_h} = \frac{\partial(-R_c)}{\partial p_h} = (1+\theta) \left\{ \int_0^{l*} \left[h(1 + \eta_{hh}) \right. \right.$$

$$\left. \left. - (1-C) \frac{\partial h(l)}{\partial C} \right] f(l)dl + h*Q(l*) \right\}$$

$$= (1+\theta) h \overline{(1 + \eta_{hh})} + (1+\theta) h*Q(l*)$$

$$- (1+\theta)(1-C) \int_0^{l*} \frac{\partial h}{\partial C} f(l)dl$$

Thus the substitution effect in part is a function of the deviation of $h(1+\eta_{hh})$ around its mean (assuming "small" values of θ), so that if the own-price elasticity of demand for h approaches zero as l increases, (28) tends to become more negative, indicating increased demand for insurance (lower C). Thus, part of the effect of p_h on demand for C depends on how the own-price elasticity for h interacts with the size of loss l. The total effect of a change in p_h is ambiguous on net, however, because of the remaining term in $\partial^2 R/\partial C\,\partial p_h$, as well as additional ambiguity introduced by larger values of θ that offset increased demand.

Loading Fees

Finally, I will analyze the effects of changes in the loading fee on demand for C. As before, several alternative structures of the premium function R can be hypothesized and their effects detailed. First, consider the function

$$R_1 = (1+\theta)\left[\int_0^{l*}(1-C)p_h h f(l)dl + (1-C)p_h Q(l*)\right]$$

Here, a change in θ produces an income effect on demand for C proportional to

(30) $\quad \dfrac{-\partial R}{\partial\theta}\left[\int_0^{l*}(-R_c - p_h h)\dfrac{\partial\lambda(l)}{\partial I}f(l)dl + \int_{l*}^{\infty}(-R_c - p_h h*)\dfrac{\partial\lambda(l)}{\partial I}f(l)dl\right]$

which has the usual income effect properties. Since R_θ is of necessity positive for this functional form of R, the income effect depends on whether there is increasing or decreasing risk aversion in income, and will have the "usual" income effect of a price change if risk aversion is such that insurance is a normal good.

The substitution effect produced by a change in θ is of the form

(31) $\quad \displaystyle\int_0^{l*}\lambda(l)\left[\left(\dfrac{-\partial^2 R}{\partial C\,\partial\theta}\right)-p_h\dfrac{\partial h}{\partial\theta}\right]f(l)dl + \int_{l*}^{\infty}\lambda(l)\left(\dfrac{-\partial^2 R}{\partial C\,\partial\theta}\right)f(l)dl$

where

$$\dfrac{\partial h}{\partial\theta} = -R_\theta\cdot\dfrac{\partial h}{\partial l}$$

and

$$-\frac{\partial^{2R}}{\partial C \partial \theta} = \frac{\partial}{\partial \theta}(-R_c) = \int_0^{l^*} \left[p_h h - (1-C)p_h \frac{\partial h}{\partial C} \right.$$

$$\left. + (1+\theta)p_h \frac{\partial h}{\partial \theta} \right] f(l)dl + (1-C)p_h Q(l^*)$$

Here, a very unusual result appears. There is a standard substitution effect that can be shown to be approximately

(32) $\quad \int_0^{\infty} \lambda(l) \cdot \frac{(-R_c)}{(1+\theta)} f(l)dl = E(\lambda) \cdot \frac{(-R_c)}{(1+\theta)} > 0$

which is positive (thus reducing demand for coverage as θ increases). But there is also an effect of changes in θ on the relative prices of insuring different states of the world, because R_θ changes available income, which changes demand for care in each state. This substitution term is of the form

(33) $\quad R_\theta \cdot \int_0^{l^*} \lambda(l)p_h \left[\frac{\partial h}{\partial I} - (1+\theta) \frac{\overline{\partial h}}{\partial I} \ f(l)dl \right]$

If $\partial h/\partial I$ increases sufficiently over losses, this term is positive, and demand for C behaves as a standard good as θ increases. But if $\partial h/\partial I$ falls as l increases, then there is a general income effect on demand for $h(l)$, and the real price of insuring states of the world tends to fall as θ increases. If this effect were sufficiently strong, demand for coverage might actually rise as θ increased, although I view this as a remote possibility. Empirically, as I shall show in the next section, demand for any measure of insurance I have used behaves "normally" with respect to changes in the loading fee, indicating that this condition does not occur in observed data with sufficient strength to produce an unusual price effect.

The second premium function I shall consider is

$$R_2 = \theta_2 + \int_0^{l^*} (1-C)p_h h(l)dl + (1-C)p_h h^* Q(l^*)$$

i.e., one with a lump sum loading fee and no marginal cost of different levels of C. Here, $R_\theta = 1$, and the usual income effects hold—if C is a "normal" good, demand for coverage falls as θ_2 rises. The only substitution effect is this unusual one just discussed with R_1, where

$$\frac{\partial(-R_c)}{\partial \theta} = -p_h \frac{\overline{\partial h}}{\partial I}$$

so this substitution effect is

$$(34) \qquad \int_0^{l^*} \lambda(l) p_h \left(\frac{\partial h}{\partial I} - \frac{\overline{\partial h}}{\partial I} \right) f(l) dl$$

which can be negative (more demand for insurance with higher θ) if $\partial h / \partial I$ falls as l increases. Thus this reversed "price effect" is also possible under this premium formulation.

The third possible premium function,

$$R_3 = \theta_3 - \theta_4 \int_0^{l^*} (1-C) p_h f(l) dl$$

is a combination of the first two, except that there is declining marginal cost of coverage. Except for the "unusual" price effect here, changes in θ_3 are equivalent to those in the function R_2, and increases in θ_4 (the marginal cost reduction factor) will tend to increase demand for coverage (lower C).

To summarize these results, recall the specific features of the insurance policy under discussion:

1. There is restricted choice of insurance parameters—only C and h^* may be chosen, rather than an actual net income transfer for each state of nature.
2. States of nature are aggregated when the premium function is written, so that effects of changes in I, p_h, and θ are linked across states of the world.

The basic findings are these:

1. The effects of income on demand for insurance depend not only on how risk aversion changes over income (as in the usual case of insurance analyzed in the literature) but on how the income elasticity of demand for medical care changes over states of the world. Hence, income elasticities of demand for health insurance cannot be used to infer behavior of the Arrow-Pratt risk-aversion measure over income changes.
2. Changes in the price of medical care produce ambiguous effects on demand for C. As p_h changes, demand for h^* changes only according to income effects. Thus if there were a compensated change in p_h, no change in demand for h^* would be expected. If the price change is uncompensated, no prediction of the effect is possible.
3. Although usual loading fees are not the "true" price of insurance, the effects of an increase in θ are generally analogous to an increase in the price of any commodity or good. A possible theoretical exception arises when considering demand for C, which may be more predominant under some premium-writing schemes than others.

3. DEMAND ESTIMATION

Demand curves for medical care have been estimated from a household survey of 2,367 families drawn in 1963 by the Center for Health Administration Studies (CHAS) of the University of Chicago. The families responded to questions about their insurance companies during the household interview, and direct verification of the parameters of the policy was made from the insurance companies. This is the only source of data I am aware of (except the 1970 survey by CHAS, not yet completed) that provides explicit data on parameters of insurance policies purchased by individual families; hence its uniqueness. Unfortunately, verification was not complete because some insurers did not respond and response was nonrandom. Thus, only families with all policies verified have been used for this study, and the data have been weighted to reproduce the actual sample means in terms of socioeconomic parameters known to affect the response rate. There remain 1,579 families in the study, 970 of which have some health insurance. An earlier study using these data (Phelps, 1973) provides more complete descriptions of the data source. Those studies established in general that there was a positive income elasticity of demand for health insurance, varying considerably by type of insurance. It was also established that health insurance was highly sensitive to the loading fee on the insurance, measured in this case by the size of the group through which insurance was obtained. A rough estimate from these data is that the elasticity of insurance with respect to changes in θ was about -0.3 to -0.5. The effects of changes in the price of medical care were ambiguous, and the results varied considerably depending on the method of estimation used. Here, I have attempted some additional analyses of these data, using new measures of the price of medical care facing each family, in an attempt to improve those estimates. I have also added measures of the wage rate facing the head of each household derived from OLS estimates of the wage rate, using fitted values for heads not employed.

The medical care price measures are obtained through instrumental variable estimation of prices for those with positive utilization. The estimating equations are in the appendix, Table 8. The dependent variables in these equations are expense/unit of service, and the explanatory variables include dummies for eight geographic regions, measures of physician and hospital supply, wages of the family head, nonwage income, and education of the head. The last variables reflect possible demand for higher-quality service with higher income, and education is a measure of efficiency in search for lower prices. Separate price equations were estimated for hospital services, for surgical care, and for total medical expense. The equations explained from 17 per cent of the variance (hospital price) to 5 per cent (total care).[10]

4. DEMAND FOR COVERAGE

From the available data in the 1963 CHAS-NORC survey, one parameter closely matches the theoretical variable C—the maximum payment per hospital day chosen by the consumer. This variable can vary from $0 (no coverage) to any positive amount. Some policies specify full coverage of semi-private rooms (or hospital wards), and for these purposes I assigned a dollar figure equal to the 95th percentile of the observed distribution of actual maximum payments. Thus the dependent variable ranges from 0 to $40, the latter figure being the largest maximum in these data.

Demand functions have been estimated using both ordinary least squares (OLS) and the limited dependent variable technique proposed by Tobin (1958), known informally as "tobit" analysis. Because of the nature of the dependent variable in these regressions, tobit analysis is preferable *a priori*. Actually, the tobit regressions produced (in three of four dependent variables) slightly higher (0.3 to 2.8 per cent higher) mean square error than the OLS estimates, the exception being demand for major medical insurance, which had the largest fraction of observations with the dependent variable at the limit. Both sets of regressions are reported here. The results are shown in Table 1, with quadratic terms for the continuous explanatory variables. I show elasticities calculated at mean values of all the x's and of y, with t ratios in parentheses. The quadratic specification is desirable on grounds of significance of the quadratic terms and will be discussed exclusively.

In the OLS equation, income is positively and significantly related to insurance demand, the elasticity being 0.22. As mentioned previously, one cannot infer from this that there is increasing risk aversion in income because of complex changes in the real price of insurance that are associated with an income change. One can, however, impute some fraction of that income elasticity to another subsidy; namely, that occurring through the income tax deductibility of insurance premiums on federal and state taxes. The

TABLE 1 Demand for Maximum Payment per Hospital Day (HOSMAX) (n = 1522)

Variable	OLS Coefficient (t statistic)	OLS Elasticity (t statistic)	TOBIT Coefficient (z statistic)	TOBIT Elasticity (z statistic)
Income	.644 E-03		.141 E-02	
	(1.61)	.22	(1.97)	.23
Income squared	−.153 E-07	(2.16)	−.577 E-07	(2.03)
	(.57)		(1.25)	
Wage	.0973		.133	
	(2.09)	.25	(1.66)	.25
Wage squared	−.304 E-03	(1.91)	−.404 E-03	(1.72)
	(1.65)		(1.28)	
Work-group size	6.756		10.438	
	(11.73)	.67	(11.46)	.86
Group size squared	−.531	(23.53)	−.838	(17.56)
	(8.08)		(8.17)	
Hospital price index	49.132		89.707	
	(4.61)	.08	(4.71)	.06
Hospital price squared	−28.768	(.69)	−53.147	(.45)
	(4.72)		(4.93)	
Estimated illness	−5.563		−9.326	
	(2.27)	.04	(2.16)	.02
Illness squared	.841	(.24)	1.415	(.114)
	(2.37)		(2.29)	
Education of head	1.885		4.164	
	(2.26)	.11	(2.78)	.22
Education squared	−.153	(.89)	−.323	(1.76)
	(1.77)		(2.15)	
Age of head	−1.593		−2.294	
	(1.89)	.16	(1.62)	.24
Age squared	.220	(2.82)	.343	(3.46)
	(2.49)		(2.30)	
Race (1=nonwhite)	−1.933		−5.588	
	(2.29)		(3.68)	
Sex of head (1=female)	2.913		4.095	
	(2.83)		(2.39)	

TABLE 1 (concluded)

Variable	OLS Coefficient (t statistic)	OLS Elasticity (t statistic)	TOBIT Coefficient (z statistic)	TOBIT Elasticity (z statistic)
Family size	−.248 (1.13)	−.06	−.483 (1.28)	−.08
Urban/Rural (1=rural)	.547 (.90)		.880 (.88)	
Welfare care (1=yes)	−2.155 (1.48)		−5.652 (2.11)	
Free care (1=yes)	1.584 (1.20)		−4.109 (1.75)	
Constant term	−29.992 (4.20)		−74.385 (5.819)	
R^2	.426		—	
F (20, 1501)	57.836		—	
X^2 (d.f.=20)	—		852.66	

net income effect is found by solving

$$\frac{dC}{dI} = \frac{\partial C}{\partial I} + \frac{\partial C}{\partial \theta} \cdot \frac{\partial \theta}{\partial I}$$

$$= \frac{\partial C}{\partial I} + \frac{\partial C}{\partial \theta} \cdot \frac{\partial \theta}{\partial MTR} \cdot \frac{\partial MTR}{\partial I}$$

or

$$\eta_{CI} = \bar{\eta}_{CI} + \frac{I}{\theta} \cdot \eta_{C\theta} \cdot \frac{\partial MTR}{\partial I/I}$$

Estimating the effect of income tax deductibility on demand for insurance requires several assumptions. First, for group insurance premiums paid by the employer, I assume that the entire amount is exempted from both income tax and payroll tax.[11] In 1963, personally paid premiums could be combined with out-of-pocket medical expense and deducted subject to a 3 per cent of adjusted gross income (AGI) limitation. Data from Mitchell and Phelps (1974) enable one to estimate how the marginal income tax rate changes with income—the estimate is that $\partial MTR(\partial I/I) = 0.1$. This estimate applies only to personally paid premiums. For employer premiums, the progression of marginal tax rate is lower because of the incidence of social security taxes; data in Mitchell and Phelps allow an estimate of $\partial \text{MTR}(\partial I/I) = 0.05$ for premiums paid by employers.[12]

For employer-group premiums, the total income elasticity is decomposed as

$$\eta_{CI} = \bar{\eta}_{CI} + \eta_{C\theta} \; \frac{\partial \text{MTR}}{\partial I/I} \cdot \frac{I}{\theta}$$

where $\bar{\eta}_{CI}$ is the total income elasticity. I have estimated $\eta_{C\theta} = -0.7$ for policies in which $\bar{\theta} \approx 0.2$. Thus $\eta_{CI} = \bar{\eta}_{CI} - 0.7(0.05)(1/0.2)$ $= \bar{\eta}_{CI} - 0.175$. Thus the tax subsidy is a substantial portion of the estimated income elasticity (see below).

For family-paid premiums, the effect is more difficult to estimate. At one extreme, if the family did not anticipate having premiums plus unreimbursed medical expenses exceeding a "deductible" of 3 per cent of AGI, there would be no effect. At the other extreme, if the family knew with certainty that such a deductible would be exceeded, the appropriate correction would be twice that computed for employer-paid premiums, since the marginal tax rate for individuals progresses faster ($\partial \text{MTR}/\partial I/I = 0.1$) when the payroll taxes are excluded. Offsetting this would be higher loading fees paid on many family premiums. The calculation must be made on the anticipations of the family, and hence cannot be computed directly—certainly the expected frequency of taking the deduction measures with error the true perception, since the family has more information about itself than is revealed by average behavior.[13] Under 15 per cent of families in 1963 actually used the medical deduction, the rate generally falling with income, so the estimate that little or no effect is present in the income elasticity estimate is probably more accurate than using the full value.

As a general summary, since about 40 per cent of premiums were paid by employers in 1963, and since that induces an upward bias of 0.1 to 0.25 in the estimated income elasticity, a rough correction factor for the estimates presented might be 0.4 times 0.1 to 0.25, or a reduction of 0.04 to 0.1.

Demand for coverage is quite sensitive to the price of insurance. In these data, the instrument for price is the group size from which the insurance was obtained. Insurance texts contain data on how premiums fall with size of total group premium, from which one can compute how the loading fee falls with the size of the group. For the scaling of group size used in these regressions, it is approximately true over the entire range that $d\ln\theta/d\ln$ (group size) $= -1$, so that the group-size elasticities should be multiplied by −1 to obtain an estimate of the own-price elasticity with respect to θ.[14] In the quadratic specification of demand for payment per day, the elasticity with respect to group size at the mean is 0.67, (t=23.53), so the elasticity with respect to θ is −0.67.

Of particular interest is the response of payment per day to the price of medical care faced by the consumer (an instrumental variable fitted from an OLS regression). In the linear equation (not shown), there is no response. In the quadratic specification, both the linear and quadratic terms are highly significant, suggesting that the relationship between demand for payment per day and hospital prices first rises and then falls as p_h increases. Thus, as might be anticipated with the complex interactions shown in (27)–(29), the effect of p_h on demand for C varies with p_h.

The tobit regression for this equation shows few significant differences. The estimated income elasticity is slightly higher (0.23), and the estimated elasticity with respect to work-group size is 0.86, rather than the 0.67 found in the OLS equation.

5. DEMAND FOR MAXIMUM COVERAGE

Three variables measure maximum coverage in these data—the maximum number of hospital days covered, the maximum surgical payment allowed in the fee schedule, and the maximum payment under a major medical insurance plan. Tables 2 through 4 present estimates of demand for each of these variables, with each of the continuous variables entered in quadratic form.

Results are similar for all three. Each is highly elastic to the loading fee, with OLS estimates of the group-size elasticity at the means of the data equal to 0.63 (hospital days), 0.67 (surgical maximum), and 0.68 (major medical insurance maximum), corresponding to elasticities with respect to θ of the negative of those values. The income elasticity for two of these maximum payment parameters is estimated to be zero, although the wage-income elasticity is positive and significant for hospital days ($\eta = 0.29$), maximum surgical payment ($\eta = 0.48$), and for major medical maximum ($\eta = 1.07$). With wage income omitted, the income elasticities are similar to those reported for wage-rate elasticities (Phelps, 1973).

The response of these variables to medical prices is interesting. The hospital maximum variable is in physical units, whereas the remaining two are in dollar units, so "no response" in the first case is a zero elasticity, and "no response" in the remaining two cases is a unitary elasticity, in which case a 1 per cent increase in p_h would cause a 1 per cent change in the maximum, leaving the "real" maximum unchanged. For the hospital days, the response is curvilinear, first increasing and then decreasing. At the mean price, the elasticity is near zero and not significant. This result, using the same data but an imputed medical price that is area-specific, is similar to one reached by Phelps (1973). The surgical maximum payment has a positive elasticity of 0.64 ($t = 2.98$), but the dependent variable is in dollar terms, so this implies a reduction in the *real* coverage maximum as prices rise. In the major medical maximum equation, the effect of medical prices is estimated to be $\eta = 1.13$ ($t = 0.91$), which is similar to results using the earlier price measure, but less precise. This result suggests a slightly increasing demand for maximum coverage with price increases.

Some secondary evidence is available on the effect of medical prices on demand for insurance. Some of the families in the sample were eligible (for various reasons) for reduced-rate or free medical care, either through welfare or for professional courtesy. Although these variables may be confounded with income (permanent income is held constant in these regressions), the tobit demand curves show systematic strong negative relationships between obtaining some free care and the demand for insurance.[15] It is possible to interpret these free-care sources as very low medical prices, in which case (at low prices) one would expect a positive relationship between medical prices and demand for coverage. This is exactly the case with the actual medical price variables, of course—the effect of price increases is first to increase, and then decrease, demand for coverage. At the average of the sample, as has been mentioned, the effect is essentially zero on demand for C, and there exists some evidence for a positive effect on demand for h^*.

The remaining variable of interest in these equations is the effect of estimated illness on demand for coverage. Particularly in community-rated insurance, it can be shown that persons with higher *anticipated* illness levels should have demands for more insurance. The estimated loss variable is an instrumental variable regression, showing in essence the average illness level for persons in a given age-sex-income class. Although this variable is of general interest, it is not a sufficient variable with which to test the problem of adverse self-selection against insurance companies. The crucial question for self-selection analysis is whether residuals in a regression study of insurance demand are correlated with residuals in a regression study of medical care demand, and it is this latter

TABLE 2 Maximum Number of Hospital Days (HOSDAY) (n=1491)

Variable	OLS Coefficient (t statistic)	OLS Elasticity (t statistic)	TOBIT Coefficient (z statistic)	TOBIT Elasticity (z statistic)
Income	.788 E-02 (1.81)	.39 (2.36)	0.174	.36 (2.36)
Income squared	−.2085 E-06 (.72)		−.7176 E-06 (1.46)	
Wage	.0507 (.12)	.29 (1.27)	−.0425 (.051)	.23 (1.16)
Wage squared	.691 E-03 (.34)		.0016 (.474)	
Work-group size	23.526 (3.69)	.63 (8.33)	65.971 (6.98)	.78 (12.13)
Group size squared	−1.147 (1.57)		−4.703 (4.39)	
Hospital price index	435.80 (3.76)	.07 (.34)	854.282 (4.23)	.02 (.09)
Hospital price squared	−258.54 (3.91)		−512.607 (4.48)	
Estimated illness	−66.298 (2.47)	−.67 (2.38)	−114.218 (2.64)	−.42 (1.64)
Illness squared	7.442 (1.93)		14.315 (2.17)	
Education of head	14.953 (1.63)	−.35 (1.78)	43.874 (2.69)	−.04 (.21)
Education squared	−1.984 (2.08)		−4.354 (2.67)	
Age of head	−3.997 (.44)	.21 (2.03)	−6.349 (.424)	.34 (3.50)
Age squared	.800 (.84)		1.754 (1.113)	
Race (1=nonwhite)	−19.854 (2.16)		−56.043 (3.44)	

TABLE 2 (concluded)

Variable	OLS Coefficient (t statistic)	Elasticity (t statistic)	TOBIT Coefficient (z statistic)	Elasticity (z statistic)
Sex (1 = female)	22.094 (1.97)		34.811 (1.94)	
Family size	2.640 (1.12)	.10	1.202 (.302)	.03
Urban/Rural (1 = rural)	3.336 (.50)		5.936 (.56)	
Welfare care (1 = yes)	−21.134 (1.36)		−68.860 (2.39)	
Free care (1 = yes)	−23.531 (1.65)		−56.413 (2.22)	
Constant term	184.02 (2.36)		−675.867 (4.94)	
R^2	.205		—	
$F (20, 1470)$	18.909		—	
X^2 (d.f. = 20)	—		544.47	

problem that TSLS estimators should be helpful in solving. Unless some measure of anticipated health status on each individual were available, studies such as those I have performed here are not likely to show strong effects of illness on demand for insurance. Notice that community-rated insurance is tantamount to hiding from the insurance company information on individual illness, so that if community rating dominated the insurance industry, even the age-sex-race-income specific illness measure I use here should have some association with demand for insurance. To the extent that experience rating predominated, one would expect illness measures to have but slight effects on insurance demand.

In the hospital maximum payment per day equation, the effect at the mean illness level is small, but the quadratic formulation shows the effect to be increasing with illness levels, so that for high expected losses, more insurance would be chosen. In the maximum hospital coverage equation, the effect is negative at mean values of expected illness, but again is increasing with losses. In the surgical maximum equation, the estimated effect is zero at mean values, but again increasing, and there appears to be no significant effect on

TABLE 3 Demand for Maximum Surgical Payment (SURMAX) (*n* = 1493)

Variable	OLS Coefficient (*t* statistic)	OLS Elasticity (*t* statistic)	TOBIT Coefficient (*z* statistic)	TOBIT Elasticity (*z* statistic)
Income	.0150 (1.80)	−.03 (.23)	.0362 (2.33)	.16 (1.00)
Income squared	−.1269 E-05 (2.25)		−.2411 E-05 (2.38)	
Wage	−.5171 E-02 (.00)	48 (2.83)	.4018 (.23)	.50 (2.28)
Wage squared	.403 E-02 (1.03)		.0038 (.55)	
Work-group size	77.971 (6.41)	.67 (17.62)	177.332 (9.04)	1.06 (14.98)
Group size squared	−4.572 (3.29)		−13.0585 (5.88)	
Surgical price index	−398.51 (1.15)	.64 (2.98)	−1049.040 (1.73)	.55 (2.03)
Surgical price squared	248.52 (1.51)		565.093 (1.94)	
Estimated illness	−142.77 (2.75)	.03 (.12)	−243.17 (2.56)	−.09 (.31)
Illness squared	21.235 (2.84)		35.295 (2.60)	
Education of head	75.111 (3.30)	.16 (1.02)	126.773 (3.07)	.35 (1.83)
Education squared	−1.46 (2.91)		−12.423 (2.63)	
Age of head	−13.121 (.76)	.13 (1.74)	−37.153 (1.23)	.27 (2.56)
Age squared	2.0496 (1.12)		5.600 (1.75)	

TABLE 3 (concluded)

Variable	OLS Coefficient (t statistic)	Elasticity (t statistic)	TOBIT Coefficient (z statistic)	Elasticity (z statistic)
Race (1 = nonwhite)	−49.507 (2.79)		−136.813 (4.09)	
Sex (1 = female)	33.091 (1.53)		70.733 (1.89)	
Family size	−2.485 (.54)	−.04	−4.288 (.51)	−.05
Urban/Rural (1 = rural)	−8.719 (.70)		−11.038 (.51)	
Welfare care (1 = yes)	−43.181 (1.41)		−121.331 (2.04)	
Free care (1 = yes)	−7.614 (.27)		−68.743 (1.31)	
Constant term	44.332 (.22)		−251.054 (.68)	
R^2	.319		—	
F (20, 1472)	36.428		—	
X^2 (d.f. = 20)	—		702.25	

demand for major medical maximum payment. Thus, the simultaneous aspect of medical demand and insurance demand would appear to be particularly acute for persons with very high expected illnesses, but not severe at mean values of illness in this population. Nevertheless, simultaneous equation methods are indicated in medical demand studies because of this association.

The tobit regressions in general show similar results for each of these three equations. The differences will be highlighted here. First, for hospital days the estimated income elasticity is positive (0.36) and significant ($z = 2.36$), where z is a unit normal variate. The elasticity with respect to work-group size is slightly higher. One surprising result is that the demand for hospital days coverage falls as a function of estimated increase in illness; the elasticity is −0.42 ($z = 1.64$). In demand for maximum surgical coverage, the

TABLE 4 Demand for Major Medical Maximum Payment (MM-MAX)

Variable	OLS Coefficient (t statistic)	OLS Elasticity (t statistic)	TOBIT Coefficient (z statistic)	TOBIT Elasticity (z statistic)
Income	−.2572 (1.13)	−.15 (.45)	.6963 (.45)	.47 (.97)
Income squared	.1713 E-04 (1.11)		.3879 E-04 (.03)	
Wage	17.7775 (.67)	1.07 (2.31)	218.9687 (1.37)	1.67 (2.63)
Wage squared	.9947 E-02 (.10)		−.4118 (.70)	
Work-group size	−172.75 (.52)	.68 (4.55)	5438.822 (3.65)	1.45 (7.82)
Group size squared	96.89 (2.57)		−249.850 (1.53)	
Medical price index	5241.1 (.59)	1.13 (.91)	21494.78 (.55)	1.77 (1.09)
Medical price squared	−1429.6 (.41)		−3252.15 (.23)	
Estimated illness	882.560 (.63)	.69 (1.19)	4039.55 (.46)	1.01 (1.26)
Illness squared	−67.399 (.33)		−220.22 (.18)	
Education of head	−503.46 (1.00)	.11 (.27)	−807.502 (.25)	−.14 (.26)
Education squared	52.827 (1.06)		55.503 (.19)	
Age of head	179.00 (.38)	−.48 (2.25)	−1764.978 (.67)	−.87 (2.59)
Age squared	−41.137 (.83)		22.441 (.08)	

TABLE 4 (concluded)

Variable	OLS Coefficient (t statistic)	Elasticity (t statistic)	TOBIT Coefficient (z statistic)	Elasticity (z statistic)
Race (1 = nonwhite)	368.12 (.77)		1668.83 (.59)	
Sex (1 = female)	840.80 (1.45)		9120.07 (2.98)	
Family size	−141.54 (1.14)	−.21	−463.855 (.66)	−.18
Urban/Rural (1 = rural)	198.55 (.59)		129.116 (.07)	
Welfare care (1 = yes)	−77.644 (.09)		−9637.624 (1.55)	
Free care (1 = yes)	−541.21 (.71)		−2133.249 (.48)	
Constant term	−6289.0 (1.07)		−1.007 E-07 (3.24)	
R^2	.171		—	
F (20, 1558)	16.096		—	
X^2 (d.f. = 20)	—		314.64	

only difference is a 20 per cent increase in the estimated own-price elasticity of demand for coverage, the elasticity with respect to work-group size being 1.06 ($z = 14.98$).

In demand for major medical insurance, the tobit regression should be and is superior to OLS because in a large fraction of the observations the dependent variable is clustered at the limit. The estimated regressions are considerably different. The income elasticity of demand for major medical maximum is 0.47 ($z = 0.97$), and the estimated elasticity with respect to wage rate is 1.67 ($z = 2.63$). Taken together, these suggest an extremely high income elasticity of demand for major medical insurance. Demand for major medical coverage is also quite sensitive to the price of medical care, with an elasticity of 1.77 ($z = 1.09$), an extremely large elasticity compared to other results found here even if precision is low. Demand for major medical coverage also rises with estimated illness, the elasticity being 1.01 ($z = 1.26$).

Taken together, these results suggest that persons facing high medical care prices, particularly those with high incomes, shift insurance coverage from basic medical care coverage (such as hospital or surgical insurance) into a major medical insurance plan. This accounts for the relatively low response of the basic hospital and surgical coverage parameters to medical care prices and the quite high response of major medical coverage. It should be recalled that these estimates are derived from data obtained for 1963, at which time less than 20 per cent of the population had major medical insurance. That ratio now exceeds 40 per cent, so these values may have changed considerably between 1963 and the present.

6. OBSERVED COINSURANCE RATES

The 1963 CHAS-NORC data also permit estimation of the observed coinsurance rates resulting from insurance policies held by the families, and from their actual medical purchases during the year. Unlike the insurance parameter equations presented above, these equations contain a considerably random component induced by variation in actual health outcomes during the year; hence, their precision is much lower than the previous estimates. The dependent variable takes on values from 0 to 1 inclusive, expressed as benefits/expenses = coverage rate. Observations with zero expenses in each category studied were deleted, since no data are available to compute a coverage rate for them. Table 5 shows maximum likelihood logistic regressions for coverage rates on total expense, hospital expense, and physician office expenses. The maximum likelihood estimator relates the dependent variable coverage to explanatory variables in a fashion analogous to normal regression, the major difference being that the error term in this maximum likelihood regression has a logistic distribution, rather than the usual normal distribution. The partial derivative is $\partial y/\partial X_i = \beta_i y \, (1-y)$ and the elasticity is $\eta_{yx_i} = \beta_i \cdot X_i \cdot (1-y_i)$.

For total expense (representing all medical outlays by the family), the average coverage rate in 1963 was 13 per cent. The equation was estimated in linear form and with quadratic terms for continuous variables. A chi-square test on the vector of quadratic terms is 24.83 (7 d.f.), rejecting the hypotheses that these coefficients are

TABLE 5 Observed Coverage Percentage (Logistic Regressions)

Explanatory Variables	All Medical Care Coefficient (z value)	All Medical Care Elasticity (z value)	Hospital Care[a] Coefficient (z value)	Hospital Care[a] Elasticity	Medical Office Visits Coefficient (z value)	Medical Office Visits Elasticity (z value)
Nonwage income	.796 E-04 (1.45)	.05 (1.30)	-.298 E-04 (1.11)	-.01	.6848 E-04 (.97)	.05 (.99)
Nonwage income squared	.1966 E-08 (.58)				-.1247 E-08 (.49)	
Wage/Week	.0181 (1.51)	.71 (1.76)	.00918 (1.66)	.31	.0254 (1.26)	.34 (.63)
Wage squared	.452 E-04 (1.01)		—		-.8464 E-04 (1.12)	
Work-group size	.5011 (4.02)	.58 (5.94)	.2532 (6.13)	.31	.6409 (3.54)	.64 (4.11)
Group size squared	-.0419 (3.06)		—		-.0563 (2.89)	
Medical price index (service-specific)	-10.24 (.56)	-1.58 (1.28)	-.840 (1.05)	-.20	.0347 (1.67)	.24 (2.08)
Price index squared	4.190 (.48)		—		-.2148 E-03 (2.08)	
Estimated illness level	1.376 (1.78)	.40 (.82)	-.3073 (1.15)	-.32	.1222 (.10)	.29 (.38)
Estimated illness squared	-.1682 (1.57)	—			-.0306 (.19)	

	(1)		(2)		(3)	
Education of head	.789 (2.58)	.09	.0400 (.37)	.05	.8974 (1.90)	−.33 (.61)
Education squared	−.0759 (2.71)		—		−.0868 (1.97)	
Age of head	−.4078 (2.06)	.04	−.0176 (.22)	−.02	.2067 (.64)	.13 (.39)
Age squared	.0427 (1.94)		—		−.0188 (.52)	
Race (nonwhite = 1)	−.164 (.62)		−.40 (.91)		−.0292 (.07)	
Sex (female = 1)	.186 (.68)		.160 (.39)		.008 (.02)	
Family size	.0865 (1.53)	.25	.0677 (.75)	.07	.1012 (1.23)	.33
Urban/Rural (rural = 1)	.0245 (.16)		−.109 (.44)		−.1088 (.50)	
Welfare care (= 1 if yes)	−.87 (1.80)	−1.48	−1.545 (2.63)	−.85	−.3645 (.56)	
Free care (= 1 if yes)	.28 (.85)		.108 (.20)		.3195 (.73)	
Constant term	−3.622 (.39)		−2.416 (1.60)		−9.000 (3.09)	
x^2 (d.f.)	107.30 (21)		75.948 (14)		54.217 (21)	
(probability)	(.00000)		(.00000)		(.00009)	
$E(y)$	.129		.717		.068	
# Observations	2328		489		1839	

[a]Non-quadratic equation given −X^2 test on quadratic coefficients is $X^2_7 = 7.88$ ($P \approx 0.4$). Hence, quadratic specification is rejected.

jointly zero; hence, the quadratic specification is presented. Three variables have effects significantly different from zero—the loading fee instrument (group size), with an elasticity at the mean of 0.58 ($z = 5.94$); receipt of welfare care, with an elasticity of -1.48 ($z = 1.80$); and wage income, with an elasticity of 0.71 ($z = 1.76$). The price of medical care had no apparent effect on demand for coverage, either in the linear or quadratic specifications. Nonwage income had an elasticity of 0.05 ($z = 1.30$), so the combined income elasticity is near 0.75. Age and education both show significant coefficients in the quadratic specification (but not the linear), but the combined effect of these variables in combination is not significant.

The coverage of hospital expenses is similar. Here, the quadratic terms are not significantly different from zero, so the linear specification is presented. The price of insurance is again the major predictor of demand, with an elasticity of 0.31 on the group-size variable ($z = 6.13$). The wage income elasticity is 0.31, under half that for total expense ($z = 1.66$), and receipt of welfare care has a negative effect ($\eta = -0.85$, $z = 2.63$). The price of hospital care had a negative but insignificant effect on demand for coverage ($\eta = -0.2$, $z = 1.05$), as is true for the expected illness variable.

In 1963 medical office visits were covered at a much lower rate than hospital care and surgical care, the average coverage being slightly under 7 per cent. However, as with hospital care, the major predictor both in terms of statistical precision and magnitude is the work-group size. This instrument for the loading fee of insurance has an elasticity of 0.64 ($z = 4.11$). This implies an own-price elasticity of demand for physician office coverage of about $-2/3$, quite elastic compared with estimates of demand for physician office care itself (Newhouse and Phelps, 1974; Phelps and Newhouse, 1974). The major difference between demand for physician office coverage and for hospital coverage is that the price of office care is positively and significantly related to demand for coverage. The elasticity is estimated to be 0.24 at the mean ($z = 2.08$). This difference between demand for physician office coverage and other types of care may well be related to the average existing coverage. As pointed out in the theoretical discussion earlier in this paper, the response of the demand for coverage to medical prices may well be nonlinear, and this presents some evidence that indeed the coverage is positively related to price of medical care when the coverage level was initially low. As coverage rises, as for example in the case of hospital care, the response to medical price may fall off.

How do these estimates compare with those using insurance policy parameters as dependent variables? In both sets of estimates, the primary predictor in terms of both explanatory power and magnitude is the price of insurance. Maximum payment parameters have an own-price elasticity of between -0.5 and -1.0, and the "coverage" types of parameter HOSMAX has an own-price elasticity of about -0.7. The coverage parameters obtained from the logistic estimates using expenditure and benefit data show own-price elasticities of about -0.4 for total medical expense, with smaller values for component expenditures (hospital, M.D. office, etc.). The value of -0.4 is about half that obtained from annual time series of aggregated benefits and expenditures (Phelps, 1973), although the mean loading fee in the time series is considerably lower than in the 1963 data used here, and the elasticity is a function of θ in the logistic specification of the dependent variable. From the time series estimates in Phelps (1973), the fitted own-price elasticity for 1963 for coverage was -0.26, considerably closer to the above estimate than the time series value taken at the mean. Similarly, the income elasticity at the mean from the time series estimate was 0.39, somewhat lower than the combined wage and nonwage elasticities taken from these results. The time series results on the effects of medical prices on demand for coverage are inconclusive, being highly sensitive to functional form employed. In the lowest mean-squared-error equation (Phelps, 1973, Table 18, LOGIT equation), the elasticity at the mean of coverage with respect to p_h was 0.83 ($z = 2.53$), suggesting a strong effect of medical prices on insurance demand. The value using 1963 levels of the explanatory variables is 0.79. This result differs considerably from the estimates found here—that medical prices have no measurable effect on insurance demand except for M.D. office coverage. The question can be raised, of course, concerning measurement error in the medical price variable used here, since it is fitted from a regression estimate of persons with positive use of medical care, and represents, in effect, the average price paid by persons in a given region and of specific socioeconomic grouping. Other medical price variables used in Phelps (1973) yield results similar to those found here, although those other variables are conceptually similar to the instrument used in this paper—they are regional averages, adjusted for income differences.

Fuchs and Kramer investigated demand for physician office care insurance using interstate aggregated data wherein the dependent variable is the absolute level of benefits (BEN). They found BEN to be highly related to income ($\eta = 0.76$ to 1.61) and also highly

TABLE 6 Summary Statistics—Insurance Policy Regressions

Variable	Mean	Standard Deviation
HOSMAX[a]	13.15	12.51
HOSDAY[b]	79.15	111.36
SURMAX[c]	203.26	242.15
MM-MAX[d]	2108.17	5709.57
Income	5897.19	3100.88
Education of head	5.16	1.67
Age of head	4.74	1.91
Medical price index	1.00	.09
Physician price index	1.06	.16
Hospital price index	.83	.18
Estimated illness	3.34	.752
Work-group size (scaled)	3.13	2.92
Free care	.068	.25
Welfare care	.059	.24
Nonwhite	.139	.34
Female head	.217	.41

[a] $n = 1522$
[b] $n = 1491$
[c] $n = 1493$
[d] $n = 1579$

own-price sensitive—on the order of -1.58 to -1.74. They also found benefits strongly negatively related to medical prices ($\eta = -0.74$, see their Table 18, Equation (D.4)). Since actual medical purchases also fall with medical prices ($\eta = -0.1$ to -0.3, tending around about -0.25), this means that coverage (BEN/EXPENSE) falls with medical prices as well, in contradiction to the large time series estimate in Phelps (1973) for total medical expenses, and to the smaller positive effect found here for M.D. office coverage. These conflicting results suggest that there still remains a considerable amount to be learned about the effects of medical prices on demand for insurance, and unfortunately, the theory provides little guidance in this matter.

Other researchers have estimated demand curves for insurance as well. M. Feldstein (1973) concluded that "a rise in the price of hospital services causes an increase in the proportion enrolled and in the total quantity of insurance." His estimated elasticity of "quantity" with respect to medical prices is 0.39, with a long-run

TABLE 7 Summary Statistics for Observed Coinsurance Regressions

Variable	Mean	Standard Deviation	Minimum	Maximum
Race (1 =nonwhite)	.134	.341	0	1
Age of head (scaled)	4.66	1.846	1	8
Education (scaled)	5.32	1.617	1	8
Sex of head (1=female)	.191	.393	0	1
Welfare care (1=yes)	.043	.204	0	1
Free care (1 −yes)	.0567	.231	0	1
Family size	3.33	1,892	1	16
Rural/Urban (rural=1)	.308	.462	0	1
Permanent income	6349.2	3047	−3795	16898
Wage income/week	116.16	37.97	−12.743	220.24
Work-group size (scaled)	3.802	3.048	1	8
Estimated illness level	3.411	.730	1.157	6.316
Nonwage income	758.42	2169	0	7000
Coverage percentage	.1278	.239	0	1
Medical prices (estimated)	1.00	.085	.767	2.382

Sample size: 2,328 families with positive medical expense (2,367 original)

For M.D. office visits, add the following:

M.D. office coverage percentage	.068	.200	0	1
M.D. office price index	7.210	7.208	.25	125.00

Sample size: 1,839 families with positive M.D. office expense

For hospitalizations, add the following:

Hospital coverage percentage	.717	.361	0	1
Hospital price index	.835	.160	.393	1.269

Sample size: 489 families with positive hospital expense

NOTE: For M.D. office and for hospital coverage percentage equations, summary statistics on independent variables differ slightly from those given for the sample of 2,328 families.

elasticity calculated to be 1.21. He also estimates an own-price effect on demand for insurance of −0.09 (and insignificant), although he estimates a strong positive relationship between an instrument for group insurance availability (percentage of employees in each state who work in manufacturing or government), and collinearity between this variable and his measure of

TABLE 8 Estimating Equations for Medical Price Variables

Variable	Medical Price Coefficient (*t* statistic)	Hospital Price Coefficient (*t* statistic)	Physician Price Coefficient (*t* statistic)
New England	−.1191	−.2621	−.0946
	(3.01)	(2.95)	(.48)
Mid-Atlantic	−.1143	−.2819	−.1265
	(4.53)	(4.93)	(1.16)
E. N. Central	−.1138	−.1642	−.2236
	(4.35)	(2.91)	(1.98)
W. N. Central	−.0595	−.2414	−.0800
	(1.92)	(3.68)	(.56)
S. Atlantic	−.0491	−.2573	.0258
	(1.76)	(4.17)	(.22)
E. S. Central	−.0636	−.3911	−.1588
	(1.69)	(4.40)	(.61)
W. S. Central	−.0573	−.1418	−.0580
	(1.81)	(2.06)	(.40)
Mountain	−.0644	−.0138	−.2022
	(1.43)	(.14)	(.96)
Wage income	.8274 E-03	.5911 E-03	−.8416 E-04
	(3.29)	(.98)	(.06)
Nonwage income	.1942 E-04	−.2823 E-05	−.3536 E-05
	(2.70)	(.16)	(.10)
Education of head	.07210	.0534	−.2523
	(3.08)	(.96)	(1.66)
Education squared	−.0056	.0040	.2267
	(2.46)	(.75)	(1.61)
M.D.'s/100,000	.7919 E-03	.00244	.00213
	(4.27)	(5.98)	(2.47)
Beds/1,000	.0013	.00918	−.00414
	(.34)	(1.21)	(.26)
Constant	.6717	.5650	1.5618
	(9.14)	(3.20)	(3.18)
R^2	.05	.17	.09
F (d.f.)	8.036 (14,222)	8.24 (14,556)	1.65 (14,229)
$E(y)$	1.00	.83	1.04

own-price may preclude precise estimation of either.[16] Given the conflicting results of my cross-section survey data studies, my aggregate time series studies, and the state cross-section studies of Feldstein, Frech, and Fuchs and Kramer, it is clear that much remains to be learned about demand for insurance, particularly about the effects of medical prices on demand. The question is of special significance because of possible supplementation of universal (if only partial) coverage that may be introduced under national health insurance. If supplementation is highly responsive to medical prices, then large demand shifts in the medical care system could be exacerbated by additional demand induced through purchase of supplemental insurance policies.

NOTES

1. It is easy to show that $h(l)$ is an increasing function of l—more illness heads for more medical care purchase—as long as the income elasticity of demand for health (H) is positive. See Phelps (1973) for proof.
2. The proof of this is in Phelps (1973).
3. It is not the case that $h(l) = \bar{h}$, the average medical care consumption in insured states.
4. In Ted Frech's comment, he points out that "moral hazard" (I interpret this to mean non-zero price elasticity) acts like a tax on the loading fee. This is true in one sense, but the analogy is not perfect. At least in formulations of an insurance premium that I have pursued, the "tax" of the non-zero elasticity applies only to a portion of a premium—that for insured states of the world under h^* (obviously), and that portion of demand that is added when C is lowered. Reducing C would increase the premium (i.e., R_c would be negative) even if η_{hC} were zero, since the insurer would pay a larger fraction of the bills. Notice also that the "tax" of the price elasticity is related to the level of insurance—it is highest when C approaches zero and when h^* is very large.
5. The optimality always holds in demand for h^* if the consumer is risk averse. That is, if (5) is zero, then the denominator of (8) is negative. However, in demand for C, the optimality is guaranteed for solutions of (4) equal to zero only if demand for h is perfectly price inelastic—the case considered by most previous analyses of insurance. When $\partial h/\partial C$ is negative, the denominator of (9) must be assumed to be negative, even if the consumer is risk averse.
6. It can be shown that R_{h^*} is not a function of income, with the insurance premium functions I consider below.
7. For notational simplicity, the dependence of λ and $r(I)$ on l is dropped here.
8. This has been observed in a multiple regression study of state market shares of the Blues; state income is positively and significantly related to market shares of Blue Cross and Blue Shield, *ceteris paribus*. (Phelps, unpublished paper.)
9. I make the simplifying assumption that

$$\frac{\partial^2 h}{\partial C\, \partial p_h} = 0$$

10. In Phelps (1973), the measure of price was derived from BLS statistics on expenditure for medical care in forty-six cities and rural areas. These data were used to construct a price index for each of the primary sampling units (PSU) from which the 2,367 families were drawn. The measure attributed the same regional price to each person living in a PSU, a measure that is considerably less person-specific than the regression estimation of price I use here.

11. If the person earns more than the base amount of the payroll (social security) tax, the appropriate marginal tax rate does not include the payroll tax rate. In 1963, the maximum earnings taxed by the payroll tax were $4,800.

12. The first equation estimated y = average marginal income tax rates. The equation estimate was $y = -0.61 + 0.09 \log (\text{income}) R^2 = 0.84, N = 19$ income
$$(t = 9.52)$$
groups. Data on income groups were obtained from IRS files. The second equation estimated used interval brackets reporting total marginal tax rates (income plus payroll), with the midpoint of income intervals used as the explanatory variable. The estimated equation was $y = -0.09 + 0.04 \times \log (\text{income}) R^2 = 0.46, N = 8$.

These data reflect 1970 incomes. Because the social security cutoff income in 1963 was lower, there may have been more progressiveness in 1963 than is indicated by the second estimate. For this reason, I use 0.05 as an estimate of $\partial \text{MTR}/\partial I/I$.

13. This problem is analogous to how a family behaves when faced with random medical expenses and is covered by an insurance policy with a deductible. For a discussion, see Keeler, Newhouse, and Phelps (1974).

14. See Mitchell and Phelps (1974) for details of this computation. In brief, the calculation is this: A relationship between loading fee and work-group size is derived from an insurance textbook. The data are then fitted with an OLS equation of the form $ln(\theta) = a_0 + a_1 ln \text{ (GROUPSIZE)}$. The estimated $\hat{a}_1$ was -0.998 ($t = 9.39$), which is $\partial \theta / \partial G \cdot G/\theta$. The inverse of this is the correction factor to convert group-size elasticities to loading fee for elasticities.

15. These coefficients were systematically lower and had smaller t ratios in the OLS regressions than in the tobit regressions presented here. In the four demand equations shown, none of the free-care or welfare-case coefficients were significant at usual significance levels in the OLS regressions, whereas the welfare coefficients are all significant at least at $p = 0.12$ and the free-care coefficients are significant in the hospital insurance demand equations with $p < 0.10$ in the tobit regression.

16. Goldstein and Pauly, in a paper presented at this conference, estimate a loading fee elasticity of -0.33, where the dependent variable is total premiums. Their data do now allow an estimate to be made of the effect of medical prices on insurance demand. Frech, in a comment on this paper, reports studies using aggregate state data, estimates an own-price elasticity for insurance very near zero, and an income elasticity of 0.17. He further reports an estimated effect of hospital prices on demand for insurance to be -0.38, quite in contrast to the figure derived by M. Feldstein using similar data. The dependent variable in Frech's work is the proportion of hospital expenses paid for by insurance, directly analogous to the hospital equation in my Table 5.

REFERENCES

1. Arrow, Kenneth J., "Uncertainty and the Welfare Economics of Health Care," *American Economic Review*, 53 (1963), pp. 941–973.

2. ———, "Optimal Insurance and Generalized Deductibles," R-1108-OEO, The Rand Corporation, February 1973a.

3. _____ , "Welfare Analysis of Changes in Health Coinsurance Rates," R-1281-OEO, The Rand Corporation, November 1973b.
4. Dickerson, O. D., *Health Insurance* (Homewood, Ill.: Richard D. Irwin, 1968).
5. Ehrlich, Isaac, and Gary S. Becker, "Market Insurance, Self-Insurance, and Self-Protection," *Journal of Political Economy*, 80 (July–August 1972), pp. 623–648.
6. Feldstein, Martin S., "Hospital Cost Inflation: A Study of Nonprofit Price Dynamics," *American Economic Review*, 61 (December 1971), pp. 853–872.
7. _____ , "The Welfare Loss of Excess Health Insurance," *Journal of Political Economy*, 81 (March–April 1973), pp. 251–280.
8. Fuchs, Victor R., and Marcia J. Kramer, *Determinants of Expenditures for Physicians' Services in the United States, 1948–68* (New York: National Bureau of Economic Research, 1972).
9. Keeler, Emmett J., Joseph P. Newhouse, and Charles F. Phelps, "Deductibles and Demand: The Theory of the Consumer Facing a Variable Price Schedule under Uncertainty," R-1514-OEO/NC, The Rand Corporation, 1974.
10. Mitchell, Bridger M., and Charles E. Phelps, "Employer-Paid Group Health Insurance and the Costs of Mandated National Coverage," R-1509-NC/OEO, The Rand Corporation, 1974. Forthcoming (1976) in *Journal of Political Economy*.
11. Mossin, Jan, "Aspects of Rational Insurance Purchasing," *Journal of Political Economy*, 76 (August 1968), pp. 553–568.
12. Newhouse, Joseph P., and Charles E. Phelps, "Price and Income Elasticities for Medical Care Services," R-1197-NC, The Rand Corporation, June 1974.
13. Phelps, Charles E., "The Demand for Health Insurance: A Theoretical and Empirical Investigation," R-1054-OEO, The Rand Corporation, 1973.
14. _____ , "Regulation of Non-Profit Health Insurers," unpublished manuscript.
15. _____ , and Joseph P. Newhouse, "Coinsurance, the Price of Time, and the Demand for Medical Services," *Review of Economics and Statistics*, 56 (August 1974), pp. 334–342.
16. Pratt, John W., "Risk Aversion in the Large and in the Small," *Econometrica*, 32 (January–April 1964), pp. 122–136.
17. Smith, Vernon, "Optimal Insurance Coverage," *Journal of Political Economy*, 76 (January–February 1968), pp. 68–77.
18. Tobin, James, "Estimation of Relationships for Limited Dependent Variables," *Econometrica*, 26 (1958), 24–36.

4 | COMMENTS

H. E. Frech III
University of California, Santa Barbara

This is a very interesting paper. It represents an attempt to properly formulate a model of demand for health insurance, making use of the fundamental insight from the Arrow-Pauly discussion of the 1960s that health insurance is characterized by moral hazard and is *not* merely an aggregation of contingent claims. This is an important enterprise because all insurance and many other financial contracts contain some sort of moral hazard. So the theory of moral hazard is important for the analysis of financial markets in general.

For policy purposes, it is important to know the relative extent of moral hazard (wherein more insurance increases the expected medical expenditure) versus adverse selection (wherein higher expected medical expenditures increase the extent of insurance). If adverse selection is relatively important, incomplete insurance and interpersonal variation in extent of insurance may reflect inefficient use of resources in trying to detect individual differences in risk and adjusting insurance contracts to minimize adverse selection. If so, a mandatory program of reasonably complete insurance for everyone may be efficient. It offers the hope of avoiding the resources spent in merely discovering individual differences in risk and adjusting contracts to such differences. Such private expenditures have a private return, but no social return. If moral hazard is relatively important, optimal insurance would be incomplete and vary a great deal on the basis of varying tastes for risk and, especially, varying elasticities of demand for the insured service (medical care).

Moral hazard works like a tax or extra loading charge on the insurance, which increases with the extent of insurance. Thus, it leads to the private choice of incomplete insurance, given the choice of various alternative insurance contracts. This private choice is socially optimal if (1) there is no alternative method of organizing the sale of insurance that will eliminate the moral hazard—the usual case—and (2) insurance is supplied competitively. Thus, moral hazard destroys the optimality of complete insurance, even if the insurance is priced at expected loss. A mandatory program of complete insurance will lead to inefficient moral hazard losses.

In the Phelps paper, moral hazard enters the model because of the form of the benefits—a subsidy for the purchase of medical care, not a simple contingent claim. This is clear in the budget constraint under insurance, his equation (2):

$$I = x + Cp_h h + R$$

Most of Phelps' results for insurance demand under moral hazard are quite reasonable. However, there is one result that seem a bit odd to me. The result would seem to hinge on the way in which the moral hazard welfare loss varies over the extent of insurance.

The result that concerns me is: The optimal limit h^* is finite if the insurance load is positively related to the size of the expected benefits. This result indicates that the marginal moral hazard loss is increasing in the extent of insurance.

The easy way to see this is to first imagine a situation in which the insurance is simply an aggregate contingent claim. In this case, the true price of deepening the coverage (raising the h^*) is simply the expected value of the loss plus some proportional load. The consumer will keep increasing h^* without limit as long as risk aversion does not fall as income decreases. This is the basis for the standard argument that the optimal insurance, in the presence of transactions costs, involves a deductible and otherwise full coverage—placing a floor on *ex post* income.

For Phelps' result, the rising real price of insurance as h^* increases must be ascribed to rising marginal moral hazard, since load is held constant or is falling. It seems clear that his model is characterized by a marginal moral hazard loss that begins at zero when there is no insurance and rises as insurance becomes more complete, finally choking off further insurance purchases at a finite upper limit.

This is counter to the views of such scholars as Mark Pauly and Martin Feldstein, who favor insurance with large deductibles and complete insurance for large losses. Furthermore, it is counter to the generally held notions about the nature of medical care. The usual view is that the elasticity of demand for relatively minor elective medical problems is large, in part because there are many reasonable ways of treating the conditions. For more serious problems, the technological possibilities are much more limited so that the ill effects of moral hazard are much reduced. Furthermore, for really large losses, the possibilities for more than usual treatment often involve experimental techniques. For these cases, a richer model than simple consumer choice of level of medical care may be useful.

In any case, the usual view is that marginal moral hazard *decreases* with increasing loss. If that view is correct, then Phelps' proof of the optimality of a finite insurance limit is no help. We are left with arguments about (1) the ability to use private and government charity as the size of loss increases and (2) a low marginal utility of wealth and/or medical care for consumers who have experienced heavy losses. The latter argument is made persuasively in Dick Zeckhauser's recent article on catastrophic insurance (1973).

As an aside, I might mention that Phelps' proof here is more general than he supposes. He states that the optimal h^* is finite only if part of the insurance load is proportional to the expected benefits. However, his proof turns on the sign of the partial derivative of the true price of insurance with respect to h^*. From his Equation (17) it is clear that his result holds if the loading, θ, is equal to zero. Thus, the optimal h^* would be finite even if insurance were available at actuarily fair rates.

In my own work, I have formulated a model of the interrelationships of health insurance regulation, health insurance markets, and health care markets that run roughly as follows. A major effect of health insurance regulation is to give nonprofit medical provider-controlled insurers (Blue Cross and Blue Shield) a competitive advantage over commercial insurers. Because of their legal status, these insurers cannot retain the monopoly rents that these regulatory advantages make possible. However, these nonprofit insurers can benefit the providers by raising the demand curve for medical services by offering only relatively complete insurance in the market. This overly complete (in terms of consumer preferences) insurance leads to increased demand for health services, as it is intended to.

In order to empirically examine the model, it is necessary to construct a model of the interactions of the insurance and medical care markets—otherwise alternative explanations (to the regulatory one) cannot be disputed. I have used state data for the year 1969, the last year for which complete data are available. The econometric model has five equations and is estimated by two-stage least squares. I will present some preliminary results that bear on Phelps' work. This is especially valuable, since econometric analyses so often are not robust over different data sets. And I basically corroborate his findings.

In this work, I have simply taken the average proportion paid by third-party payers as the measure of the extent of insurance. Also, my work is limited to hospital care. The demand equation determining the extent of insurance in my system is (standard errors in parentheses):

(1) $I = 0.518 - 0.0540 \text{ PRINS} + 0.00012 \text{ INC} - 0.0065 \text{ PHOS} + 0.404 \text{ BCMSR}$,
        $\quad\quad\quad\quad (0.404) \quad\quad\quad (0.00004) \quad\quad (0.0032) \quad\quad\quad (0.210)$

$n = 46$

where

$\quad\quad\quad\quad I$ = proportion of hospital expenses paid by insurers
$\quad\quad$ PRINS = price of insurance
$\quad\quad\quad$ INC = per capita disposable income
$\quad\quad$ PHOS = price of hospital care (endogenous)
$\quad$ BCMSR = Blue Cross market share (endogenous)

The coefficient of variation is not reported because it is meaningless in two-stage estimation.

Phelps found an income elasticity of demand for health insurance of about 0.23. In my equation, that elasticity is slightly lower, about 0.17. Furthermore, the standard error is less than half the estimated coefficient.

Turning to the estimated price elasticity of demand for insurance, the estimated elasticity in my data is very low, −0.004 when defined the same as Phelps' variable. Feldstein (1973) also found a very low price elasticity in his work, using somewhat similar data. Phelps finds a much higher price elasticity of −0.5. The reconciliation seems to lie in the high collinearity between income and price in state data. High income states have larger employment groups and thus lower insurance prices.

I find a strong negative influence of the price of hospital care on the extent of insurance, with an elasticity equal to about −0.38. This is the opposite of what Feldstein (1973) found. The standard error is less than half the estimate in absolute value. Phelps found essentially no effect when he entered the price of hospital care in a linear fashion, but a significant effect when he used a more flexible quadratic formulation. I tried that in my equation, but the squared term did not do well, in part because of collinearity problems.

Another variable that I tested was the expected illness, measured by the average hospital expenditures of the state. There was virtually no effect on insurance demand. My results, as do Phelps', clearly show that the adverse selection problem in health insurance is not terribly important. This finding makes the case for compulsory relatively complete health insurance a more difficult one to make. This may be the most important finding in all this work.

At this point I cannot fail to mention that the Blue Cross market share, holding constant market influences, tends to increase the extent of insurance held by consumers. This is consistent with the main argument of my work.

Phelps raised the question of how insurers price their product. He believes that load is roughly proportional to the amount of the expected benefits, but does not have the necessary data to examine the question. The question is of some interest since it will certainly affect consumer choice. Information on insurance pricing might also be useful in evaluating some of the differences between Blue Cross and commercial insurer behavior. My data allow me to directly investigate the matter. Following are regressions of per capita insurance load (LD, LDBC, LDC) on expected benefits (BEN, BENBC, BENC) for all insurers, Blue Cross insurers, and commercial insurers, respectively. The equations were estimated across states for 1969. In the overall regression, BCMSR is also entered to standardize for the lower load of Blue Cross firms. Both BCMSR and the benefit measures are treated as endogenous variables.

(2) $LD = 21.396 + 0.178 \text{ BEN} - 39.763 \text{ BCMSR}$ $n = 41$
          (3.434)   (0.076)   (9.414)

(3) $LDBC = -4.607 + 0.103 \text{ BENBC}$ $n = 41$
              (4.540)   (0.032)

(4) $LDC = 9.657 + 0.216 \text{ BENC}$ $n = 41$
             (4.590)   (0.072)

The results seem quite reasonable and bear out Phelps' hunches. Much of the loading charge is proportional to the expected benefits. In the case of Blue Cross insurance, for which selling expenses are low, the bulk of the loading charge seems to be proportional.[1] A more interesting study, for which I do not have adequate data, would examine the marginal load for large group insurance alone. One would expect very low marginal loads and great similarity between Blue Cross and the commercial insurers.

NOTES

1. Measurement error in the number of insureds would lead to an upward bias in the marginal load. Checking for this by running the regressions in terms of total load, rather than per capita, showed the problem to be nonexistent for Blue Cross insurance and of minor importance for commercial insurance. A more important problem, especially with commercial insurance, is the aggregation of insurance plans with great variation in selling cost, which shows up as load in my data.

REFERENCES

1. Feldstein, M. S., "The Welfare Loss of Excess Health Insurance," *Journal of Political Economy*, 81 (March–April 1973), pp. 251–281.
2. Zeckhauser, R. J., "Coverage for Catastrophic Illness," *Public Policy*, 21 (Spring 1973), pp. 149–172.

Lester B. Lave

Carnegie-Mellon University

The paper I am to discuss is a good one, displaying authoritative knowledge in economic theory, econometrics, and health care. It is entirely appropriate, if somewhat unfortunate, that the author should be gaining firsthand knowledge of the health care industry, as well as of the health care insurance industry, instead of being able to attend the conference. In our conversation yesterday, he assured me that his back problem was actually a way of gaining better information about his subject, for which he is to be commended.

The paper is actually two papers. There is a theoretical paper, which looks at how an individual maximizes utility when confronted with an insurance policy that has a fixed coinsurance rate and a maximum payment. There also is an empirical paper that looks in detail at a 1963 survey and attempts to isolate the price and income elasticities of medical care as well as a host of other effects.

It is unfortunate that the two papers are combined. In order to keep the size of the paper down, Phelps has had to skimp on the details in presenting both his theoretical and empirical results. This means that each of them is extremely difficult to understand. The other problem is that, frankly, the empirical part of the paper has little or nothing to do with the theoretical part. For example, insurance is regarded as compensating an individual for the financial penalty of illness in the theoretical part, yet the financial penalty of illness includes not only the payment to providers for medical care received, but also lost income stemming either from absence from work or permanent disability. Although the income in the model is a permanent income, there are still significant losses owing to disability or death; yet, the insurance that he considers in the empirical part of the paper is merely insurance to compensate for medical expenses. There is no provision for replacing lost income.

I find myself vaguely dissatisfied with the results of the theoretical analysis. Without being able to pinpoint exactly where the dissatisfaction arises, I would point out that some of the conclusions seem to contradict what I see in the world. For example, if an individual is very wealthy, relative to the risk that he bears, he will insure only if the tax incentives of insuring are greater than the loading on the insurance policy or if his individual probability of loss means that the insurance costs less than its actuarial value. Notice that there are in fact tax breaks that attend the purchase of medical insurance and also that almost all medical insurance policies are community rather than individual rated. It seems to me that these facts are central in any theoretical examination of the purchase of insurance.

The purpose of insurance is to mitigate the financial loss stemming from an untoward event. To what extent does an individual (or society) desire to isolate his wealth from the effects of illness? How far is society willing to go to ensure that no individual ever has to live with a correctable health problem? Only the most risk-averse individual would insure so that his wealth was completely independent of untoward events. However, insofar as society bears residual responsibility for mitigating the financial and other consequences of disaster, it might choose to increase the incentives to purchase insurance.

Aside from income redistribution effects, the purpose of health insurance is to remove any financial barrier that might deter an individual from having a correctable medical problem treated. Notice that there are a host of difficulties in determining which health states are "correctable," especially since treatment involves risk. More important, there is no way of rationing medical care so that it goes only to those people it can help. To get 100 people with correctable problems who would not currently seek care to seek it, one would have to lower access and other costs so much that perhaps 5,000 extra people would seek care. Nor is it obvious that iatrogenic disease would not harm more than 100 of the 5,000 people induced to seek care. Although it might be good political rhetoric to declare that no individual shall ever have to live with a correctable health state, it does not make good sense to attempt to implement such a platitude.

Some years ago, Robert Solow and John Kenneth Galbraith argued in the *Public Interest* about how competitive the economy was, the welfare implications of consumer sovereignty, and other matters. Although I thought the discussion was amusing, I was struck the day before yesterday while driving on the Bayshore Freeway by how well Janis Joplin had said it all—"Lord, I need a Mercedes Benz." How much medical care do we *need*? Unlike the Mercedes Benz, we presumably believe that medical care is necessity more than luxury. The theoretical models presented in the papers at this conference assume that medical care is efficacious and a matter for public concern. As Dr. Berg commented, some parts of medical care such as screening and asymptomatic check-ups are of doubtful value; it is equally doubtful that other types of medical care are efficacious on the margin. Would one extra office visit a year improve health? Thus, I wonder if, on the margin, medical care is not more palliation than cure. If so, the Grossman investment model that approaches medical care as restoring the health stock lost to disease (or as improving the health stock) is true on average, but not on the margin. On the margin, I equate Joplin's Mercedes Benz with medical care as being pure consumption. The analogy extends to the unintended harmful effects of each in the form of accidents and iatrogenic disease.

It behooves us to look not only at what people believe they need, but also at whether they are correctly informed. Medical care is perhaps the extreme case in which an individual's observations on the amount of care that he needs are shaped by the providers of that service. It seems to me that we are misleading ourselves and society by happily grinding away at complicated, maximum problems that are based on the assumption that medical care is highly efficacious on the margin. Before we collaborate in pushing expenditures to $200 billion per year, I think we must inquire about whether additional expenditures on medical care would be effective.

I have no quarrel with the empirical contributions of the various papers presented at this conference. Alas, it seems that policymakers are going to go ahead with some national health insurance plan whether medical care is efficacious or not. (My quarrel is with pumping more money into the current system, not with national health insurance per se.) The least that we can do for policymakers in these circumstances is to give them some estimates of the increased demand that the lower prices will call forth. Need I add that while we're giving them these positive results, we should continually warn them not to delude themselves that this additional expenditure on medical care is other than a U.S.-built Mercedes Benz.

PART TWO

Effects of Health Insurance on the Market for Health Services

5

JAN PAUL
ACTON
The Rand Corporation

Demand for Health Care among the Urban Poor, with Special Emphasis on the Role of Time

1. INTRODUCTION

This study examines the demand for medical services by type of provider with particular emphasis on the role of time as a determining factor. The demand for health and medical services has attracted considerable interest in recent years because of the dramatic increase in health expenditures and because of substantial cost inflation in that sector. Although the causes of this rise in demand and cost inflation are complex to analyze, there is reason to believe that the substantial spread of reimbursement insurance in the last twenty years has played a major role by reducing the out-of-pocket money price the consumer faces in buying medical care.[1] Health research is focusing more and more on the economic determinants

This report was sponsored by the New York City Health Services Administration and the U.S. Office of Economic Opportunity as R-1151-OEO/NYC. I would like to thank Y. Ben-Porath, D. DeTray, A. Ginsberg, M. Grossman, H. Luft, C. Morris, J. Newhouse, L. Orr, C. Phelps, R. Zeckhauser, and the two discussants for useful comments and suggestions at various stages of this work. The views expressed here are those of the author and not necessarily those of The Rand Corporation or its sponsors.

of this demand, explicitly including third-party expenses.[2] Surprisingly, there has been almost no discussion of alternative rationing mechanisms that might become effective if money prices continue to decrease in importance as a result of spreading third-party reimbursement. Since there is every reason to believe that money prices will continue to decline in relative importance because of (1) the secular trend in third-party coverage, (2) the rising opportunity cost of time, (3) increases in time required to receive care, and, perhaps most important, (4) the prospect of national health insurance, it is necessary to examine other factors that may control demand.

This paper suggests that travel time and waiting time may replace money prices as the chief determinant of demand.[3] First, a model of the demand for medical services is developed with time explicitly included as part of the price of the goods purchased. From the model we predict that the time-price elasticity of demand for medical services will exceed the money-price elasticity as out-of-pocket money prices decrease, and also that changes in time prices will have a greater effect on demand for free medical services than on the demand for non-free services. We can further predict a differential effect of earned and non-earned income on the demand for medical services. A rise in non-earned income increases the demand for medical services; the effect of a rise in earned income cannot be predicted because it produces both an income and a price effect (by raising the opportunity cost of time).

The data used to test the predictions of this model were taken from two household surveys conducted in New York City. The city is a particularly good laboratory to estimate the importance of time prices and possible behavior under national health insurance because of the long-standing availability of free ambulatory and inpatient care through municipal hospitals and clinics. Thus, we get some notion of the steady-state behavior of a population with free, governmentally sponsored care available. Demand equations are estimated for four types of medical care: public ambulatory, private ambulatory, public inpatient, and private inpatient. In addition to a number of controlling variables for health and sociodemographic status, the important explanatory variables include travel and waiting times for alternative sources of care, and earned and non-earned income. The results indicate that in low-income neighborhoods of New York City, time-price elasticities already exceed the money-price elasticity of demand for care.

The paper concludes with a number of implications for policy with regard to locating health facilities, queuing practices at ambulatory facilities, and the possibility of substituting income subsidies for subsidies for medical services.

2. CONSUMPTION MODEL OF THE DEMAND FOR MEDICAL SERVICES

Details of the model and its implications are described in Appendix 3;[4] the major predictions are summarized here. The model concentrates on the role of money prices, time prices, and earned and non-earned income in determining the demand for medical care. The empirical section concentrates on demand for care from public and private providers of ambulatory and inpatient care. For simplicity, the formal model is developed in terms of only one provider of services, but the implications for several providers can easily be drawn.

Assume that two goods enter the individual's utility function: medical services, m, and a composite, X, for all other goods and services. Assuming fixed proportions of money and time to consume m and X and the full income assumption, the model can be represented as follows:

Maximize

(1a) $\quad U = U(m,X)$

subject to

(1b) $\quad (p + wt)m + (q + ws)X \leq Y = y + wT$

where

$U =$ utility
$m =$ medical services
$X =$ all other goods and services
$p =$ out-of-pocket money price per unit of medical services
$t =$ own-time input per unit of medical services consumed
$q =$ money price per unit of X
$s =$ own-time input per unit of X
$w =$ earnings per hour
$Y =$ total (full) income
$y =$ non-earned income
$T =$ total amount of time available for market and own production of goods and services

First, notice that the consumption of medical services, m, does not affect the amount of time available for production, T.[5] Second, p is the out-of-pocket expenditure for a unit of medical services, incorporating any deductible and coinsurance rate the individual faces from insurance. It would be appealing to make these insurance parameters endogenous, but data limitations do not permit the estimation of demand for insurance along with the demand for services.[6] Third, the manner in which the goods produce utility is not specified. Some researchers have included "health" in the utility function and allowed health to be produced by combining medical services with other inputs.[7] Health enters because of a demand for the "healthy days" it will cause. The interested reader may consult Phelps (1972) or Grossman (1972a) for these alternative motivations of the demand for medical services. For present purposes, an understanding of this mechanism is not necessary. The simpler formulation used here yields most of the same predictions as the other specifications. Furthermore, the data do not allow us to estimate the manner in which medical services are translated into health.

Effects of a Change in Price

Assumptions sufficient to make money function as a price in determining the demand for medical services are also sufficient to make time function as a price.[8] Therefore, the first prediction derived from this model is that if medical services are a normal good, time will function as a price, producing negative own-time/price elasticities of demand and positive cross-time/price elasticities.

One of my chief interests in this study is the relative importance of money and time prices in determining the demand for medical services. If we let π equal the total price per unit of medical services (that is, $\pi = p + wt$), then the elasticity of demand for medical services with respect to money price is

$$(2a) \qquad \eta_{mp} = \frac{p}{\pi} \, \eta_{m\pi}$$

and the elasticity with respect to time price is[9]

$$(2b) \qquad \eta_{mt} = \frac{wt}{\pi} \, \eta_{m\pi}$$

That is, the elasticity with respect to one component of the price equals the elasticity with respect to the total price weighted by the share of the total price owing to that component. Comparing these two elasticities yields the second prediction from the formal model; namely, that

$$\eta_{mt} \gtreqless \eta_{mp}$$

as $wt \gtreqless p$. Clearly, as p falls to zero and wt does not, the time-price elasticity will exceed the money-price elasticity. In other words, as the out-of-pocket payment for a unit of medical services falls, because of either increasing insurance coverage or the availability of subsidized care, demand becomes relatively more sensitive to changes in time prices. Furthermore, this implies that the demand for free medical services should be more responsive to changes in time prices than demand for non-free services, because time is a greater proportion of total price at free than at non-free providers.

Effects of a Change in Income

Exogenous changes in income can arise either from a change in earnings per hour or from a change in non-earned income. The two effects are not, in general, equal. The assumptions that are suffi-cient to make money function as a price are also sufficient to mean that an increase in non-earned income will produce an increase in the demand for medical services. So the first prediction about income is that there will be a positive non-earned income elasticity of demand for normal goods.

The effects of a change in the wage rate cannot be determined *a priori* because of offsetting influences. An increase in earnings per hour produces an income effect, which acts to increase demand. It also raises the opportunity cost of time, which reduces demand for time-intensive activities. The net effect on the demand for medical services depends on the time intensity of the price of medical services relative to the time intensity of the price of all other goods and services. We can break the effects of a change in the wage rate, w, into an income effect and a substitution effect:

$$(3) \qquad \frac{\partial m}{\partial w} = (T - mt - Xs)\frac{\partial m}{\partial y} - \frac{\lambda s\,(q + ws)\,(p + wt) - \lambda t\,(q + ws)^2}{|D|}$$

where $|D|$ is a determinant of the matrix of coefficients from the maximization equations. The first term is an income effect and is, by assumption, positive. The second term is the substitution of m for X because of a change in w. We can establish that the substitution term is positive if and only if

(4)
$$\frac{ws}{(q + ws)} > \frac{wt}{(p + wt)}$$

that is, if the time price is a larger proportion of the total price for the composite good, X, than it is for medical services, m. The substitution effect is necessarily negative for free sources of medical care since the condition in Equation (4) will not be met as long as there is a non-zero monetary price for X; that is, an increase in the wage rate will always cause a substitution effect away from the free good. Of course, the net effect of a change in wages may still be to increase the demand for medical services if the income effect exceeds the substitution effect. Intuitively, however, the effect of a wage change on the demand for free medical services is primarily a price effect (and therefore is likely to be negative) and the effect of a wage change on the demand for non-free sources is primarily an income effect (and therefore is likely to be positive).

Predictions from Other Formal Models

The simplified consumption model is adequate to generate empirically verifiable hypotheses for the variables of primary interest in this study. The Grossman (1972a, 1972b) investment model provides additional predictions regarding the effects of education and age. Grossman enters health into the utility function and lets health be produced by combining medical and other inputs. He argues that if education raises health productivity (e.g., more highly educated persons are more skillful in combining medical inputs to produce health) and if the price elasticity of demand for health is less than 1, then when all other things are accounted for, he expects to find a negative relation between education and the amount of medical services demanded.[10]

The second implication of the Grossman formulation involves investment in health over the life cycle. If the price elasticity of demand for health is less than 1, then the effect of age on the demand for medical care is positive if the depreciation rate on health rises with age and is negative if it falls with age. In general, we may suspect that the depreciation rate increases over the life cycle, causing a positive effect of age on the consumption of medical care. However, the evidence presented below (and in

Acton, 1973) suggests that in poor populations, substantial depreciation in the health stock may be occurring early in life.

3. THE DATA BASE

In this section I discuss the source of the data used for estimation, the definition of the variables used for analysis, and the expected effect of these variables. The data used came from two household surveys conducted in 1968 by the National Opinion Research Center (NORC) for the Office of Economic Opportunity (OEO). The surveys were conducted in Brooklyn, New York, to establish baseline characteristics on the population before the Red Hook and Charles Drew (in Bedford-Stuyvesant/Crown Heights) Neighborhood Health centers were established. Both surveys were conducted on straight probability samples of the target population. (I will refer to them as Red Hook and Bedford-Crown.) In the completed survey, approximately 1,500 households, containing almost 5,000 individuals, had been interviewed in each study. The completion rates were 82 and 81 per cent for the two samples, respectively, and there is no evidence of bias in the incomplete interviews.[11]

An advantage in using survey data is that it provides much more detail about the variables of interest than the use of aggregate data. Consequently, it allows more precise estimates of the relationships. A weakness of survey data is that it relies chiefly on self-reporting by the individual for some of the most important variables (especially medical utilization and income). Since the actual amounts are usually under-reported, the coefficients may be biased. As long as the under-reporting (or over-reporting) is proportional, the elasticities will be unaffected.[12] Consequently, the empirical section concentrates on the elasticities of the important variables.

Selected Characteristics of the Red Hook Population

The Red Hook population contains about 25,000 persons. The racial breakdown is 26 per cent Puerto Rican, 43 per cent "other white," and 30 per cent black. It is a relatively stable neighborhood (77 per cent had lived in the Red Hook area for more than five years); average family size is 4.7 persons. The average income is $5,030 per year. In twenty per cent of the households at least one member was receiving welfare, and 23 per cent fell below the OEO poverty line. The mean age is 27.3 years and the mean educational level is 6.8 years in the full sample.

Approximately 33 per cent of the Red Hook population saw a physician in the outpatient department (OPD) of a municipal hospital or a free-standing clinic during the year, and 48 per cent saw a physician in his private office. The average number of visits for users of these physicians is 5.2 and 3.8 per year. In the preceding year, over 9 per cent of the survey population was hospitalized at least once, and, on the average, hospitalized persons spent 14.6 days in the hospital during the year. Almost 14 per cent of the population reported having at least one chronic health condition limiting activity. There is a strong negative correlation between number of chronic conditions and family income, with the under $3,000 individuals reporting five times as many chronic conditions as the over $7,000.

Selected Characteristics of the Bedford-Crown Population

The general characteristics of the Bedford-Crown survey are similar to the Red Hook population and can be summarized quickly. Bedford-Stuyvesant/Crown Heights is a predominantly black neighborhood. Blacks constitute 84 per cent of all residents, Puerto Ricans, 7 per cent, and "other white," 9 per cent. The mean income is $5,599. In Bedford-Crown, almost 20 per cent of the families fall below the OEO poverty line and in 24 per cent at least one member was receiving welfare. Average household size is 4.3 persons. Females head 41 per cent of the Bedford-Crown households; only 32 per cent of households were so headed in Red Hook. The mean age is 25.2 and educational level is 7.3 years in the full sample.

Although almost 15 per cent of respondents reported at least one chronic health condition that limited activity, medical utilization appears generally lower in Bedford-Crown than in Red Hook. Broken down by type of physician visit, 29 per cent saw a physician at the OPD of a municipal hospital or a clinic (5.0 visits per year), and 40 per cent saw a physician in his private office (3.9 visits). The hospitalization rate was similar to what it was in Red Hook. Less than 8 per cent of the population was hospitalized for an average of 15.3 days per person.[13]

Definition of Variables Used and Expected Effect

This subsection discusses the nature of the variables used for the empirical analysis and their expected effect on the demand for medical services. For reference, Appendix 1 lists the variables in alphabetical order and provides a brief definition and the mean values. The four dependent variables cover the volume of ambulatory and inpatient care. The number of physician visits in an OPD or clinic is OPDC and the number of private office visits is PRIV. Days of hospitalization in public (municipal) and private (voluntary or proprietary) hospitals are DAZPUB and DAZPRIV. The discussion here will focus on explanatory variables by type—time price, income, sociodemographic, and so forth—and the interpretation that may be given to them.

Price Variables

Although the surveys conducted by NORC provide us with both travel time and waiting time information, the respondents were not queried about the money prices paid for medical services. I will consider the bias the omitted money-price variables may cause in the estimation after discussing the time variables, but the problem is not severe since the appropriate monetary price for free care is zero anyway.

The questions about travel time and waiting time were similar in form. After determining the usual source of medical care (general practitioner, specialist, clinic, etc.) NORC asked: "How long does it usually take you to get there (the way you usually go)?" (The travel times used for this analysis are for a round trip.) In the Red Hook Survey NORC asked a similar question about usual waiting time. NORC then asked if there were a most trusted source of medical care, and if so, what it was (same options as usual source). Again, a waiting time question was posed in Red Hook. For analysis, it was necessary to associate these times for usual and trusted sources with the dependent variables OPDC and PRIV. This was accomplished by creating travel time variables, TOPDC and TPRIV, and two waiting time variables, ATOPDC and ATPRIV. The waiting time to usual source of care was used for creating the TOPDC variables if the usual source was an OPD or clinic; if it was not, and the trusted source was an OPD or clinic, then the travel time to a trusted source was used. Similarly, if the usual source was a private practitioner, then that time information was used to create TPRIV and ATPRIV. If the usual source was not a private practitioner, but the trusted source was, the trusted source information was used. When trusted and usual providers were of the same type, the time information for the usual source was used. When the above algorithm failed to assign a value to one or more of the time variables (typically because usual and trusted sources of care were both private and TOPDC and ATOPDC were therefore not available), the mean value for those who reported a time was used.[14]

Depending on the particular application of the results, the chief interest may be in the effect of the time variables themselves, or there may be more interest in the effect of the time variables multiplied by the opportunity cost of the unit of time. Each of the four time-price variables is multiplied by the earned income per minute for working persons to create four alternative time-price variables: CTOPDC, CATOPDC, CTPRIV, and CATPRIV. If the person is not working or there is no earned income reported for the family, 1 cent per minute is used as the value of time.[15]

The travel and waiting time data were reported in intervals. For purposes of estimation, I used interval midpoints. The highest value (recorded as an open interval) was calculated by smoothing a cumulative distribution function through the interval midpoints and estimating an intercept. The mean value for travel time to the sources of care generally requiring no out-of-pocket money expenditure, TOPDC, was 72.9 minutes in Red Hook and 64.0 minutes in Bedford-Crown. The corresponding mean travel time for private physician visits, TPRIV, which generally required a money payment, was 44.6 minutes for Red Hook and 48.8 for Bedford-Crown. The greater mean value for travel time to "free" sources of care provides preliminary evidence to support the theoretical model developed above; people seem to be substituting time payments for money payments in their demand for care. The mean waiting times from Red Hook are 59.1 minutes for ATOPDC and 73.7 minutes for ATPRIV. Although waiting time appears to be longer at private providers, the total time required to receive free care still exceeds that for non-free care.

The expected effect of the time variables should be clear from the theoretical development. TOPDC and ATOPDC are the own-time prices for OPDC and the cross-time prices for PRIV. They should have a negative effect on utilization at OPDC and a positive effect on PRIV. Similarly, TPRIV and ATPRIV are the own-time prices for PRIV and cross-time prices for OPDC and should act accordingly. The absence of money-price information acts to bias the estimated effect of time prices associated with non-free sources of care. If there is a negative correlation between money prices and time prices, then the absence of money prices in the regression will bias the coefficient on TPRIV upward. This will bias upward (toward zero) the effect of own-time price in the PRIV equation and bias downward the effect of cross-time prices in OPDC.

For a number of reasons, the demand for medical services may be more responsive to changes in travel time than to changes in waiting time. Travel frequently requires a monetary expense that varies with distance or time; distant facilities require a higher (and unobserved) financial payment. Waiting time does not entail this implicit monetary charge. Furthermore, all other things equal, it may be more pleasant to spend a given amount of time waiting than travelling. Both effects lead us to expect a greater elasticity of demand for travel time than for waiting time.

Income

Earned (EARN) and non-earned (NEARN) income were asked in the survey instrument by household. The mean earned income reported in Red Hook was \$4,110 and non-earned income was \$920 per year. The earned and non-earned incomes for Bedford-Crown were \$4,532 and \$1,067, respectively. The theoretical model showed an unambiguously positive non-earned income elasticity of demand for medical services. The model was developed with medical services as only one good. When there are four components for public and private ambulatory and inpatient care, some may act as inferior goods. In particular, there may be a negative income elasticity of demand for OPDC and DAZPUB. The elasticity with respect to earned income was indeterminate because an increase in earned income also increased the opportunity cost of time.

Relatively few problems were encountered in the income measures in this data file. The figures for earned and non-earned income apply to each member of the family. This differs from the procedure used to create the variables CTOPDC, CATOPDC, CTPRIV, and CATPRIV, wherein earned income was attributed only to working members of the family.[16]

Age

The age term is entered as AGE and AGE^2 to allow for nonlinearity in the demand for medical services. The Grossman (1972) formulation suggested a positive correlation between age and the depreciation rate on health. The nonlinear specification allows detection of variations in the depreciation rate through the life cycle. In particular, Acton (1973) suggested that the city's poor population may be experiencing significant depreciation early in life.

Insurance

The insurance information is coded in categories that are not mutually exclusive. For ambulatory care, I was forced to create a variable, NOAMB, taking the value 1 if the person unambiguously had no ambulatory coverage. In Red Hook, this meant he either had no insurance at all or Medicare without the doctor coverage and without private insurance. In Bedford-Crown, this meant only that there was no coverage at all. For inpatient care, two dummy variables, CAID and CARE, could be created to indicate if the person had Medicaid or Medicare. Ideally, I would have liked to have the specific deductible and coinsurance rates of the person faced at the margin, but this was totally beyond the available data.

NOAMB should have a positive sign in the equation for OPDC and a negative sign in the PRIV equation, if their effects are significant. If we assume that, all other things the same (such as out-of-pocket payment), people would prefer to be in a non-governmental hospital, then CAID and CARE should have a negative sign in the equation for DAZPUB and a positive sign in the DAZPRIV equation. Indeed, it is the popular impression in New York City that the availability of Medicare and Medicaid caused an exodus of patients from city municipal hospitals to the private and voluntary hospitals.

Health Status

Several measures of health status are available that seem to be equally effective in explaining use.[17] I chose CHRON, the number of chronic health conditions that limit activity, because it was available in both surveys. Other variables that could have been used in one data file or the other include number of days in bed last year; number of days in bed or indoors last year; and self-perceived health status (excellent, good, fair, poor). When I ran regressions with these alternative measures, they all appeared with the anticipated sign and were highly significant (t ratios on the coefficient in excess of 4) and the remaining coefficients were quite stable.

CHRON is expected to appear with a positive sign in all equations. Persons with chronic conditions are more likely to suffer losses to their health stock during the year, making (at least partial) replacement more likely.[18] This is the gross effect of a decrement in health status. It may be that sufficient decrements in health will have a significant income effect, causing a shift to less expensive forms of care. The chief influence of this income effect should be captured in the income coefficients (which is one reason why they will be entered nonlinearly). If a differential effect on health status persists, it will probably be reflected in a greater coefficient in the OPDC and DAZPUB equations than in the other two equations.

Hospitalization

Days of both public (DAZPUB) and private (DAZPRIV) hospital care were entered in the ambulatory equations to measure decrements in the health stock that occurred during the year. As such, they should act like the health status measures; the more days of hospitalization, the more likely the person is to consume ambulatory care.[19] This should produce positive coefficients on DAZPUB and DAZPRIV in both the OPDC and PRIV equations. In general, those who received public inpatient care should be more likely to consume public than private ambulatory care. Those who received private hospital care are more likely to consume private ambulatory care, other things being equal. At least two factors could lead to a positive coefficient on DAZPRIV in the OPDC equation. First, many people have insurance that covers inpatient care but not outpatient care (Medicare without Part B is an example).[20] These people may seek inpatient care in private hospitals and ambulatory care in public facilities. Second, there may be an income effect of a long hospitalization in a private facility that causes the person to shift to the public sector for his ambulatory care.

Education

The highest grade completed is coded in years (EDUC). If the hypothesis is correct that more highly educated persons are more efficient producers of health (along with appropriate price elasticities), then there should be a negative coefficient in all four equations. If, on the other hand, more highly educated persons prefer private rather than public providers, then we should have a negative coefficient in the OPDC and DAZPUB equations. The coefficient in the PRIV and DAZPRIV equations would then be biased toward zero because of the offsetting effects of the efficient effect and the preference.

Race

Two dummy variables, BLACK and PR (Puerto Rican), were created. Since many of the factors expected to affect demand are already entered (particularly, income and health status), the coefficients on these two variables should reflect differences owing to preferences for a particular type of provider or to discrimination faced by members of particular races.

Sex

A dummy variable, MALE, was created, taking the value 1 if male and zero otherwise. The expectation, based on the aggregate consumption by sex (and ignoring childbearing as the explanation), is that males will be less intensive users of the system. This may, however, reflect a higher opportunity cost of time that is not controlled for in aggregate data; the current test should shed some light on the partial effect of sex, given value of time. An interesting additional hypothesis to test with this data base is that once they become ill, men will tend to remain under care longer (in a public system that does not require a significant monetary payment at the margin) because they have let their health stock deteriorate more than women have. Thus, we may find a positive coefficient on MALE in DAZPUB.

Household Size

The final variable is household size (HSIZE). All other things being the same, larger households will have a lower income per capita, reducing the demand for care at non-free sources. On the other hand, taking a lifetime view of family decision making, the number of children is an object of choice, making total family income the relevant variable and causing HSIZE to be relatively insignificant.

4. ESTIMATION TECHNIQUES AND RESULTS

Before discussing the results of the estimation, let me comment on estimation techniques. Whenever a non-negligible proportion of the observations of the dependent variable takes on an extreme value (either high or low), the assumptions underlying ordinary least squares (OLS) regression break down. Intuitively, the reason is that OLS requires equal variance in the error terms associated with the dependent variable, regardless of the values of the independent variables. When the dependent variable is constrained (say, it must be greater than or equal to zero), then the variance is reduced near zero. Indeed, in this example, we can never consider negative values.

Such is the case in the estimation here; we never consider negative consumption of medical services. Furthermore, a large proportion of the population reports a zero consumption of any one particular type of service. This general problem was addressed by Tobin (1958), who developed a maximum likelihood estimator for such data (called the tobit estimator). The technique estimates an index from which the probability of a non zero purchase and the expected value of that purchase can be determined, given the explanatory variables. As the data approach the assumptions underlying OLS estimation, the tobit results approach OLS results.

In the theoretical model developed in Section 2, a general utility function was used. For purposes of estimation, I have deliberately not specified a particular utility function in order to put as few restrictions as possible on the results. Instead, I have entered important explanatory variables in linear and quadratic form. The system can be viewed as the first two terms of a Taylor expansion around whatever is the true model.

The results of the tobit estimation are given in tables 1 and 2. For reference, the OLS estimation results are presented in Appendix 2. For reasons just discussed, the tobit estimations receive all our attention. In general, the coefficients presented in tables 1 and 2 are very significant.[21] Furthermore, their signs and relative magnitudes lend support to the theoretical implication derived in Section 2. Since it is difficult to make a quick judgment of the net effect of variables entered in quadratic form, table 3 gives the elasticities of the expected value locus of the four dependent variables with respect to all quadratically estimated explanatory variables, calculated at the mean values.

The Time Variables

The effects of time can be measured either from table 1, in which travel and waiting times are multiplied by a measure of the opportunity cost of time, or from table 2, in which time is entered in natural units only. As shown in Appendix 3, the elasticity of demand with respect to time equals the elasticity with respect to

TABLE 1 · TOBIT Regression Results with Time Weighted by the Wage Rate (C · Time)

	Red Hook Dependent Variables								Bedford-Crown Dependent Variables							
	OPDC [Eq. (1)]		PRIV [Eq. (2)]		DAZPUB [Eq. (3)]		DAZPRIV [Eq. (4)]		OPDC [Eq. (5)]		PRIV [Eq. (6)]		DAZPUB [Eq. (7)]		DAZPRIV [Eq. (8)]	
Independent Variables	Coef.	t val.	Coef.	t val.	Coef.	t val.	Coef.	t val.	Coef.	t val.	Coef.	t val.	Coef.	t val.	Coef.	t val.
CHRON	3.79	12.56	1.88	8.74	17.66	4.10	11.58	10.86	5.32	15.06	3.18	11.79	16.07	5.78	10.76	6.27
EDUC	-.262	4.58	-.0164	.43	1.85	1.63	.441	1.81	-.167	2.41	.121	2.49	-.603	.85	1.29	3.20
MALE	-.705	1.89	-1.79	7.25	5.24	.70	-1.32	.81	-2.06	4.86	-1.87	6.06	2.88	.66	-8.28	3.19
PR	3.72	7.76	-1.29	4.01	8.53	.85	-.735	.35	4.20	3.81	-4.26	5.58	16.46	1.27	9.08	1.51
BLACK	3.66	8.29	-1.27	4.38	3.73	.41	-6.20	3.08	3.96	4.73	-3.29	6.75	22.52	2.14	3.08	.65
HSIZE	-.369	3.71	-.489	7.30	-.863	.43	-1.31	2.88	-.182	1.60	-.194	2.30	.264	.25	-.800	1.16
AGE	.048	1.19	.039	1.41	.810	.90	.484	2.46	.0053	.10	.0340	.90	1.92	3.02	.632	1.80
AGE2 ×10⁻³	-.679	1.30	-.608	1.71	-9.78	.76	-6.45	2.27	-.595	.85	-.207	.41	-25.99	2.69	-8.77	1.69
CTOPDC	-.921	1.70	.905	2.23	29.16	2.85	.176	.07	-.895	2.65	-.0171	.07	-8.24	2.17	-4.34	2.10
CTOPDC2	.0139	.25	-.0698	1.85	-1.76	1.71	-.0458	.17	.0722	2.99	-.0074	.38	.930	3.39	.126	.78
CATOPDC	-2.46	3.34	-.515	.97	-46.0	3.40	-2.92	.81								
CATOPDC2	.296	3.31	.0562	.93	4.98	2.77	.349	.80								
CTPRIV	1.159	3.65	-.0174	.09	10.73	1.12	1.20	.92	.286	1.02	-.147	1.08	10.82	1.41	3.00	1.56
CTPRIV2	-.0374	1.87	.0154	1.38	-1.40	.94	-.0304	.37	-.0154	1.03	.0051	1.37	-2.85	1.65	-.154	1.14
CATPRIV	.743	1.86	-.481	2.48	-10.64	1.66	-2.96	2.24								
CATPRIV2	-.0626	1.55	.0186	1.35	.408	.87	.204	2.26								
NOAMB	-1.19	2.60	-1.28	4.25					-.416	.83	.0324	.09				
EARN ×10⁻³	.236	1.82	.0813	1.19	2.24	.72	.990	1.80	.0020	.02	.282	3.83	.795	.64	.765	1.24
EARN2 ×10⁻⁷	-.312	2.96	.0262	.61	-3.24	1.01	-.610	1.43	.0213	.52	-.0784	2.32	-1.39	1.72	-.0663	.27
NEARN ×10⁻³	.248	.82	.289	1.40	7.87	1.03	-.667	.50	2.21	6.50	-.824	3.22	.135	.04	4.02	1.88
NEARN2 ×10⁻⁷	.0278	.05	-.0922	.24	-17.56	1.05	3.55	1.57	-3.20	5.19	.547	1.18	.343	.06	-5.96	1.53
DAZPUB	.110	3.18	-.0701	2.08					.131	4.47	.0120	.45				
DAZPRIV	.221	9.14	.0438	2.37					.199	6.54	.124	5.12				
CARE					15.17	.68	11.48	2.32					.839	.05	11.65	1.35
CAID					9.08	.93	8.67	4.09					15.53	2.95	9.17	2.74
CONST	-4.33	5.60	1.13	2.24	-189.76	10.63	-48.71	13.62	-9.30	8.38	-1.31	1.75	-147.98	10.87	-84.65	12.67
Prob. Y>limit |X = X̄	.2803		.4144		.0128		.0684		.2686		.3369		.0227		.0512	
Chi²	724		347		68		258		562		485		117		143	
(d.f.)	(23)		(23)		(22)		(22)		(19)		(19)		(18)		(18)	

TABLE 2. TOBIT Regression Results with Time Entered

| | Red Hook Dependent Variables | | | | | | | | Bedford-Crown Dependent Variables | | | | | | | |
| Independent Variables | OPDC [Eq. (9)] | | PRIV [Eq. (10)] | | DAZPUB [Eq. (11)] | | DAZPRIV [Eq. (12)] | | OPDC [Ec. (13)] | | PRIV [Eq. (14)] | | DAZPUB [Eq. (15)] | | DAZPRIV [Eq. (16)] | |
	Coef.	t val.	Coef.	t val.	Coef.	t val.	Coef.	t val.	Coef.	t val.	Coef.	t val.	Coef.	t val.	Coef.	t val.
CHRON	3.84	12.90	1.87	8.82	16.92	3.94	11.55	10.87	5.43	15.20	3.28	12.26	16.75	5.97	10.79	6.27
EDUC	-.262	4.60	-.028	.764	2.05	1.82	.428	1.77	-.154	2.23	.0940	1.96	-.599	.84	1.22	3.01
MALE	-1.33	3.72	-1.57	6.67	.921	.13	-2.33	1.48	-2.19	5.24	-1.91	6.30	1.26	.30	-9.34	3.65
PR	3.44	6.93	-.992	3.03	-1.99	.20	-3.38	1.53	3.92	3.56	-4.06	5.34	14.60	1.12	9.46	1.57
BLACK	3.55	7.88	-1.28	4.42	-5.19	.56	-7.65	3.74	3.51	4.18	-2.69	5.54	20.63	1.95	4.76	1.07
HSIZE	-.287	2.94	-.503	7.70	.274	.14	-1.09	2.44	-.132	1.17	-.188	2.27	.521	.49	-.646	.95
AGE	-.005	.12	.043	1.63	.376	.43	.381	1.98	-.0148	.29	.0284	.79	1.79	2.84	.533	1.55
AGE2 $\times 10^{-2}$	-.017	.33	-.059	1.73	-.571	.46	-.548	1.96	-.0360	.52	-.0145	.30	-2.47	2.55	-.778	1.52
TOPDC	-.197	9.34	.108	5.95	.485	.96	.184	1.62	-.201	6.69	.190	6.49	-.889	3.35	-.200	1.04
TOPDC2 $\times 10^{-3}$	.817	9.50	-.447	6.02	-.690	.36	-.738	1.62	1.10	7.26	-1.07	7.02	4.53	3.41	.859	.88
ATOPDC	-.201	5.01	.052	1.59	-1.69	2.25	-.263	1.31								
ATOPDC2 $\times 10^{-2}$	.160	4.93	-.059	2.19	1.53	2.63	.265	1.67								
TOPRIV $\times 10^{-2}$	.065	4.10	-.067	6.89	.135	.41	.148	2.21	.0439	2.57	-.090	7.32	.264	1.38	-.225	2.28
TOPRIV2 $\times 10^{-3}$	-.239	2.62	.443	7.71	.286	.16	-.620	1.60	-.302	2.93	.538	7.96	-1.77	1.54	1.64	3.11
ATPRIV	.029	1.19	-.156	10.47	.438	.89	-.279	2.80								
ATPRIV2 $\times 10^{-2}$	-.009	.55	.104	10.15	-.337	1.01	.198	2.90								
NOAMB	-.859	1.88	-1.42	4.78	-1.89	1.12	.316	.72	-.556	1.31	.257	.74				
EARN $\times 10^{-3}$	-.045	.40	.110	1.95	1.08	1.48	-.229	.84	-.131	1.50	.253	4.14	-.687	.52	.173	.32
EARN2 $\times 10^{-7}$	-.139	1.64	-.009	.29	6.42	.87	-.894	.67	.0842	2.52	-.084	3.23	-.352	.36	-.0252	.12
NEARN $\times 10^{-3}$	.210	.70	.289	1.42	-1.38	.87	.377	1.68	2.07	6.03	-.707	2.78	-.543	.16	3.76	1.75
NEARN2 $\times 10^{-4}$	.024	.45	.024	.66					-.300	4.85	.0266	.58	.0910	.16	-.608	1.55
DAZPUB	.083	2.42	-.041	1.24					.127	4.38	.0113	.43				
DAZPRIV	.226	9.50	.043	2.38					.202	6.69	.122	5.09				
CARE					16.32	.74	12.33	2.50					1.55	.09	12.88	1.49
CAID					9.06	.94	8.62	4.05					15.53	2.90	8.93	2.65
CONST	7.00	3.88	1.16	.88	-190.99	4.97	-49.31	5.74	-2.40	1.32	-6.73	4.39	-115.63	6.16	-70.59	6.27
Prob. Y>limit $|X=\bar{X}$	.2472		.3533		.0095		.0741		.5396		.3275		.0337		.0404	
Chi²	954		679		84		266		6.8		608		113		148	
(d.f.)	(23)		(23)		(22)		(22)		(19)		(19)		(18)		(18)	

TABLE 3 Elasticities of Expected Value of Dependent Variable, Evaluated at the Mean[a]

Independent Variables	Red Hook Dependent Variables								Bedford-Crown Dependent Variables							
	OPDC		PRIV		DAZPUB		DAZPRIV		OPDC		PRIV		DAZPUB		DAZPRIV	
	[Eq. (1)]	t val.	[Eq. (2)]	t val.	[Eq. (3)]	t val.	[Eq. (4)]	t val.	[Eq. (5)]	t val.	[Eq. (6)]	t val.	[Eq. (7)]	t val.	[Eq. (8)]	t val.
CTOPDC	-.199	2.14	.185	2.26	1.427	3.14	.005	.02	-.162	2.43	-.011	.22	-.445	1.73	-.410	2.39
CATOPDC	-.327	3.18	-.083	.94	-1.663	3.41	-.186	.77								
CTPRIV	.153	3.78	.002	.06	.302	1.10	.077	.97	.047	.99	-.030	1.04	.246	.86	.214	1.60
CATPRIV	.126	1.85	-.110	2.64	-.550	1.76	-.252	2.14								
EARN	-.014	.30	.078	2.37	-.073	.28	.152	1.60	.015	.29	.172	4.10	-.111	.56	.210	1.57
NEARN	.037	1.16	.046	1.84	.177	.93	-.001	.01	.251	6.60	-.136	4.06	.012	.09	.193	1.90
AGE	.049	.74	.028	.55	.312	.87	.273	1.97	-.096	1.20	.107	1.67	.821	2.98	.315	1.56

Independent Variables	Red Hook Dependent Variables								Bedford-Crown Dependent Variables							
	OPDC		PRIV		DAZPUB		DAZPRIV		OPDC		PRIV		DAZPUB		DAZPRIV	
	[Eq. (9)]	t val.	[Eq. (10)]	t val.	[Eq. (11)]	t val.	[Eq. (12)]	t val.	[Eq. (13)]	t val.	[Eq. (14)]	t val.	[Eq. (15)]	t val.	[Eq. (16)]	t val.
TOPDC	-.958	8.08	.640	5.14	1.241	1.64	.415	1.45	-.619	4.56	.629	4.16	-.994	2.65	-.394	1.06
ATOPDC	-.120	1.12	-.202	1.82	.301	.61	.224	.91								
TPRIV	.332	5.08	-.252	5.28	.316	.87	.310	2.55	.137	1.83	-.337	5.82	.224	.93	-.216	1.25
ATPRIV	.196	2.73	-.050	.94	-.193	.48	.070	.53								
EARN	-.110	2.54	.086	2.73	-.182	.82	.039	.47	-.040	.86	.147	4.08	-.229	1.39	.046	.38
NEARN	.039	1.16	.046	1.68	.158	.79	-.014	.20	.244	6.13	-.128	3.75	-.019	.15	.180	1.69
AGE	-.064	.95	.057	1.07	.077	.21	.166	1.26	-.133	1.65	.098	1.47	.695	2.74	.243	1.20

[a] The t values test the significance of the above at the mean.

time weighted by the opportunity cost of time. There are likely to be biases in each set of coefficients such that the true elasticities with respect to time prices are greater in absolute value than those estimated. Consider first the specification with time weighted by the opportunity cost of time (table 1). Since the opportunity cost of time had to be imputed to nonworking persons and is not entirely precise even for working persons, the wage rate is measured with error. This error will bias the coefficients on the time variables in table 1 toward zero. Thus, the true elasticities will be greater (in absolute value) than those implied by the first specification. Consider the alternative specification employing time in natural units (table 2). In light of the model developed in Appendix 3, $w \cdot t$ is the correct variable, so that regressions employing t alone constitute an omitted variable bias. If w and t are negatively correlated (as seems reasonable), the coefficients estimated in Table 2 will also be biased toward zero.[22] In general, the elasticities implied by the coefficients in table 2 exceed in absolute value those implied by table 1, suggesting that the bias resulting from the error in measuring the opportunity cost of time is greater than the bias caused by omitting it from the specification. I shall discuss both specifications; almost all the remaining coefficients are quite stable between tables 1 and 2. The chief exceptions are the income coefficients—which are discussed in the next subsection—but even so, their elasticities are reasonably stable. The other apparent instabilities (PR and BLACK in the DAZPUB equations) reflect coefficients that were not significantly different from zero in either specification. Since both sets of estimated elasticities understate the true elasticity, I will concentrate on the generally larger ones implied by table 2.

Let us first concentrate on the travel time-price elasticities for ambulatory care using time in natural units. The elasticities are given in table 4. In this table we find support for many of the hypotheses generated in Section 2. Travel time is indeed functioning as a normal price, producing negative own-time/price elasticities and positive cross-time/price elasticities. Furthermore, the magnitude of the own-time/price elasticities exceeds that of own-money/price elasticities reported by other researchers. Using disaggregated data from several sources, Phelps and Newhouse (1973) derive money-price elasticities for private care on the order of −0.15 in the range of 25 per cent to 0 per cent coinsurance—well below (in absolute value) the −0.25 to −0.337 estimated here for private care and −0.6 to −1.0 estimated for public care. Even using the much higher elasticities for all ambulatory care of between −0.5

TABLE 4   Travel Time-Price Elasticities for Ambulatory Care [equations (9), (10), (13), and (14)]

| | Red Hook | | Bedford-Crown | |
	TOPDC	TPRIV	TOPDC	TPRIV
OPDC	−.958	.332	−.619	.137
PRIV	.640	−.252	.629	−.337

and −1.0 reported by Rosett and Huang (1971), Feldstein (1971), and Davis and Russell (1972), the travel-time elasticities appear to be of at least a comparable size.

The hypotheses developed above also suggested that demand should be more responsive to changes in TOPDC than to changes in TPRIV—which is the case. In both Red Hook and Bedford-Crown, the own-travel time-price elasticities with respect to TOPDC exceed those for TPRIV by a factor of two or three times. Similarly, the cross elasticities for TOPDC are significantly greater than those for TPRIV. The elasticities calculated for the C·TIME variables support the conclusions drawn for the TIME variables above. Found in table 3 are negative own-price elasticities, positive cross-price elasticities, and larger responses to CTOPDC and CTPRIV. The one exception is Equation (6), in which there is a negative cross-time/price elasticity of demand for PRIV with respect to CTOPDC.

The effect of waiting time is similar to travel time as a determinant of demand. But, as predicted, the elasticities with respect to waiting time are smaller (in absolute value) than the elasticities with respect to travel time. The own-waiting time-price elasticities of demand for OPDC and PRIV are −0.120 for ATOPDC and −0.050 for ATPRIV. The cross elasticities are 0.196 for ATPRIV and −0.202 for ATOPDC. The last figure, giving a negative cross-price elasticity of demand for PRIV with respect to ATOPDC, is the only violation of the theoretical implications developed above.[23] Otherwise, waiting time also functions as a normal price, with demand being more responsive to changes in waiting time at OPD's and clinics than it is to waiting times at private physicians' offices.

We can draw some limited inferences about the effect of time prices on the demand for inpatient care. We do not have a direct measure of the time prices associated with hospitalization. The effects of travel and waiting times for outpatient care should be interpreted primarily as cross prices to inpatient care—the more time one must spend getting ambulatory care, the more likely one should be to demand inpatient care. To a limited degree, we may wish to consider TOPDC as a measure of travel time to public hospitals—the DAZPUB variable—because all municipal OPD's are located in a hospital. In Red Hook equations (3), (4), (11), and (12), inpatient and outpatient care seem to be operating as substitutes. The longer one must wait for ambulatory care, the more likely one is to use inpatient care. The opposite appears to be true in Bedford-Crown. It is not clear why this difference exists at this level of analysis, but it may be compatible with the hypothesis that residents of Bedford-Crown are seeking care only for the more serious health conditions, and in those cases, inpatient and outpatient care are complements.[24]

Income

The theoretical model predicted that the elasticity of demand for all forms of medical services with respect to non-earned income should be positive unless public care is an inferior good, in which case the elasticity is negative in OPDC and DAZPUB. The sign of the elasticity with respect to earned income was indeterminate because of offsetting effects of income and the time price, although I suggested that it should be lower for free sources than for non-free sources of care. Broadly speaking, the empirical results in table 3 support these hypotheses. With few exceptions, a positive elasticity with respect to non-earned income was found in all equations. With respect to earned income, a generally positive elasticity was found for private care and a negative elasticity for public care. There is little evidence to support the hypothesis that public care is an inferior good (that is, that the elasticity of demand for OPDC and DAZPUB with respect to NEARN is negative). Although the signs of the income elasticities are reasonably stable between Red Hook and Bedford-Crown, the size varies and the whole set of findings must be regarded as provisional.

A word on alternative specification of the equations is in order. Instead of using earned and non-earned income as explanatory variables, I also estimated the entire set of equations using only total income—entered as income and income squared.[25] This alternative specification was used because I thought there might be a high degree of collinearity between EARN and NEARN and the waiting and travel time variables, especially when they were weighted by earned income. This alternative specification left the remaining coefficients virtually unchanged (to the third decimal place) and the significance of INC and INC2 was roughly the same as either EARN and EARN2 or NEARN and NEARN2. The other point worth mentioning about alternative specifications is the effect of the C·TIME versus the TIME variables on the income elasticities. Although the EARN elasticities vary somewhat, the elasticities with respect to NEARN are identical in the two specifications.

In Red Hook, there is substantial support for the hypothesis that medical services are normal goods, producing an elasticity of demand with respect to non-earned income of about 0.04 or 0.05 for ambulatory care and 0.16 for inpatient care.[26] The elasticities with respect to earned income are positive for private sources of care and negative for public sources, supporting the suggestion that they should be smaller for the free sources of care because a change in the wage rate has a greater price effect in demand for free care. In net, the price effect of a wage change dominates in the demand for public care and the income effect dominates in the demand for private care.

The Bedford-Crown results produce elasticities somewhat less in conformity with the predictions of the model and there are two sign reversals of corresponding elasticities between the C·TIME and TIME specifications. I will discuss only aberrations from the picture just described for Red Hook. In equations (6) and (14), there is a negative non-earned income elasticity of demand for private physician care that appears robust, suggesting that public care is a normal good and private ambulatory care is an inferior good. When I discuss the effects of race on demand for care, there is some suggestion of discrimination, and part of the effect may appear here. The two sign reversals occur for earned income in equations (5) and (13) and for non-earned income in equations (7) and (15). The latter may be explained by the critical point lying near the mean of the data, but the former is not so easily accounted for.

Otherwise, the general pattern of effects of income on demand for care that was reported in Red Hook holds in Bedford-Crown. The only support in either set of regressions for the hypothesis that public care is an inferior good is in Equation (15), in which the non-earned income elasticity of demand for DAZPUB is −0.019.[27]

From the estimated elasticities with respect to non-earned income we can calculate the approximate magnitude of the full wealth elasticity. The full wealth elasticity equals the non-earned income elasticity multiplied by the increase of the share of full wealth attributable to non-earned income.[28] Let full earned income (wT) be the earning of a person employed full time and assume that all employed persons are working full time.[29] Then the implied full wealth elasticity of demand is 0.202 for OPDC and 0.251 for private care in Red Hook.[30]

In discussing the remaining effects, I will concentrate on the specification with the time variables in natural units, equations (9)–(16).

Age

The human capital formulation predicts a positive correlation of the demand for care and rate of depreciation on the health stock (if the price elasticity of demand for health is less than 1). We can infer where in the life cycle depreciation is greatest by examining the age coefficients. The age curve is either monotonically decreasing (equations (9) and (13)) or is an inverted U shape (equations (10), (11), (12), (15), and (16) all peak between thirty-two and thirty-six years). Both patterns support the conclusion that there are substantial decrements in health early in life for these populations. The only curve that is monotonically rising is the demand for private physician care in Bedford-Crown (equation (14)), and its coefficients are not significantly different from zero.

Insurance

The greatest effect of insurance is seen in the demand for hospital care. In all cases, the estimated coefficients are positive, although the coefficients in the DAZPUB equations (equations (3), (7), (11), and (15)) are not statistically significantly different from zero in general. The significant effects support the popular image that Medicare and Medicaid caused an increase in the demand for private hospitalization. We cannot conclude, however, that this lowers demand for public hospital care (which should have produced significant negative coefficients in the DAZPUB equations). The picture with respect to insurance for ambulatory care is less certain, no doubt because of the imprecise definition of the explanatory variable NOAMB. The only statistically significant results (at 5 per cent or lower, equations (2) and (10)) show people with no ambulatory insurance demanding less care from private physicians.

Hospitalization

By and large, people who reported being hospitalized were likely to be users of ambulatory facilities. As suggested, people who reported public hospitalization were more likely to use public ambulatory care than private ambulatory care (the coefficients for DAZPUB in the PRIV equations (2), (6), (10), and (14) were either negative or not significantly different from zero). Those who reported private hospitalization were significantly more likely to use both public and private ambulatory care.

Health Status

The health status variables are the most consistently significant predictors of demand for care. Greater numbers of chronic health conditions produce higher utilization of all forms of medical services (with t ratios ranging from 4 to over 16). We suggested that poorer health stock might produce an income effect, causing greater demand for free than for non-free care from those with chronic conditions. The evidence is consistent with this hypothesis.[31]

Education

It was postulated that if educated persons were more efficient producers of health and the price elasticity of health is less than 1, then the coefficient on education would be negative. On the other hand, those with higher education might have developed a taste for more health services, particularly non-free services. The two effects together should yield a negative coefficient on EDUC in the OPDC and DAZPUB equations and coefficients biased upward in PRIV and DAZPRIV. This pattern is found in the estimated demand for ambulatory care. There is a significant negative coefficient on education in the demand for OPDC and clinic services. The mixed effect of efficiency and taste is shown by coefficients biased upward in equations (2), (6), (10), and (14). In the demand for inpatient care, education has a positive effect in all but one case, when its t value is 0.84.

Race

Generally, the coefficients on the race variables are very significant for ambulatory care but not significant for inpatient care. The relations are compatible with an interpretation that blacks and Puerto Ricans either have an aversion to private care or that they face discrimination in private ambulatory care. There are significant negative coefficients on both BLACK and PR in the PRIV equations and significant positive coefficients in OPDC. There is a definite substitution of public for private care, all other things held constant. The coefficients in the hospital equations are less significant, but when their t value exceeds 1.96 they support the conclusion of substituting public for private care.

Sex

Gross consumption figures lead us to expect a negative coefficient on the dummy variable for MALE in all demand equations. The possible exception would be a positive (or at least greater) coefficient in the DAZPUB equation if men had let their health stock deteriorate more and thus, once hospitalized, would be confined longer. These two expectations are supported in all the estimated relations, although the positive coefficient in the DAZPUB equations is not significantly different from zero.

Household Size

Finally, all other things held the same, HSIZE should produce a negative coefficient in paid sources of care. For reasons that are not entirely clear, there is also frequently a negative coefficient on HSIZE in the public sources of care. It may be that the larger family size is increasing the opportunity cost of everyone's time (especially that of the parents) and thus reducing all use of services.

5. CONCLUSION AND SELECTED POLICY IMPLICATIONS

Conclusion

The objective of this study was to measure the major factors influencing demand for medical services. In particular, we were looking for a mechanism that might replace money prices in determining demand as money price out of pocket diminished. There was considerable theoretical and empirical support for the suggestion that time prices would fill that role. Travel and waiting time appear to be operating as normal prices, producing a negative own-price elasticity and a positive cross-price elasticity of demand for medical services. As predicted, elasticities were greater with respect to times associated with free care than with times associated with non-free care. The magnitude of the own-elasticity with respect to travel time is -0.6 to -1.0 for public outpatient care and between -0.25 and -0.34 for private outpatient care. These elasticities are significantly greater than the money-price elasticities of about -0.15 over the range 0 to 25 per cent coinsurance reported by Phelps and Newhouse (1972) for a Palo Alto group and equal or exceed the higher values reported by Feldstein (1971), Davis and Russell (1972), and Rosett and Huang (1973). The estimated elasticities with respect to travel time weighted by earnings are in the order of -0.15 to -0.2 for OPDC care and nearly zero for private care but, as discussed, these estimates are biased significantly toward zero. Furthermore, as predicted, demand is more sensitive to changes in travel time than to changes in waiting time, producing elasticities several times as large for travel as for waiting time. The conclusion is clear that time is already functioning as a rationing device for demand in this New York population, and its importance seems to exceed that of money prices.

From the theoretical model, we derived a prediction of positive elasticity of demand with respect to non-earned income. A picture of mixed statistical significance was found, but when significant, elasticities were around 0.04 to 0.05 for ambulatory care and 0.15 to 0.20 for inpatient care. The sign of the earned income elasticity of demand could not be predicted *a priori* because of the offsetting income and price effects of a wage change, but a change in the wage rate was expected to act more like income effect on the demand for non-free care. In fact, negative elasticities were found for free care and positive elasticities for non-free care, roughly of the same absolute magnitude as the non-earned income elasticities.

Selected Policy Implications

A number of policy considerations are suggested by the significant elasticities found for time prices and earned and non-earned income. The most important involves the distribution of medical services as out-of-pocket monetary expenses are reduced, either because of continued spread of health insurance or because of the enactment of some federal health insurance scheme. Persons with a lower opportunity cost of time will take more advantage of a reduction of out-of-pocket monetary costs than those with higher opportunity cost of time because their time prices are lower. This conclusion holds even with no differential subsidy of monetary costs and no supply response to an increase in demand. Moreover, there is likely to be a supply response to a shift in demand that increases the time needed to receive medical services (increased waiting time or perhaps increased travel time owing to more referrals).[32] This will increase further the relative shift in favor of those with lower opportunity cost of time (although the increase in the vector of time prices will reduce aggregate demand over what it would be with no supply response). In any case, the general effect of a reduction in personal monetary prices will be to shift the distribution of medical services.

Among the important additional policy considerations, if one wishes to increase aggregate demand for services, are shortening travel time to medical facilities, shortening waiting time, and considering the degree to which income subsidies might be substituted for subsidized purchase of medical services.

Clinic Location

A significant own-time/price elasticity of demand was found for outpatient department and clinic services with respect to travel time. A number of policy options are available to the government for altering travel time, ranging from improved transportation facilities to the building of new clinics and health centers. The travel time elasticities show that moving centers "closer" in time will increase the demand for care at those centers. For instance, when the city, OEO, or another agency is thinking about opening a new clinic to serve a target population, it may want to consider building a number of smaller clinics that are substantially closer, on the average, to the individuals, rather than building one large clinic to serve the population.[33] Faster means of transportation to more distant facilities may achieve the same goal. This observation should not be interpreted as a recommendation to create more clinics or to create smaller clinics. Obviously the decision rests on a number of factors, such as the cost of building centers of various sizes, the benefit of serving additional persons, and the alternative means of achieving the same goals. One alternative means of achieving the goal of increased service is to reduce waiting time in existing and new facilities.

Shorter Queues

There are two points to consider about waiting time and the demand for care. First, it is a popular impression that patients have to wait considerably longer in outpatient departments of hospitals than in private physicians' offices. The reported waiting times for 1968 show that, for this population, mean waiting time was less at OPD's and clinics than in private physicians' offices. The second point, however, is that longer waiting times do discourage use, and mechanisms that reduce waiting time should increase use. For instance, appointments rather than unscheduled visits in OPD's might prove successful in reducing waiting time. This implication is not limited to the city. Many hospitals across the nation use a system of giving all the patients a morning appointment (say 9:00) or an afternoon appointment (say 1:30). If this algorithm results in a wait, on the average, of ninety minutes and an alternative scheduling (say appointments on the hour for 9, 10, or 11) reduces the average wait to thirty minutes, the elasticities reported in table 3 suggest that this will increase demand approximately 12 per cent.[34]

Tradeoffs of Subsidized Care and Income Supplements

Many people have expressed concern over the level of medical services consumed by the poor and conclude that a variety of measures are needed to improve access. In one form or another, most boil down to a subsidized provision of services, whether through social insurance schemes such as Medicaid or various national health insurance proposals, or through direct provision of care as in neighborhood health centers or the requirement that Hill-Burton hospitals provide charity care. Seldom considered is the extent to which changing the income distribution will meet the desire to subsidize the medical purchase (Davis, 1972).

The equations reported in tables 1 and 2 put us in a position to address this question of substituting income maintenance for subsidized medical care to achieve a given increase in health consumption. Although it will not meet the objective of risk spreading, income maintenance will increase aggregate medical care demand for the poor. Since income maintenance is a non-earned source of income, the elasticity of demand for medical care with respect to changes in non-earned income is used.[35] Two of the prominent health insurance proposals, the administration's comprehensive health insurance proposal (CHIP) and the Kennedy-Mills bill, have similar income-related coinsurance features and demonstrate the tradeoff with income maintenance. The Red Hook results in table 3 indicate that a $1,000 increase in non-earned income for a family with a current (1968) non-earned income of $450 and earned income of about $4,100 will produce a 6.3 per cent increase in the demand for private practitioners' care per member. This change is probably a lower bound on the increase, since the non-earned income elasticity may be biased downward by a transitory component. If the money-price elasticity of demand for ambulatory medical services is around −0.15 over the range under consideration,[36] and the out-of-pocket expenditure is reduced from 25 per cent of money price to 15 per cent (the upper limit on CHIP's coinsurance rate and the rate for a family with income of $2,500–5,000), then the demand for private care will increase by 8 per cent. Clearly, one means of achieving the objective of increased aggregate medical consumption by the poor is income supplementation, and the magnitude of the change may be very comparable over the range of subsidy and income guarantee under consideration.

APPENDIX 1

Definitions of Variables Used and Their Mean Values[37]

AGE = Age in years. Means = (27.3, 25.2).

AGE2 = AGE^2. Means = (1,200, 1,006).

ATOPDC = Waiting time, on the average, at municipal outpatient departments (MDOPD) or free-standing clinics (CLIN), in minutes. Available for Red Hook only. Mean = (59.1).

ATOPDC2 = $ATOPDC^2$. Mean = (3,717).

ATPRIV = Waiting time, on the average, in a private physician's office, in minutes. Available for Red Hook only. Mean = (73.7).

ATPRIV2 = $ATPRIV^2$. Mean = (6,530).

BLACK = Dummy variable equaling 1 if Negro or indeterminate, or other than Puerto Rican, Mexican-American, American Indian, or other white. Means = (0.30, 0.84).

CAID = One if the person has Medicaid coverage and is under 65 years of age; zero otherwise. Means = (0.32, 0.36).

CARE = One if person has Medicare coverage; zero otherwise. Means = (0.07, 0.04).

C·TIME = For all time variables prefixed by C it is the corresponding variable without the prefix C multiplied by the opportunity cost of time. The opportunity cost of time is measured by the earnings per minute of family workers if the individual is working and is set to 1 cent per minute if the individual is not working or if there is no reported earned income for the family.

CATOPDC Mean = ($1.17).

CATOPDC2 Mean = (3.61).

CATPRIV Mean = ($1.39).

CATPRIV2 Mean = (5.32).

CTOPDC Means = ($1.42, $1.57).

CTOPDC2 Means = (5.46, 6.66).

CTPRIV Means = ($0.88, $1.24).

CTPRIV2 Means = (2.98, 6.76).

CHRON Number of reported chronic health conditions that limit activity. Means = (0.20, 0.21).

DAZPRIV = Number of days hospitalized in last year in a nongovernmental hospital. Means = (1.07, 0.69).

DAZPUB = Number of days hospitalized in last year in a city or other governmental hospital. Mean = (0.30, 0.50).

EARN = Earned family income in last year. Means = ($4,110, $4,532).

EARN2 = $EARN^2$. Means = (35388091, 45129544).

EDUC = Highest grade completed, in years. Means = (6.8, 7.3).

HSIZE = Number of persons in individual's household. Means = (4.7, 4.3).

MALE = One if male, zero if female. Means = (0.46, 0.44).

NEARN = Non-earned family income in last year. Means = ($920, $1,067).

NEARN2 = $NEARN^2$. Means = (3326386, 3996932).

NOAMB   = One if the person unambiguously has no insurance coverage for ambulatory care; zero otherwise. Means = (0.21, 0.23).

OPDC   = Number of visits in last year to a physician in outpatient department of a municipal hospital or to a clinic not connected to a hospital. Means = (1.68, 1.46).

PR   = One if Puerto Rican; zero otherwise. Means = (0.26, 0.07).

PRIV   = Number of visits in last year to a physician in his private office. Means = (1.83, 1.56).

TOPDC   = Travel time, on the average, to and from municipal outpatient department or free-standing clinic, in minutes. Means = (72.9, 64.0).

TOPDC2 = $TOPDC^2$. Means = (6,085, 4,424).

TPRIV   = Travel time, on the average, to and from private physician's office (PRIV), in minutes. Means = (44.6, 48.8).

TPRIV2 = $TPRIV^2$. Means = (3,096, 3,521).

APPENDIX 2

Results of Ordinary Least Squares Estimation

TABLE 1 OLS Regression Results with Time Weighted by the Wage Rate (C·Time)

Independent Variables	Red Hook Dependent Variables								Bedford-Crown Dependent Variables							
	OPDC		PRIV		DAZPUB		DAZPRIV		OPDC		PRIV		DAZPUB		DAZPRIV	
	Coef.	t val.	Coef.	t val.	Coef.	t val.	Coef.	t val.	Coef.	t val.	Coef.	t val.	Coef.	t val.	Coef.	t val.
CHRON	2.27	17.27	1.37	11.22	.495	4.65	2.70	17.30	2.52	17.71	1.95	14.43	1.08	6.80	1.14	7.42
EDUC $\times10^{-2}$	-10.02	4.53	-.262	.128	.783	.413	4.24	1.53	-4.62	1.91	-1.27	.550	-3.58	1.26	.0317	1.16
MALE	-.137	.949	-.709	5.30	.471	3.93	.182	1.03	-.259	1.72	-.575	4.02	.503	2.97	-.0313	.190
PR	.556	2.96	-.557	3.19	.0803	.497	-.157	.664	.0829	.220	-1.33	3.73	.552	1.29	.672	1.62
BLACK	.622	3.65	-.473	3.00	-.0348	.240	-.502	2.37	.260	.996	-1.09	4.38	.352	1.19	.304	1.06
HSIZE	-.076	1.99	-.186	5.25	-.062	1.94	-.087	1.85	-.0740	1.83	-.028	.724	.087	1.88	-.004	.0903
AGE	.062	3.85	.0162	1.08	.0112	.711	-.0179	.772	.0394	2.08	.042	2.34	.048	1.96	.024	.998
AGE2 $\times10^{-3}$	-.818	3.92	-.113	.584	-.0673	.288	.301	.878	-.540	2.13	-.425	1.76	-.418	1.14	-.236	.663
CTOPDC	.124	.565	.081	.399	.621	3.41	-.175	.654	-.246	2.09	.062	.552	-.167	1.26	-.148	1.15
CTOPDC2 $\times10^{-2}$										1.77	-.081	.092	1.43	1.37	.186	.184
CATOPDC	-1.88	.941	-.247	.133	4.41	2.65	1.17	.482	1.65							
CATOPDC2 $\times10^{-1}$	-.712	2.45	-.053	.196	-.619	2.56	.243	.685								
CTOPRIV	.716	2.20	.0422	.140	.653	2.41	-.192	.483	.051	.709	-.153	2.25	-.0276	.344	.0716	.921
CTOPRIV2 $\times10^{-2}$	.224	1.99	.135	1.30	-.102	1.09	.112	.818								
CATPRIV	-.854	1.24	.139	.217	.313	.544	-.500	.592	-1.76	.872	.289	1.51	-.024	.105	-.152	.493
CATPRIV2 $\times10^{-2}$	-.0020	.017	-.151	1.38	-.197	2.01	-.265	1.85								
NOAMB	.0857	.102	.319	.408	.811	1.15	1.51	1.46			.012	.071				
EARN $\times10^{-4}$	-.234	1.35	-.434	2.69					.0647	.369						
EARN2 $\times10^{-8}$	.0264	.065	.590	1.56	-.075	.221	.0027	.0053	.0581	.160	1.11	3.20	.366	.876	.640	1.58
NEARN $\times10^{-4}$	-.151	.577	-.185	.762	.0737	.338	-.0596	.186	.0274	.170	-.309	2.01	-.166	.912	-.084	.473
NEARN2 $\times10^{-8}$	1.13	.946	.834	.753	1.89	1.82	-2.00	1.31	7.16	5.98	-.277	.244	1.24	.883	2.89	2.12
DAZPUB $\times10^{-8}$	-1.34	.627	-.153	.077	-2.07	1.14	4.31	1.62	-10.73	5.18	.075	.038	-2.35	.992	-4.48	1.95
DAZPRIV	.0299	1.80	-.0278	1.81					.059	4.52	.0086	.687				
CARE	.135	11.95	.0285	2.72	-.304	.722	.464	.754	.0961	7.11	.0898	6.99	-1.18	1.81	.715	1.13
CAID					.062	.387	.534	2.26					.293	1.27	.293	1.31
CONST	1.48	5.02	2.60	9.52	.035	.141	.918	2.53	.782	2.08	1.66	4.65	-1.16	2.72	-.780	1.89
									.1187		.0866		.0165		.0190	

TABLE 2 OLS Regression Results with Time Entered

Independent Variables	Red Hook — OPDC Coef.	t val.	Red Hook — PRIV Coef.	t val.	Red Hook — DAZPUB Coef.	t val.	Red Hook — DAZPRIV Coef.	t val.	Bedford-Crown — OPDC Coef.	t val.	Bedford-Crown — PRIV Coef.	t val.	Bedford-Crown — DAZPUB Coef.	t val.	Bedford-Crown — DAZPRIV Coef.	t val.
CHRON	2.27	17.40	1.34	11.17	.476	4.50	2.69	17.26	2.53	17.81	1.98	14.71	1.08	6.83	1.14	7.43
EDUC	-.099	4.53	-.0076	.378	.011	.562	.042	1.52	-.045	1.86	-.020	.853	-.036	1.29	.026	.955
MALE	-.289	2.09	-.618	4.84	.409	3.54	.144	.845	-.304	2.05	-.586	4.17	.462	2.77	-.068	.422
PR	.386	1.99	-.472	2.64	-.143	.862	-.358	1.46	.047	.126	-1.22	3.42	-.516	1.21	.693	1.67
BLACK	.505	2.92	-.482	3.02	-.200	1.36	-.585	2.70	.210	.800	-.893	3.58	.319	1.07	.371	1.29
HSIZE	-.055	1.46	-.186	5.36	-.054	1.73	-.080	1.72	-.061	1.53	-.027	.704	.093	2.04	.0047	.106
AGE	.048	3.09	.018	1.25	.0047	.303	-.022	.959	.0302	1.65	.039	2.28	.043	1.77	.020	.852
AGE2 $\times10^{-3}$	-.680	3.36	-.112	.600	-.022	.095	.326	.960	-.432	1.75	-.396	1.69	-.365	1.00	-.205	.582
TOPDC	-.046	4.90	.028	3.20	.0055	.710	.0094	.821	-.052	4.23	.0434	3.72	-.037	2.66	-.0051	.376
TOPDC2 $\times10^{-3}$	.217	5.69	-.119	3.37	.037	1.16	-.043	.906	.286	4.59	-.237	4.00	.151	2.14	.033	.481
ATOPDC	-.046	2.56	.017	1.05	-.031	2.05	-.012	.551								
ATOPDC2 $\times10^{-3}$	.348	2.42	-.175	1.32	.323	2.68	.196	1.11								
TOPRIV	.133	2.22	-.178	3.21	.0031	.061	.202	2.74	-.0060	.094	-.300	4.96	-.0036	.050	-.085	1.22
TOPRIV2 $\times10^{-1}$	-.404	1.13	1.49	4.53	-.114	.383	-1.08	2.48	-.083	.235	1.68	5.02	.124	.312	.692	1.79
ATPRIV $\times10^{-2}$	.624	.688	-5.90	7.24	.319	.421	-2.13	1.91								
ATPRIV2 $\times10^{-4}$	-.234	.378	3.89	6.84	-.355	.689	1.33	1.75								
NOAMB	-.151	.876	-.474	2.97	-.283	.992			.027	.157	.089	.536				
EARN $\times10^{-4}$	-.588	1.73	.531	1.69	.168	1.07	-.191	.455	-.376	1.23	.962	3.31	-.0434	.122	.446	1.30
EARN2 $\times10^{-8}$	.157	.836	-.147	.845	1.94	1.87	-.0037	.016	.188	1.48	-.284	2.35	-.0083	.058	-.105	.748
NEARN $\times10^{-4}$	.953	.801	.675	.614	-1.89	1.04	-1.94	1.27	6.59	5.50	-.039	.034	1.15	.818	2.81	2.06
NEARN2 $\times10^{-8}$	-.763	.358	-.609	.310	-.251	.602	4.37	1.64	-10.10	4.88	-.628	.320	-2.29	.964	-4.58	1.99
DAZPUB	.021	1.28	-.018	1.20					.058	4.45	.0102	.826				
DAZPRIV	.136	12.12	.029	2.68					.097	7.16	.088	6.90				
CARE					.088	.547	.513	.835					-.110	1.68	.810	1.28
CAID					.116	.188	.542	2.29					.274	1.18	.288	1.28
CONST	4.19	5.67	3.04	4.46			.622	.684	2.96	4.31	.675	1.03	.543	.698	-.438	.581
R^2	.1453		.0885		.0235		.0754		.1221		.0945		.0177		.0193	

APPENDIX 3

Detail of the Formal Model of Demand for Medical Services

The formal model is developed in terms of a two-good utility function, medical services, m, and a composite good, X, and has people pay in both money and time for each good. If the proportion of money and the price per unit of the good remains fixed and the full wealth assumption is used, the objective is to maximize

(A-1a) $\quad U = U(m,X)$

subject to

(A-1b) $\quad (p + wt)m + (q + ws)X \leqslant Y = y + wT$

where the variables are defined as on p. 167. I assume that all equations are twice differentiable and that the first derivatives of the utility function are positive, the second derivatives, negative, and the cross derivatives are positive.[38] The conditions for maximizing utility are found by forming the Lagrangian expression

(A-2) $\quad L = U(m,X) + \lambda \left[m(p + wt) + X(q + ws) - y - wT \right]$

Differentiating with respect to the three unknowns, m, X, and λ, and setting these equal to zero yields the first-order conditions for a maximization:

(A-3a) $\quad \dfrac{\partial L}{\partial m} = U_m + \lambda(p + wt) = 0$

(A-3b) $\quad \dfrac{\partial L}{\partial X} = U_x + \lambda(q + ws) = 0$

and

(A-3c) $\quad \dfrac{\partial L}{\partial \lambda} = m(p + wt) + X(q + ws) - y - wT = 0$

where by definition

$$U_m \equiv \frac{\partial U}{\partial m} \text{ and } U_x \equiv \frac{\partial U}{\partial X}$$

Effects of a Change in Price

To calculate the effect of a change in the out-of-pocket money price of m on the demand for m, we must differentiate the system of equations (A-3) with respect to p, yielding:

(A-4a) $\quad U_{mm}\,\dfrac{\partial m}{\partial p} + U_{mX}\,\dfrac{\partial X}{\partial p} + (p+wl)\dfrac{\partial \lambda}{\partial p} - -\lambda$

(A-4b) $\quad U_{Xm}\,\dfrac{\partial m}{\partial p} + U_{XX}\,\dfrac{\partial X}{\partial p} + (q+ws)\dfrac{\partial \lambda}{\partial p} = 0$

and

(A-4c) $\quad (p+wt)\,\dfrac{\partial m}{\partial p} + (q+ws)\dfrac{\partial X}{\partial p} = -m$

If we designate the determinant of the matrix of coefficients $|D|$, then

$$|D| = \begin{vmatrix} U_{mm} & U_{mX} & (p+wl) \\ U_{Xm} & U_{XX} & (q+ws) \\ (p+wt) & (q+ws) & 0 \end{vmatrix}$$

(A-4d)

$$= U_{mX}\,(q+ws)(p+wt) + U_{Xm}\,(q+ws)(p+wt)$$
$$- U_{XX}\,(p+wt)^2 - U_{mm}\,(q+ws)^2$$

Assuming that U_{XX} and $U_{mm} < 0$ and that U_{Xm} and $U_{mX} > 0$, then $|D|$ is unambiguously positive. We can solve for $\partial m/\partial p$ by Cramer's rule:

(A-4e) $\quad \dfrac{\partial m}{\partial p} = \dfrac{\begin{vmatrix} -\lambda & U_{mX} & (p+wt) \\ 0 & U_{XX} & (q+ws) \\ -m & (q+ws) & 0 \end{vmatrix}}{|D|}$

$$= \dfrac{-mU_{mX}(q+ws) + mU_{XX}\,(p+wt) + \lambda(q+ws)^2}{|D|}$$

Since λ is necessarily negative by (A-3a) and (A-3b), $\partial m/\partial p$ is unambiguously negative. Medical services, m, is acting as a normal good; with a higher money price, people demand less.

Similarly, we can calculate the effect of a change in the time price of m on the demand for m. Differentiating with respect to t yields .

(A-5a) $\quad U_{mm}\,\dfrac{\partial m}{\partial t} + U_{mX}\,\dfrac{\partial X}{\partial t} + (p+wt)\dfrac{\partial \lambda}{\partial t} = -\lambda w$

(A-5b) $\quad U_{Xm}\,\dfrac{\partial m}{\partial t} + U_{XX}\,\dfrac{\partial X}{\partial t} + (q+ws)\dfrac{\partial \lambda}{\partial t} = 0$

and

$$\text{(A-5c)} \quad (p + wt) \frac{\partial m}{\partial t} + (q + ws) \frac{\partial X}{\partial t} = -mw$$

Using Cramer's rule again,

$$\text{(A-5d)} \quad \frac{\partial m}{\partial t} = \frac{\begin{vmatrix} -\lambda w & U_{mX} & (p + wt) \\ 0 & U_{XX} & (q + ws) \\ -mw & (q + ws) & 0 \end{vmatrix}}{|D|}$$

$$= \frac{-mw\, U_{mX}\,(q + ws) + mw\, U_{XX}\,(p + wt) + \lambda w\,(q + ws)^2}{|D|}$$

which is also unambiguously negative. That is, time is also functioning as a price in determining the consumption of m.

For reference, it is interesting to calculate the total price elasticity of demand for m. Differentiating equations (A-3) with respect to $(p + wt)$, we find

$$\text{(A-6a)} \quad U_{mm} \frac{\partial m}{\partial (p + wy)} + U_{mX} \frac{\partial X}{\partial (p + wt)} + (p + wt) \frac{\partial \lambda}{\partial (p + wt)} = -\lambda$$

$$\text{(A-6b)} \quad U_{Xm} \frac{\partial m}{\partial (p + wt)} + U_{XX} \frac{\partial X}{\partial (p + wt)} + (q + ws) \frac{\partial \lambda}{\partial (p + wt)} = 0$$

and

$$\text{(A-6c)} \quad (p + wt) \frac{\partial m}{\partial (p + wt)} + (q + ws) \frac{\partial X}{\partial (p + wt)} = -m$$

So,

$$\text{(A-6d)} \quad \frac{\partial m}{\partial (p + wt)} = \frac{\begin{vmatrix} -\lambda & U_{mX} & (p + wt) \\ 0 & U_{XX} & (q + ws) \\ -m & (q + ws) & 0 \end{vmatrix}}{|D|}$$

$$= \frac{-mU_{mX}\,(q + ws) + mU_{XX}\,(p + wt) + \lambda\,(q + ws)^2}{|D|}$$

Thus, we find that

$$\text{(A-6e)} \quad \frac{\partial m}{\partial (p + wt)} = \frac{\partial m}{\partial p}$$

The three price elasticities are related in the following manner:

(A-7a) $\quad \eta_{m(wt)} = \eta_{mt} = \dfrac{wt}{(p + wt)}\ \eta_{m(p + wt)}$

and

(A-7b) $\quad \eta_{mp} = \dfrac{p}{(p + wt)}\ \eta_{m(p + wt)}$

Consequently, it follows that

$\qquad \eta_{mp} \gtreqless \eta_{mt}$

as

$\qquad p \gtreqless wt$

Effects of a Change in Income

The effects of a change in earned and non-earned income are systematically related, but they are not, in general, the same. The effect of a change in non-earned income is straightforward to calculate. Differentiating equations (A-3) with respect to y yields:

(A-8a) $\quad U_{mm}\dfrac{\partial m}{\partial y} + U_{mX}\dfrac{\partial X}{\partial y} + (p + wt)\dfrac{\partial \lambda}{\partial y} = 0$

(A-8b) $\quad U_{Xm}\dfrac{\partial m}{\partial y} + U_{XX}\dfrac{\partial X}{\partial y} + (q + ws)\dfrac{\partial \lambda}{\partial y} = 0$

and

(A-8c) $\quad (p + wt)\dfrac{\partial m}{\partial y} + (q + ws)\dfrac{\partial X}{\partial y} = 1$

Thus,

$$
\text{(A-8d)}\quad \frac{\partial m}{\partial y} = \frac{\begin{vmatrix} 0 & U_{mX} & (p + wt) \\ 0 & U_{XX} & (q + ws) \\ 0 & (q + ws) & 0 \end{vmatrix}}{|D|}
$$

$$
= \frac{U_{mX}\,(q + ws) - U_{XX}\,(p + wt)}{|D|}
$$

which is unambiguously positive. The demand for medical services is normal; with more non-earned income, people demand more.

We can see the effect of a change in the earnings per hour by differentiating with respect to w:

(A-9a) $\quad U_{mm} \dfrac{\partial m}{\partial w} + U_{mX} \dfrac{\partial X}{\partial w} + (p + wt) \dfrac{\partial \lambda}{\partial w} = -\lambda t$

(A-9b) $\quad U_{Xm} \dfrac{\partial m}{\partial w} + U_{XX} \dfrac{\partial X}{\partial w} + (q + ws) \dfrac{\partial \lambda}{\partial w} = -\lambda s$

and

(A-9c) $\quad (p + wt) \dfrac{\partial m}{\partial w} + (q + ws) = -mt - Xs + T$

Cramer's rule yields:

(A-9d) $\quad \dfrac{\partial m}{\partial w} = \dfrac{\begin{vmatrix} -\lambda t & U_{mX} & (p + wt) \\ -\lambda s & U_{XX} & (q + ws) \\ T - mt - Xs & (q + ws) & 0 \end{vmatrix}}{|D|}$

$$= \frac{(T - mt - Xs)U_{mX}(q + ws) - (T - mt - Xs)U_{XX}(p + wt) - \lambda s(q + ws)(p + wt) + \lambda t(q + w\ldots}{|D|}$$

The effects of a change in the wage rate can be broken down into an income effect and substitution effect:

(A-9e) $\quad \dfrac{\partial m}{\partial w} = (T - mt - Xs)\dfrac{\lambda m}{\partial y} - \dfrac{\lambda s(q + ws)(p + wt) - \lambda t(q + ws)^2}{|D|}$

The first term, the income effect, is by assumption positive. The sign of the substitution effect depends on the relative time intensity of the goods m and X. If the time component of total price is larger for X than it is for m, there will be a positive substitution from X to m. That is, the substitution term is positive if and only if

(A-10a) $\quad \dfrac{ws}{(q + ws)} > \dfrac{wt}{(p + wt)}$

It is easy to show that the substitution effect is negative if medical care is "free." Substituting $p = 0$ into (A-10a), canceling common terms, and multiplying through by $(q + ws)$ yields

(A-10b) $\quad ws < (q + ws)$

Therefore, the substitution effect is negative.

NOTES

1. See Newhouse and Acton (1974) for a discussion of this point.
2. See especially Davis and Russell (1972), Feldstein (1971), Phelps (1973), Phelps and Newhouse (1973), and Rosett and Huang (1973).
3. If demand increases in response to spreading insurance, in addition to increases in waiting and travel time, the supply responses may be to (1) increase the number of referrals to other providers, (2) cause a postponement in treating some conditions, or (3) change the quality of services being provided. Increased referrals and postponement are alternative forms of greater time costs. In this study, I am concentrating directly on the role of waiting and travel time. The importance of time in determining demand was explored by Becker (1965); its importance in medical care, by, among others, Leveson (1970), Holtman (1972), and Auster and Ro (1972). In her comments, Mrs. Campbell correctly points out that "waiting time" in this survey probably does not include the amount of time spent in an examination room unattended or the time in transit between different tests or parts of the facility. This more detailed information would be interesting to explore but was unavailable in this survey. If such additional "hidden" time charges are independent of or proportional to time in the waiting room, the elasticities are unaffected; if they are negatively correlated, then the empirical results are misleading. She also comments that increased referrals or postponement of appointments may be an important supply response to spreading coverage—with which I agree. I do not agree that its absence in these equations limits their value for policy assessment. Unless one can demonstrate that suppliers will discriminate systematically in their patterns of postponement and referrals, then the waiting time and travel time results reported below are partial effects that should be observed regardless of these other effects.
4. Similar models can be found in Grossman (1970), Becker (1965), and Acton (1973).
5. See Grossman (1972) for a formulation accommodating this feature.
6. See Phelps (1973) for a theoretical and empirical treatment with insurance endogenous.
7. See Lancaster (1966) for a similar formulation of demand in terms of the attributes of a good.
8. Although they are more restrictive than necessary, sufficient assumptions are that the first derivatives of the utility function with respect to a good are positive, that the second derivatives are negative, and that the cross-partial derivatives are positive.
9. As shown in Appendix 3, $\eta_{m(\pi t)} = \eta_{mt}$. These elasticities are approximate only in the long run if insurance premiums are adjusted to reflect the changes in utilization.
10. In the consumption model, given a neutral effect of education on all household activities, the elasticity with respect to wealth must also be less than 1 to have a negative effect on education; Grossman (1972a, pp. 36–37).
11. NORC conducted ten baseline surveys for OEO. The Bedford-Crown survey was the second survey and Red Hook the third. The survey instrument improved somewhat, so occasionally we have useful information on the Red Hook sample that is not available for Bedford-Crown. A description of the Bedford-Crown study, along with the survey instrument and selected findings, is available in Richardson (1969a). A similar report on the Red Hook study is

Richardson (1969b). Selected findings for the first three NORC studies (Atlanta and the two Brooklyn surveys) are presented in Richardson (1970).

12. Let k proportion of the variable x be reported, then the estimated (price) elasticity $\eta_{xp} = \partial kx/\partial p)(\bar{p}/k\bar{x}) = (\partial x/\partial p)\,(\bar{p}/\bar{x})$, the same elasticity that would have been estimated with correct reporting.

13. Conversations with OEO officials have indicated that the acceptance of the neighborhood health centers has been different from the two populations. The Red Hook population is changing its behavior by coming to the center for early care and preventive medicine. In Bedford-Crown, the population comes in chiefly for treatment of advanced and chronic conditions. There may be some persistent differences in the two populations that will be reflected in the analysis below. It could simply be a different acceptance of the neighborhood health centers. The Bedford-Crown center is located in a very rough neighborhood and, purportedly, taxi drivers refuse to travel there. This does not appear to be true for the Red Hook neighborhood.

14. The use of a mean value rather than zero for these nonresponses was necessary to avoid the implausible situation that higher own-time prices are associated with lower utilization except for zero utilization when own-time prices are zero. A predicted value of own-time price might have been used, but that option is deferred for further analysis. It was necessary to use the mean value for about three-fourths of the times associated with free care and about one-fourth of the times associated with non-free care in both samples.

   Using the mean to replace missing values reduced the efficiency in estimating that coefficient, but Charles Phelps demonstrated that use of the mean for some observations does not bias the remaining coefficients if the mean is uncorrelated with the remaining variables. Consider the bivariate case in which m observations on x_i are known and the next p are replaced with the mean (their true value is $\bar{x}_1 + u_i$). The OLS estimator of β is $b = \{\sum_m (xy) + \sum_p [(x + u)y]\}/[\sum_m x^2 + \sum_p (x + u)^2] = \{\sum_m [(xx\beta) + x\epsilon] + \sum_p [(x + u)(x\beta + \epsilon)]\}/[\sum_m x^2 + \sum_p (x + u)^2]$. The measurement error for the subset, p, of observation is $u_i = (\bar{x} - x_i)$ so that $\sigma^2_{u_p} = \sigma_{x_p}$ and $\sigma^2_{x + u_p} = 0$, where the subscripts on variances indicate the subsample to which they relate. The probability limit of b can be shown to be plim $b = (\sigma^2_{x_m} + \sigma^2_{x_p} + \sigma_{xu_p})\beta/(\sigma^2_{x_m} + \sigma^2_{(x + u_p)})$. Since, in subsample of size p, $\sigma^2_{x_p} + \sigma^2_{u_p} + 2\sigma_{xu_p} = 0$ and $\sigma^2_{x_p} = \sigma^2_{u_p}$, it follows that $-\sigma_{xu_p} = \sigma^2_{x_p}$ and plim $b = (\sigma^2_{x_m} + 0)\beta/(\sigma^2_{x_m} + 0) = \beta$.

15. It is necessary to use a non-zero value for the opportunity cost of a unit of time if travel and waiting time are to play a role in determining demand for a specific provider by nonworking persons. Otherwise, we are assuming that, in effect, the person is indifferent whether he travels a short distance for care or travels a great distance. Furthermore, physician visits by children frequently cause an adult to spend time accompanying them. The value of 60 cents per hour for this group is arbitrary, but it can be motivated to some degree as a plausible value for the cost of hiring a babysitter. The value of 60 cents is lower than any observed value of earnings per hour in either sample (which was over $1 per hour). A number of researchers have taken a much more detailed look at valuing the time of persons out of the labor force (see, for instance, Gronau, 1973a and b, and references cited). I did not feel a more complicated approach was justified in the current application because of limited information about time allocation of individual family members.

16. I took the total reported income and subtracted the elements that were non-earned to create the earned income variable. In a few cases, the sum of

non-earned incomes exceeded the stated total income (typically, zero was recorded for total, but a monthly social security income was reported). In these cases, the amount created by summing up the components was used.

17. Ideally, health status lagged one period would be used. It was not available, but its absence is not too serious since the underlying stock of health is highly correlated from one year to the next.

18. In addition, people with more chronic health conditions probably have a lower stock of health to begin with, so that it takes more medical inputs to achieve a given replacement of health than it would if they had started with a greater stock. This argument assumes that the function transforming medical inputs to health has decreasing returns to scale.

19. To some degree, inpatient and outpatient care may be substitutes for each other, but I expect their complementary nature to dominate. I checked the sensitivity of the remaining coefficients to the inclusion and exclusion of these hospital variables and found the coefficients practically unchanged.

20. If everyone's insurance coverage were known in detail, this would not be a problem; but NOAMB is an imperfect measure, as indicated above.

21. The t statistics are asymptotic tests in the tobit framework. With samples of 5,000, they probably are good guides to significance. Furthermore, the chi² statistics test the hypothesis that the vector of coefficients is zero; they, too, are highly significant.

The reader should not attach too much importance to the equations for public hospitalization since the number of non-zero observations is very small.

22. Figure 1A shows the quantity of care demanded as a function of either t or wt. People who appear to have high time inputs to the purchase of care (indicated on the line marked t) tend to have proportionately lower values of wt because of the negative correlation of w and t. Conversely, those who appear to have low time inputs tend to have higher opportunity costs of time and therefore proportionately higher values of wt. The same result holds for the cross-time prices indicated in Fig. 1B. Thus, the true elasticity with respect to wt will be greater than that implied by the regression on t alone.

FIGURE 1a
Relation between own-time prices and quantity

FIGURE 1b
Relation between cross-time prices and quantity

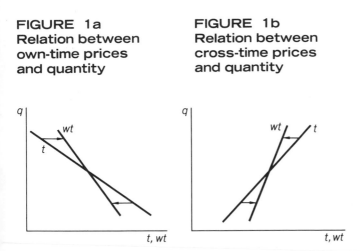

23. This apparent contradiction may be because the estimated maximum occurs where ATOPDC = 45 minutes. The mean, used for calculating the elasticity, is 59 minutes, which is one standard deviation above the critical point.
24. Using a 1965 survey of users of the municipal hospitals' OPDs (specifying a simultaneous equation system with public and private ambulatory care and public hospitalization all endogenous), I found complementarity in public ambulatory and inpatient care. See Acton (1973).
25. This comparison was carried out using OLS—whose results approach tobit asymptotically—because patterns of significance and collinearity were found to carry over well to tobit results.
26. These estimated elasticities may be biased downward by a transitory component in non-earned income. The negative elasticity for private hospital days, equations (4) and (12), is caused by the elasticity's being calculated at the mean of the data ($920), which was just to the left of the minimum of our estimated relationship ($939 in Equation (4) and $1,183 in Equation (12), which is within one-seventh of a standard deviation of the mean). For approximately half the sample, the non-earned income elasticity has the expected positive sign. For most other equations, the critical point is not within one standard deviation of the mean of the data.
27. Michael Grossman pointed out that, in general, we can expect to find lower elasticities with respect to earned income in equations (9)–(16) than in equations (1)–(8). Consider the simplified form of a demand equation,

(4a) $\quad m = a + bp + cY$

where $p = wt$ and $Y = y + wT$. We expect $b < 0$ and $c > 0$. Substituting into (4a) yields

(4b) $\quad m = a = bwt + cwT + cy$

similar to equations (1)–(8). With wt held constant, the coefficient, c, on full earnings should be positive. When we estimate

(4c) $\quad m = a' + b't + c'wT + dy$

the coefficient c' could be negative. The elasticities reported in table 3 generally support this prediction that the earning elasticities in equations (9)–(16) are lower than those in equations (1)–(8).
28. Since $(\partial m/\partial Y) = (\partial m/\partial y)$, it follows that $\eta_{mY} = (\partial m/\partial Y)(\overline{Y}/\overline{m}) = (\partial m/\partial y)$ $(\overline{Y}/\overline{m}) \cdot (\overline{Y}/\overline{y}) = \eta_{my}(\overline{Y}/\overline{y})$.
29. If the reader wishes to make other assumptions about the definition of full wealth, then the elasticities can be adjusted accordingly. For instance, if T is taken as referring to a twenty-four-hour day instead of a forty-hour work week, the full wealth elasticities reported here should be scaled up by 4.2.
30. The corresponding elasticities for the Bedford-Crown sample, 1.317 and −0.714, reflect the estimated coefficients on NEARN, and the comments made above apply.
31. It is probably not worth conducting a rigorous test of this hypothesis, which requires calculation of the covariance among equations, but it seems valid.
32. This supply response is likely for a number of reasons. First, it may be optimal from the point of view of the provider to have a queue to even out the variation in demand that he experiences, without having to invest in significant excess capacity. A shift in demand will generally cause the optimal queue length to change (for instance, the opportunity cost of an idle moment of the supplier's facility is higher). Second, the suppliers may not be profit maximizers, so that

they do not respond to a shift in demand by charging the highest possible monetary prices but instead allow time prices to increase. In particular, physicians may be income satisfiers rather than maximizers. See Newhouse (1970), Frech and Ginsburg (1972), and Newhouse and Sloan (1972) for a discussion of physician pricing behavior. Third, there may be a conscious attempt to redistribute services by discriminating in favor of those with a lower opportunity cost of time. See Nichols, Smolensky, and Tideman (1971) for a discussion of the first and third points.

33. One form might be for several satellite clinics to be associated with a more centrally located referral clinic.

34. This is an arc elasticity based on the elasticity calculated at the mean.

35. This calculation ignores substitution effects induced by changes in the marginal tax rate implicit in the income maintenance proposals.

36. The actual money-price elasticity may be even lower than this. See Newhouse and Phelps (1973) for a discussion of the price elasticities in several published reports.

37. The mean values are reported first for Red Hook and second for Bedford-Crown.

38. These assumptions are sufficient to imply that both goods are normal and that a rise in their price will reduce demand.

REFERENCES

1. Acton, Jan Paul, "Demand for Health Care When Time Prices Vary More Than Money Prices," R-1189-OEO/NYC, The Rand Corporation, May 1973b.

2. Auster, Richard, and Kong-Kyan Ro, "The Demand for Hospital Care by Hospitalized Individuals," Mimeographed paper presented at the Winter Econometrics Society Meetings, Toronto, 1972.

3. Becker, Gary, "A Theory of the Allocation of Time," *Economic Journal*, 75 (September 1965), pp. 493–517.

4. Davis, Karen, "Health Insurance," in Charles Schultze *et al.* (eds.), *Setting National Priorities: The 1973 Budget* (Washington, D.C.: The Brookings Institution, 1972), pp. 213–251.

5. _____ , and Louise Russell, "The Substitution of Hospital Care for Inpatient Care," *Review of Economics and Statistics*, 54 (May 1972), pp. 109–120.

6. Feldstein, Martin S., "An Econometric Model of the Medicare System," *Quarterly Journal of Economics*, 85 (1971), pp. 1–20.

7. Frech, H.E., and Paul B. Ginsburg, "Physician Pricing: Monopolistic or Competitive: Comment," *Southern Economic Journal*, 38 (1972), pp. 573–577.

8. Gronau, Reuben, "The Intrafamily Allocation of Time: The Value of the Housewife's Time," *The American Economic Review*, forthcoming.

9. _____ , "The Effects of Children on the Housewife's Value of Time," *Journal of Political Economy*, 81 (March–April 1973b), pp. 168–199.

10. Grossman, Michael, *The Demand for Health: A Theoretical and Empirical Investigation* (New York: National Bureau of Economic Research, 1972a).

11. _____ , "On the Concept of Health Capital and the Demand for Health," *Journal of Political Economy*, 80 (March–April 1972), pp. 223–255.

12. Holtman, A.G., "Prices, Time, and Technology in the Medical Care Market," *Journal of Human Resources,* 7 (Spring 1972), pp. 179–190.
13. Lancaster, Kevin, "A New Approach to Consumer Theory," *Journal of Political Economy,* 74 (April 1966), pp. 132–157.
14. Newhouse, Joseph P., "A Model of Physician Pricing," *Southern Economic Journal,* 37 (October 1970), pp. 174–183.
15. _____, and Jan Paul Acton, "Compulsory Health Planning Laws and National Health Insurance," in Clark Havighurst (ed.), *Regulating Health Facilities Construction* (Washington, D.C.: The American Enterprise Institute, 1974).
16. _____, and Charles E. Phelps, "On Having Your Cake and Eating It Too: A Review of Estimated Effects of Insurance on Demand for Health Services," R-1149-NC, The Rand Corporation, April 1974.
17. _____, and Frank A. Sloan, "Physician Pricing, Monopolistic or Competitive: Reply," *Southern Economic Journal,* 38 (April 1972), pp. 577–580.
18. Nichols, D.E., and T.N. Tideman, "Discrimination by Waiting Time in Merit Goods," *American Economic Review,* 61 (June 1971), pp. 312–323.
19. Phelps, Charles E., "The Effects of Coinsurance on Demand for Physician Services," R-976-OEO, The Rand Corporation, June 1972.
20. _____, "Demand for Health Insurance: A Theoretical and Empirical Investigation," R-1054-OEO, The Rand Corporation, July 1973.
21. _____, and Joseph P. Newhouse, "Coinsurance and the Demand for Medical Services," R-964-OEO/NYC, The Rand Corporation, July 1973.
22. Richardson, William C., *Charles Drew Neighborhood Health Center Survey Bedford-Stuyvesant–Crown Heights, Brooklyn, New York* (Chicago: NORC, University of Chicago, 1969a).
23. _____, *Red Hook Neighborhood Health Center Survey Brooklyn, New York* (Chicago: NORC, University of Chicago, 1969b).
24. _____, "Measuring the Urban Poor's Use of Physicians' Services in Response to Illness Episodes," *Medical Care,* 8 (1970), pp. 132–142.
25. Rosett, Richard N., and Lien-Fu Huang, "The Effects of Health Insurance on the Demand for Medical Care," *Journal of Political Economy,* 81 (March–April 1971).
26. Tobin, James, "Estimation of Relationships for Limited Dependent Variables," *Econometrica,* 26 (1958), pp. 24–36.

5 ‖ COMMENTS

Rita Ricardo Campbell
Hoover Institution on War, Revolution and Peace

As some of you may know, I have been involved in the public policy area in regard to the financing and delivery of medical care and am not an econometrician. I greatly appreciate, therefore, the efforts of econometricians, as represented by the paper of Jan Acton, and by others at this conference, to determine the effect of net price on the demand for health care.

Acton's econometric analysis and empirical data about the role of time as part of the net price paid by the consumer or potential patient, I feel, is long overdue in discussions about the allocation and quality of the delivery of medical care in the U.S. In other countries, where the financing and system of medical care are more nationalized, the role of "waiting" in allocation has been more obvious and is recognized. For example, Professor Spek of the University of Gothenburg defines "demand" for that portion of health care in Sweden that is completely free, as follows:

> *Demand* (active, effective) for public care is that part of the need for care which is represented by those individuals who come in touch with the system of public care with a desire for consultation and treatment, and who are willing to wait if this cannot be provided at once. In each period, demand takes the form of queueing or results in *consumption. . . .*[1]

This is a definition of demand wholly in terms of time.

When third-party payments cover two-thirds of the U.S. total personal health care bill, money price cannot be considered the primary allocation factor and especially not in those areas of care—hospital and surgical—wherein third-party payments are 92 per cent and about 70–75 per cent, respectively. In an earlier published discussion of methods other than a price to allocate medical care, I asked, "Would the distribution of scarce medical resources be more optimal if all financial barriers to securing care were removed and no special categories were set up?" and stated that "there is as much logic to implying a high correlation between income and need for medical care throughout the income distribution ranges as there is to implying a high correlation between a low opportunity cost of time and need for medical care."[2] It is with this public policy approach that I have read Dr. Acton's paper, which develops a consumption model and analyzes two sets of specific data re the urban poor to test his model, which includes as variables time prices, money prices, earned and unearned income, and as the outcome measure, physician visits.

To discuss the role of opportunity costs of time, it is necessary to consider all different kinds of time involved in consuming health care. Although Acton's model includes "waiting" and travel time,[3] it does not cover all forms of consumption of time involved in getting medical care nor does it distinguish between week days and weekends or after usual work hours.

In addition to the waiting time in a physician's outer office, there may be considerable waiting in the actual examination room before seeing an M.D. This "waiting" does not appear to be included—probably the data are unavailable—yet in some clinics and group practices it may be a sizable "hidden" form of waiting.

There is also the amount of time spent not in waiting but in consuming health care, such as is involved in having examinations, X-rays, tests, and the like. This consumption of time may be less important in initial decisions by the consumer to seek medical care, because he may be ignorant of the subsequent amount of time involved, which is largely controlled by the provider. The more knowledgeable consumer does, however, consider this potential "time" in deciding whether or not to have a postponable operation, or even more routine care, such as an eye examination. However, from an even broader point of view, and as stated by Michael Grossman in his *Demand for Health* (NBER Occasional Paper No. 119), although "a demand curve for the time spent producing health [by the consumer] could also be developed, data pertaining to this input are, in general, not available" (p. 41).

A third concept involving waiting is the time one has to wait for an appointment. To relegate to a footnote, as does Acton, suppliers' responses of "increased referrals and postponement" as an alternative form of greater time costs to the consumer is insufficient for public policy decision making. The quality of medical care and the resource costs of providing it are affected by structuring the demand for medical care through imposing long waits for appointments. For example, to the degree that HMO's or prepaid group practice use an appointment system, and most do, they can consciously curtail demand by delaying appointments six weeks or two months or more for check-ups and especially for specialists' care wherein explanations of delay may be more acceptable to the consumer, whose ignorance exceeds in this matter the physician's. The quality of care is less with long waits than with short waits. To the extent that the "waiting" induces subscribers to seek care elsewhere, total costs to a prepaid group are lowered. Data on voluntary outside utilization of physician services by members of a prepaid group are sparse and scattered and the reasons for the outside utilization are largely unexplored. To what degree outside use of services occurs, which otherwise would not require out-of-pocket expense to the patient because of various forms of waiting, I do not know.

Acton's paper does not incorporate into the analysis these various types of "time," probably because the empirical data are unavailable. Econometric modeling to encompass more kinds of waiting may encourage better data collection. From the point of view of public policy, the different types of waiting time cannot be ignored and some recognition should be given these variables even if they are not in the formal model.

Recent empirical studies emphasize the importance of these, possibly nonmeasurable, inputs as follows: "Patient waiting time was longer for nonwhites, females, poor people, and the elderly; waiting time was not related to practice size but varied proportionately with use of allied health personnel, . . ."[4] in the fee-for-service sector, solo and group.

To determine potential utilization, a state planning agency, New York,[5] recommends that a new prepaid group practice or HMO obtain answers to such questions as: "How many waiting rooms should there be and where should they be located? (1) What will be the average length of a patient visit? (2) How many people will there be at one time in each waiting area? . . ." and further, "How many consultation and examination rooms will be needed for each physician?" Obviously, HMO's, and for that matter any physician, can structure demand by the way they answer these and other questions. Additionally, HMO's decide how many physicians per 1,000 enrollees, number of hospital beds per 1,000 enrollees, and so on, will be provided.

An interesting evaluation of the California Medical Group (CMG) prepared for the Teamsters and Food Employers Security Trust Fund in Los Angeles[6] criticizes that group as having physician and hospital bed ratios far lower than Kaiser's, which are lower than the average in California, and comments, "over the years, Trust Funds have become increasingly aware of subscriber dissatisfaction with Kaiser services. Difficulties making appointments, lengthy waits to see physicians even with appointments, and hurried, impersonal physician contacts are common complaints" (p. 9). For those who are Kaiser supporters, the evaluation report recommended turning down CMG and retaining Kaiser because obviously CMG's proposed much lower physician and hospital bed enrollee ratios would increase complaints.

The general approach of quality control in prepaid groups has, in the past, relied almost entirely on providing the subscriber with an alternative choice at time of enrollment, and subsequently once a year. This works to control quality only if at least one of the alternatives provides an acceptable standard of quality of care. This may not always be the case and there is a need for some type of continuing review of ambulatory delivery of medical care as well as of in-hospital care. At a minimum is input control through careful assessment of the quantity of the medical care inputs in relationship to the anticipated demand and their quality; e.g., numbers of primary physicians and specialists, initial training and continuing education, and the like.

The Institute of Medicine's[7] proposal to use selected tracers, wherein medical inputs and health outcomes are directly related, as in iron-deficiency anemia or middle ear infection, is worth exploring by economists who are trying to develop better health outcome measures than mortality and morbidity rates or, as in Acton's study, the number of physician visits. The latter is used in this study without being subdivided into different types of visits nor qualified by number of minutes. The omission of any reference to the importance of the use of the telephone visit by persons in higher income levels as a means of avoiding waiting is disappointing.

Whether Acton's conclusions re the "urban poor" that "travel and waiting time appear to be operating as normal prices . . ." and that "time is already functioning as a rationing device for demand in this New York population, and its importance seems to exceed that of money prices, . . ." can be carried over to other sectors of society as defined by income levels in urban and suburban areas is doubtful, even if one accepts his fairly rigid assumptions. The percentage of third-party payments of total health care costs, levels and ratios of earned and unearned incomes, use of telephone and of appointment schedules, level of knowledge re medical care, and so on, differ at different income and educational levels.

Probably the most important policy inference discussed by Dr. Acton, and time limits my discussion of it, is under "Tradeoffs of Subsidized Care and Income Supplements," in which he states that "income maintenance will increase aggregate medical demand for the poor" because it is non-earned income, and concludes that "the magnitude of the change may be very comparable over the range of subsidy and income guarantee under consideration."

NOTES

1. J. E. Spek, "On the Economic Analysis of Health and Medical Care in a Swedish Health District," in M. M. Hauser (editor), *The Economics of Medical Care,* University of York Studies in Economics, 7 (London: George Allen and Unwin, 1972), p. 265.
2. Rita R. Campbell, *Economics of Health and Public Policy* (Washington, D.C.: American Enterprise Institute, June 1971), p. 69.
3. Additionally, for a given person living in a city, travel time from home to the physician's office may vary greatly, depending on whether it is undertaken during rush hours or not and also whether one has available a private car or must depend on public transportation, with possibly inconvenient schedules and transfers.
4. The AMA and USC joint studies using AMA's data, as reported in *Health Services Research,* (Winter 1973), p. 326.
5. New York State Health Planning Commission, *Group Practice* . . . by Anne Bush, September 1971, pp. 39, 40.
6. California Council for Health Plan Alternatives, December 6, 1972.
7. National Academy of Sciences, *A Strategy for Evaluating Health Services,* D.M. Kessner, Project Director, Washington, D.C., 1973.

Harry J. Gilman
University of Rochester

I generally agree with Acton's arguments about the desirability of measuring the role of time in the demand for medical services. I also admire most of his econometric work. I do not, however, like his data, or the use to which he puts these data. I am therefore extremely uneasy about his findings, particularly his principal findings of fairly high time-price elasticities of demand and extremely low or nonexistent income elasticity of demand for medical services.

Measurement problems aside, casual empiricism suggests that the demand for medical services is a function of costs other than money prices, in addition to money prices. Even if we ignore the behavior of lower-income groups and concentrate instead on groups having completely free medical coverage as part of the pay package (families of military personnel are an example), we suspect that their demand for medical services are less than what they would be if they faced only zero money prices. For if the zero money prices represented the marginal costs, individuals facing such costs would increase the consumption of medical services until the value of the last unit consumed, say, the value of their last visit to the doctor, equaled zero. Since we do not observe such consumption behavior, it is reasonable to assume that the money prices do not represent the total cost of medical services.

It does not follow, however, that one can expect the time-price elasticities of demand to be much higher (by a factor of 4 or 5) than the money-price elasticities of demand. Moreover, the nonmonetary constraints need not be exclusively or even largely those imposed by the two specific variables used in this study, travel to and waiting time in the office. Other important variables that have been omitted from this study are waiting time for appointments (queuing time) and quality of medical services. I suspect that there is a positive correlation between the out-of-pocket costs and the quality of medical services. Furthermore, if queuing time were positively correlated with waiting time in the office, the time-price elasticities of demand would be biased upward, or away from zero, rather than downward, as claimed by Acton.

The travel and waiting time variables used in this study have the added deficiency of being endogenous to the equations. This is particularly true in the equations for the demand for private medical care.

Acton's data consist of questionnaire responses elicited from individuals and families living in two well-defined neighborhoods in New York City. These responses do not include information on money prices paid for medical services or on the quality of medical services received. They do show variability in travel and waiting time as well as variability in the number of visits to the doctor and in the number of days of hospital care. Acton expects and finds an inverse correlation between travel and waiting time and, say, the number of visits to the doctor. He reasons correctly that more time spent for medical care increases the time price of such care. He concludes from that, in my judgment incorrectly, that this negative correlation between time and use of medical care is a measure of the time-price elasticity of demand. This is an incorrect conclusion because the individuals in these neighborhoods have a choice of private physicians. This choice includes the location of the physician and therefore the distance and time of travel from home as well as the length of the waiting period. If an individual chooses a physician associated with more travel and waiting time over one requiring less travel time, it must mean that the total cost for this physician is lower, for a given quality, than is the total cost of the lower time-price physician. In the presence of voluntary choice, therefore, the negative relationship between time and quantity *cannot* be used, by itself, to estimate the time-price elasticities of demand.

Acton's arguments about the changing role of money versus time prices over time also ignore the secular increase in the amount of time available as sick leave, thereby reducing an individual's time costs of medical services. This trend is paralleled by a cross-sectional pattern of sick leave benefits opposite to that of opportunity costs. Therefore, his conclusions about the relative roles of time prices among income groups are probably also incorrect.

These several factors lead me to believe that his time-price elasticities of demand are, to say the least, extremely unreliable. His unstable but extremely low income elasticities of demand are also highly questionable. They are inconsistent with the rising demand for medical services over time as reflected in the behavior of price indexes, doctors' incomes, and the growth of employment in the medical services industry.

At fault here may be the poor quality of his dependent variable. In one case, this variable is simply the number of visits to a doctor. However, higher or rising income may have a greater effect on the quality of the doctor visited or on the quality of a visit to a given doctor than it does on the number of visits to a given doctor. This would be in line with the findings in a number of studies on the demand for durable goods, including the demand for children. All of these studies found a substantially higher quality income elasticity of demand than quantity income elasticity of demand.

To some extent the quality effects could have been reflected in a shift from free to non-free physician's services, with rising income. Acton's study finds no such income effect. However, it is my impression that his dependent variable does not truly differentiate, as claimed, between free and money-price services.

6

ROBERT P.
INMAN
University of Pennsylvania

The Family Provision of Children's Health: An Economic Analysis

1. INTRODUCTION

The healthiness of children can be a major source of consumption and investment benefits for a society. In the U.S., for example, we spend nearly $1 billion annually on pediatric services and publicly allocate $800 million yearly (1970) for predominantly children-directed health care.[1] In this paper my purpose is to propose and to statistically test a model of the family as a provider-protector of the health of its children. Since our society is interested in protecting and enhancing the state of health of our children, and since the family is the primary social unit for child care, analysis such as that

The paper is dedicated to the memory of Robert Eilers, past Director of Leonard Davis Institute of Health Economics. The author appreciates the financial assistance of the Leonard Davis Institute and a grant from Wharton Economic Forecasting Associates. The data used in this study were kindly made available by the National Academy of Sciences, Institute of Medicine, from the survey "Contrasting Forms of Health Care Delivery" financed by the Ford Foundation. Robert Eilers, Robert Pollak, Walter Tunnessen (M.D.), Jeffrey Harris (M.D.), David Kessner (M.D.), Ross Anthony, Patricia Inman, and Andrew Reschovsky were all most helpful at various stages of this project. I also appreciate the careful comments of Michael Grossman, David Salkever, and Lee Benham on an earlier version of this paper.

presented here becomes indispensable for sound social policy. The results developed below are offered as a beginning step toward a policy model of children's health.

Section 2 is a brief outline of a concept of "healthiness" for statistical and policy analysis and contains a description of a model of the demand for health care wherein the effects on healthiness of health care activities (e.g., doctor visits, good nutrition, rest) are uncertain. The model yields a demand for health care activities with the usual price and income specifications plus a relationship between quantities consumed and the means and variances of the effects of health activities on healthiness.

In Section 3 this model of the demand for health care activities is applied to the family's decisions to buy preventive and curative doctor service and to allocate parents' time for the protection of children's health. "Production functions" of the family's provision of children's health are specified, and models of the demand for child health care by working and nonworking mothers are presented.

In Section 4 there are econometric estimates of the health care production and demand models proposed in Section 3 for one major class of childhood diseases—ear, nose, and throat (ENT) infections. The production model shows that parents' time and doctor visits do have, on average, a positive effect on children's health but that the final outcome is extremely uncertain. The relationship of the health care technology to mother's education and the source of physician services (public or private) is explored. Estimation of the demand model provides price and income elasticities as well as a test of the uncertainty model of Section 2.

Section 4 contains a few *tentative* policy conclusions. National health insurance with shallow coverage, as well as most policies operating through the economic variables of prices and income, appear to have only minor positive effects on children's ENT health. Changes in medical technology, parent health knowledge, and the patterns of adult-child interaction appear to be more promising avenues for improved children's health.

2. HEALTH CARE DEMAND WHEN OUTCOMES ARE UNCERTAIN

Unlike many consumption activities in which consumers know exactly what they are getting for their dollars, the consumption of health-related services can be extremely uncertain. We rarely know what the exact effects of a doctor visit, a night's rest, or a "well-balanced" meal will be on our physical healthiness. At best we have expectations and a sense of the range of possible results. This section outlines a consumer model of health care demand that incorporates these uncertain effects on health of health care consumption activities. The model forms the basis for our empirical analysis of the family's provision for children's health.

The individual (or family) is assumed to derive satisfaction from three basic sets of consumption goods—non-health-related consumer goods (denoted by the vector y), health-related consumer goods (x), and a vector of *measurable* attributes of *physical* healthiness (A).[1] The new element here is the formal inclusion of physical healthiness into the consumer's allocation problem.[3]

The elements of the vector of health attributes (A) are cardinal measures of (physical) health-related human characteristics.[4] Height, weight, body temperature, blood pressure, white blood count, serum protein level, eye acuity, and hearing range are all candidates for membership in A. In addition to such continuous measures of the body's physical state, the health-attribute vector may also include elements whose values are 0 or 1 to signify the absence or presence of qualitative characteristics. The 0, 1 elements of A might measure the presence or absence of such characteristics as inguinal hernia, stenoused (narrowed) cardiac value, or a fractured femur. Clearly, some configurations of the elements of A will be preferable to others.

The consumer has control over some, perhaps most, of the elements of A through his consumption of health-related goods and services (x). In a certain world, the level (or presence) of an attribute, A_t, will be a function of the initial level of health attributes (A_0) and the current consumption of x:

(1) $\quad A_t = f_t(x, A_0)$

where $\partial A_t/\partial x_i > 0$ and $\partial A_t/\partial x_i < 0$, respectively, define "health-enhancing" and "health-reducing" goods and services.

In an uncertain world, however, the selection of x will not be sufficient to define A unmistakably. First, independent of A_0 and of the chosen levels x, the individual may be exposed to random, health-related incidents that will alter A_t. These exogenous influences on healthiness—accidents over which the individual has no control—are represented here by the continuous random variable, $\tilde{u}_t$.[5] There is a second source of uncertainty, however, which is at least equally important, the uncertainty regarding the health consequences of changes in any specific health-related good or service. Even knowing A_0, x, and $\tilde{u}$, the consumer often cannot predict perfectly the marginal health effectiveness of changes in x_i ($i = 1 \ldots N$). Indeed, medical science may not even know the exact marginal impact of each input. These uncertain input effects can be represented by a vector of continuous random variables, $\tilde{v}_t$, whose typical element is $\tilde{v}_{it}$. The random variables $\tilde{v}_{it}(i = 1 \ldots N; t = 1 \ldots T)$ represent the technological uncertainty of using health care inputs $x_i(i = 1 \ldots N)$ to affect attributes $A_t(t = 1 \ldots T)$. Given such uncertainty, the health attribute production function must be generalized to:

(1a) $\tilde{A}_t = f_t(x, A_0, \tilde{u}_t, \tilde{v}_t)$

Here, A_t itself is a random variable whose distribution, conditional on x and past attributes A_0, is defined by $f(\cdot)$ and the distributions of $\tilde{u}_t$ and the $\tilde{v}_{it}$'s.[6]

The consumer's allocation behavior can now be characterized by the selection of a vector x and a vector y that maximize expected utility, where health attributes, $\tilde{A}$, are random variables conditional on x. The commodities in y are assumed to affect satisfaction directly and with certainty. The health-related goods—in addition to their (uncertain) effects on A—may also generate direct and certain consumer satisfaction. For example, food, cigarettes, and exercise can provide direct consumption benefits. Doctor visits can be a source of comfort and emotional support; hospitals often provide very attractive "hotel" services. Health-related goods (x) play a dual role. Expected utility therefore assumes the general form:

(2) $V = \int \ldots \int U[\, y, x, \tilde{A}(x)]\, \cdot f(A_1 \ldots A_T) \cdot dA_1 \ldots dA_T$

Consumers are assumed to purchase x and y so as to maximize V subject to constraints on their time and income.

Assuming that V is a continuous concave function, that the income and time constraints are linear, and that the distributions of $\tilde{u}_t$ and $\tilde{v}_{it}$ are independent and members of the class of two parameter distributions, a vector of health care demand functions of the form:

(3) $x_i = \phi_i(p_x, p_y, I \mid \mu_1 \ldots \mu_T, \sigma^2_{u_1} \ldots \sigma^2_{u_T}; \beta_{11} \ldots \beta_{NT}, \sigma^2_{v_{11}} \ldots \sigma^2_{v_{NT}}; A_0)$

can be specified, where p_x is the vector of prices (including a wage as the price of leisure) for x, p_y is the vector of prices for y, I is exogenous income, and A_0 is the vector of initial attribute levels. The parameters μ_t and $\sigma^2_{u_t}$ define the "location"(e.g., mean) and the "spread" (e.g., variance), respectively, for the distributions of

$\tilde{u}_t$; β_{it} and $\sigma^2_{v_{it}}$ define the location and spread of the distribution of $\tilde{v}_{it}$.[7]

Given the vectors μ, σ^2_u, β, and σ^2_v, the demand schedules in (3) display the usual Slutsky properties with respect to exogenous shifts in prices and income. No general *a priori* predictions about the demand effects of changes in the elements of μ, σ^2_u, β, or σ^2_v, are possible, however.[8] The effect on health care consumption of changes in an uncertain health care technology is an empirical issue. Sections 3 and 4 provide one set of answers in the context of the family's provision for its children's health.

3. THE FAMILY'S PROVISION FOR ITS CHILDREN'S HEALTH: A MODEL SPECIFICATION

The model developed here, and formally tested in Section 4, is an application to children's health of the demand analysis presented in Section 2. Specifically, the model is an attempt to structure the family's decisions to spend income and parents' time on three child health-related goods and services—curative care ("illness-motivated") doctor visits, preventive care ("check-up") doctor visits, and parents' time with children.

The focus of the model is on the mother. She is assumed to be the decision-maker for and the family's provider of child health services. It is her scarce time that is used in raising the child and her preferences define the family's choices for child health care. She is assumed to be predominantly interested in her and her family's direct consumption benefits of having healthy children.[9]

Four facts of the family's environment will be taken as given when the mother decides on the level and mix of child health care activities—(1) the level of health insurance coverage, (2) the family's usual provider of doctor care, (3) the mother's work status, and (4) the number of children in the family. Each of the four factors may, of course, influence the level of doctor visits and parents' time with children (we will test for this), but the factors themselves are assumed to be unaffected by changes in the consumption of the three health care commodities. I will discuss the validity and implication of these assumptions when the statistical results are reported in Section 4.

The model will be tested against data from a National Academy of Science, Institute of Medicine, survey of Washington, D.C., families. The survey includes detailed information on children's utilization of health care facilities, family socioeconomic information, and, important for this study, the results of a thorough ear, nose, and throat examination by an independent NAS team of physicians.[10] The sample is composed predominantly of black children between the ages of six months and twelve years from lower- and middle-income families (see the Data Appendix).

The analysis will be developed in two steps. First, a health attribute production function corresponding to (1a) will be specified (Part A, below) and estimated for children's ear, nose, and throat diseases (Part A, Section 4). Next, the results of the production function model will be integrated into our demand equation specifications (Part B, below) and these demand equations will be estimated (Part B, Section 4). The demand results will offer a first test of the health care demand specification presented in Equation (3) of Section 2.

A.

The health attribute production function specified here is for children's ear, nose, and throat infections. Table 1 summarizes the prevalence rates for the major ENT diseases in the NAS sample population. Approximately 11 per cent of the children were found

TABLE 1 Prevalence of ENT Diseases in NAS Children Survey

	Prevalence
Ear Infections	
Acute Serous Otitis Media	.0603
Acute Suppurative Otitis Media	.0145
Acute External Otitis Media	.0052
Nose Infections	
Acute Nasopharyngitis (common cold) plus Acute Rhinitis	
Throat Infections	
Acute Tonsillitis	.0017
Acute Pharyngitis (sore throat)	.0005
Total	.1077

to be suffering from some ENT disease, the major source of illness being ear infections. This study will concentrate on two aspects of this disease pattern—(1) a "clean bill" of ENT health with no diagnosed ENT infections at the time of medical examination (denoted by NOSICK), and (2) the absence of diagnosed inner ear infection (denoted by NOEARINF).[11] In both cases the dependent health attribute is specified as a dichotomous sick (0) or not sick (1) variable. In effect we are trying to explain the probability that a child from the sample will have an ENT disease.

The functional form chosen for the NOSICK and NOEARINF attribute models is the logit specification, which can be written as:

$$(4) \qquad ln\left(\frac{p_t}{1-p_t}\right) = lnA_0 + \sum_i \tilde{v}_{it} \cdot x_i + \tilde{u}_t$$

where p_t is the child's probability of NOSICK or NOEARINF, A_0 is a measure of the child's initial health state, x_i is the child's consumption of health care commodities, and the $\tilde{v}_{it}$'s and $\tilde{u}_t$ are random coefficients reflecting the uncertainty of the health care process. In the work that follows, $\tilde{v}_{it}$ is assumed to be normally distributed with mean β_{it} and variance $\sigma^2_{v_{it}}$ whereas $\tilde{u}_t$ is assumed to be normally distributed with mean 0 and variance $\sigma^2_{u_t}$.[12]

The child's initial health state, A_0, is summarized by three variables. The presence (EARSCAR = 1) or absence (EARSCAR = 0) of significant scarring of the tympanic membrane describes the child's history of inner ear infections. A history of three or more colds a year (COLDHIST = 1, otherwise 0) is also used to measure a susceptibility to ENT infections. In addition, the age of the child (AGE) is included in our health attribute model. Previous epidemiological studies have shown that older children are less susceptible to inner ear infections.[13]

The health care goods that are assumed to influence a child's chances of ENT infections are the number of preventive doctor visits (DOCPRV) in the past year, the number of curative doctor visits (DOCCUR) *for ENT infections* in the past six months, and the average number of hours per day one or both parents spend with the child in play or conversation (PARTIME/N).[14] Family income per person (INCPC) is used as a single measure of the quality of the family's *material* environment. Unlike studies of adult healthiness, in which income and health are simultaneously determined, it is reasonable to assume for this study of children's ENT health that there is only the one direction of causation—from income to health.

DOCPRV, DOCCUR, PARTIME/N, and INCPC are expected to enhance health and therefore are positively related to the child's probability of NOSICK and NOEARINF. EARSCAR and COLDHIST should be negatively related and the child's AGE positively related to the probability of the healthy state.

The two fundamental premises of the health care production-demand model of Section 2 were (1) that the effects of health inputs on health outputs will differ across inputs and be uncertain, and (2) that consumers will adjust their consumption in response to perceived changes in this health technology.

It is hypothesized here that the average effects of health inputs (DOCPRV, DOCCUR, PARTIME/N) on health outputs (NOSICK, NOEARINF) and the variability of these effects will depend on the education of the mother and the professional source of health care. There is some sociological evidence to suggest that more highly educated parents follow a physician's advice more closely and are more likely to know the warning signals of illness than are parents with less education.[15] For both reasons we anticipate the average effect (β_{it}) of care to rise and the uncertainty $(\sigma^2_{v_{it}})$ to fall as the mother's education rises.

The provider of medical services may also influence β and σ^2_v. The doctor's role is not only to diagnose illness and dispense office care but to educate patients and encourage good curative and preventive health practices. The provider format that permits continued personal physcian care is more likely to succeed in this education-encouragement task. All else equal, patients receiving care from solo private physicians or small-group practitioners may therefore face higher β's and lower σ^2_v's than patients receiving care from public clinics or outpatient services.

To test for the differential effects of education and provider type on the means and variances of health care inputs, our health attribute production functions will be estimated for four subsamples of the NAS survey population: (1) a low education (mother's education less than eight years)-public (clinic and outpatient) provider sample, (2) a high school education (mother's education nine–twelve years)-public provider sample, (3) a high school education-private (solo and group) provider sample, and (4) a college-private provider sample.

In Section 4, Part A, I will present and discuss estimates of the production function of children's ENT health.

B.

The mother's allocation problem, as characterized in Section 2, is to spend family income and parents' time on non-health goods and

DOCCUR, DOCPRV, and PARTIME in order to maximize family satisfaction, of which the uncertain ENT health of the children forms an integral part. The basic demand specification for the three health goods is given by (3) and elaborated by the following extensions.

Income and Prices

The demand model tested here distinguishes between working and nonworking mothers, and separate demand systems will be estimated for each. Both mothers face income and time constraints, but the specification of the two constraints for the two types of mothers differs and this difference generates testably distinct demand models.

Both working and nonworking mothers are limited to 24-hour days, 365 days a year. Their scarce time can be allocated to activities without the children (t_L), time with the children (PARTIME), time invested in providing doctor visits for the children (t_v), and, for the working mother, time on the job (t_w). The time required for doctor visits (t_v) is defined by the number of visits multiplied by the time cost per visit (TIMCOST). The time cost per visit equals the travel time to and from the physician plus waiting time at the office or clinic.[16] As I have assumed that the family's source of physician care is predetermined, TIMCOST is exogenous in this analysis and plays the role of a parameter in the household's consumption technology—t_v = TIMCOST*(DOCPRV + DOCCUR). The yearly time constraint is therefore:

$$(5) \qquad T = t_L + \text{PARTIME} + \text{TIMCOST*(DOCPRV + DOCCUR)} + t_w$$

where $t_w > 0$ for working mothers and $t_w = 0$ for nonworking mothers. Assuming mother needs eight hours a day to herself for personal health and sanity, $T = 16*365 = 5,840$ hours.

The income constraint (INC) facing the working and nonworking mother is defined by the level of husband's earnings (h, assumed exogenous) plus family nonwork income (z, also exogenous). For the working wife there is an additional source of income equal to working time (t_w) times her (exogenously set) hourly wage (WIFWAGE).[17] Thus, the yearly income constraint is given by:

$$(6) \qquad \text{INC} = h + z + \text{WIFWAGE*}t_w$$

where again $t_w > 0$ for working mothers and $t_w = 0$ for nonworking mothers.

The purchase of non-health-related goods and services (y) costs

p_y per bundle, whereas a preventive or curative doctor visit costs a doctor's fee per visit (DOCFEE).[18] The family's income constraint limits the purchase of y and DOCPRV and DOCCUR by:

(6a) $INC = p_y \cdot y + DOCFEE^* (DOCCUR + DOCPRV)$

Maximizing the mother's expected utility subject to the time (5) and income (6a) constraints yields (a la Section 2) a health care demand system for nonworking mothers $(t_w = 0)$ of the form:

(7) $PARTIME = f_0(p_y, DOCFEE, TIMCOST, INC|\cdot)$

(8) $DOCPRV = g_0(p_y, DOCFEE, TIMCOST, INC|\cdot)$

(9) $DOCCUR = h_0(p_y, DOCFEE, TIMCOST, INC|\cdot)$

and for working mothers $(t_u > 0)$ of the form:

(10) $PARTIME = f_w(p_y, FULINC, FULFEE, WIFWAGE|\cdot)$

(11) $DOCPRV = g_w(p_y, FULINC, FULFEE, WIFWAGE|\cdot)$

(12) $DOCCUR = h_w(p_y, FULINC, FULFEE, WIFWAGE|\cdot)$

where $FULINC = h + z + T^*WIFWAGE$, and $FULFEE = DOCFEE + WIFWAGE^*TIMCOST$. As the NAS survey of households does not give estimates of h and z, FULINC is approximated by $(T\text{-}2,000)^*WIFWAGE + INC$ under the assumption that all working mothers work forty hours a week for fifty weeks each year. The direction and extent of bias this assumption introduces in our estimate of income effects are discussed in Section 4.

The specification of the working-mother model in (10)–(12) has implicitly assumed that the woman is free to vary working hours, t_w, to meet her preferences. This may or may not be true. If the woman is constrained to work $\bar{t}_w$ hours or not at all, the working-mother's time constraint changes to:

(5a) $T - \bar{t}_w = T_H = t_L + PARTIME + TIMCOST^*(DOCCUR + DOCPRV)$

where T_H measures available time for "home" activities. The income constraint reduces to a fixed $INC = h + z + WIFWAGE^*\bar{t}_w$. Under this assumption of rationed work hours, the derived demand system for the working wife becomes:

(10a) $PARTIME = f_{wr}(p_y, INC, DOCFEE, TIMCOST, T_H|\cdot)$

(11a) $DOCPRV = g_{wr}(p_y, INC, DOCFEE, TIMCOST, T_H|\cdot)$

(12a) $DOCCUR = h_{wr}(p_y, INC, DOCFEE, TIMCOST, T_H|\cdot)$

The "rationed" (10a)–(12a) and the "equilibrium" (10)–(12) working-wife models will be compared in Section 4.

The Demand Effects of an Uncertain Health Care Technology

Estimates of the ENT health attribute production function will provide estimates of the average impact of care and the variability or uncertainty of that impact on ENT health for each of the three inputs for each of the four wife education-provider type subsamples. The estimates of the average effects (β_{it}) of curative doctor care (MEANDOCC), preventive doctor visits (MEANDOCP), and parents' time (MEANPART) are given by the corresponding estimated regression coefficients from logit model in (4). Estimates of the uncertainty of input effects ($\sigma_{r_{it}}^2$) are provided by the square of the corresponding regression coefficient's standard error, normalized to a common sample size, and will be denoted by VARDOCC, VARDOCP, and VARPART, respectively. These estimates of means (β_{it}'s) and variances ($\sigma_{r_{it}}^2$'s) from each of the four subsamples will then be used as child-specific independent variables in the demand models (7)–(12a) to test for the effects of changes in health care technology on the demand for health-related goods and services.

An *a priori* motivation for this specification of the β's and σ_r^2's in our demand model is to assume that the mother behaves as a Bayesian. Starting with an uninformative (flat) prior distribution on the β's, she observes a sample of children passing through the health care system—her own children and her neighbors'—and subjectively "estimates" a posterior distribution. This posterior distribution will correspond to the distribution of our maximum likelihood estimates of the parameters of the logit health care technology. The sample of children used to obtain each mother's posterior distribution is assumed to come from that mother's education-provider subgroup.[19]

The Child's Health

The healthiness of a child at the time of the mother's decision to consume health services is also expected to influence household allocations. A child with a history of past illnesses may be more susceptible to ENT diseases and thus induce closer monitoring by parents and doctor. Using a history of colds (COLDHIST = 1, 0 otherwise) as an indicator of susceptibility, we expect COLDHIST to be positively related to PARTIME, DOCPRV, and DOCCUR. In addition, a child who displays current symptoms of illness will be more likely to be taken to the doctor for curative care. Our survey provides information on children's complaints of dizziness, earaches, loss of hearing, and plugged ears (EARPAIN = 1, 0 otherwise), which we expect to be positively related to the decision to seek curative care (DOCCUR).

How the mother reacts to health susceptibility and complaints of her children may be a function of the characteristics of the child and the family. Specifically, we test for the effects of child age (AGE), sex (MALE), and the number of other children in the family under twelve (N) on the mother's decision to seek care given the presence of COLDHIST or EARPAIN.

Parent Preferences and Health Attitudes

Parents' attitudes toward the medical care system as well as their view of children's role in the family should also influence the family's demand for child health care. Such attitudes are introduced as (1,0) dummy variables. One might expect parents who profess to have faith in the curative power of doctors (DOCFAITH = 1) to be more likely to use curative care, perhaps at the expense of preventive care and parents' time. Parents who consider their health to be good or excellent (PARHEAL = 1) are presumably enjoying the benefits of healthiness and therefore wish to protect the health of their children—either to further protect their own health or because healthy parents and healthy children are complements for many consumption activities. Future-oriented parents (FUTURE = 1)—indicated by disagreement with the statement "Nowadays a person has to live pretty much for today and let tomorrow take care of itself"—might presumably be sensitive to the investment as well as the consumption benefits of health care and thus increase health-enhancing activities. Also included are variables to reflect possible difference in reference group norms in regard to the importance and/or effectiveness of health care—(BLACK = 1) if the family is black and (RELIGION = 1) if the family attends religious services once or more a week. The final family variable tested is whether the mother is currently married (MARD = 1, 0 otherwise). There may be some sharing of child-raising tasks, thereby reducing the *individual* time costs of the activities causing an increase in demand.

The Demand System's Error Structure

The demand specification is completed by the assumption of an additive influence of a random error term (w_i) in each demand equation, where:

(13) $E(w_i) = 0, E(w_i^2) = \sigma_{wi}^2$

The error term from demand equation i (say, DOCCUR) is distributed $N(0, \sigma_{wi}^2)$ and need *not* be independent of the error term from demand equation j (say, DOCPRV), distributed as $N(0, \sigma_{wi}^2)$. That is, $E(w_i, w_j) \neq 0$ is assumed for this health care demand system.

4. THE FAMILY'S PROVISION FOR ITS CHILDREN'S HEALTH: MODEL ESTIMATION

The results of the model's estimation are summarized below. Part A presents and discusses the estimation of the ENT health attribute production functions. Part B summarizes the testing of our model of the demand for child health care.

A.

Table 2 presents the maximum likelihood estimates of the parameters of the logistic specification for the NOSICK and NOEARINF health attributes for the four education-provider subsamples of our child population. The maximum likelihood estimation procedure converged in all case within ten iterations. The test statistic for the overall significance of the production model, -2 log (likelihood ratio), is distributed as χ^2 with seven degrees of freedom and is reported in the final column. The χ^2 values are all highly significant except for the high school private subsample. For this subsample, we can reject the null hypothesis that all β_{it}'s are in fact zero at the 0.84 confidence level for the NOSICK equation but at only the 0.5 level for the NOEARINF equation.

The parameter estimates for the child's health history (EARSCAR, COLDHIST) are negative, as expected, and generally exceed their standard errors. Also, as expected, older children (AGE) have fewer colds, fewer ear infections, and are generally healthier. Family income per person (INCPC) is never a significant determinant of children's ENT health, though there is some reason to believe this measured effect of income is biased toward zero. (see below, Note 22).

The parameter estimates for curative doctor visits (DOCCUR) were developed in two stages to remove a possible simultaneity between DOCCUR and the presence of illness. DOCCUR informa-

TABLE 2 Health Attribute Production Functions

								—Dependent Variable: NOSICK—	
Sample	PARTIME/N	DOCPRV	DOCCUR	INCPC	EARSCAR	COLDHIST	AGE	CONSTANT	χ^2 (DOF = 7)
Eighth grade–public	3.59[b]	−1.23[b]	4.37[a]	−.44	−1.31[a]	−.51	.33	−3.13	14.05
(n = 136)	(1.65)	(.55)	(2.70)	(.42)	(.78)	(.88)	(.17)	(2.93)	
High school–public	−.01	.01	1.46[b]	−.06	−1.16[b]	−.62[b]	.26[b]	−.05	34.89
(n = 718)	(.3)	(.15)	(.71)	(.17)	(.48)	(.27)	(.07)	(.83)	
High school–private	.11	.04	−.32	−.12	−1.19	−.14	−.15[a]	2.11[a]	10.43
(n = 469)	(.41)	(.24)	(1.03)	(.21)	(.83)	(.38)	(.10)	(1.32)	
College–private	−.45	.47[b]	.45	−.05	−.71	.68	.34[b]	−.42	30.23
(n = 369)	(.32)	(.23)	(.45)	(.17)	(1.03)	(.40)	(.08)	(.81)	

								—Dependent Variable: NOEARINF—	
Sample	PARTIME/N	DOCPRV	DOCCUR	INCPC	EARSCAR	COLDHIST	AGE	CONSTANT	χ^2 (DOF = 7)
Eighth grade–public	5.80[b]	−1.62[b]	4.11	−.59	−1.36[a]	−.71	.24	−2.41	14.58
(n = 136)	(2.51)	(.75)	(3.29)	(.59)	(.84)	(1.15)	(.20)	(3.54)	
High school–public	.30	.10	.69	−.27	−1.61[b]	−.61[b]	.32[b]	.68	42.21
(n = 718)	(.37)	(.19)	(.88)	(.20)	(.52)	(.33)	(.09)	(1.06)	
High school–private	.45	−.37	.23	.18	−1.49	.70	.15	1.97	6.45
(n = 469)	(.74)	(.35)	(1.48)	(.38)	(1.12)	(.70)	(.16)	(2.01)	
College–private	−.16	.66[b]	−.04	.13	−1.18	.35	.36[b]	−.24	23.32
(n = 369)	(.41)	(.29)	(.56)	(.22)	(1.09)	(.50)	(.10)	(1.01)	

NOTE: Standard errors within parentheses.
[a] Coefficient significantly different from zero at the 0.90 level for a two-sided asymptotic t test.
[b] Coefficient significantly different from zero at the 0.95 level for a two-sided asymptotic t test.

tion was obtained from a family questionnaire administered from December 1970 to April 1971. The medical examinations of the children to determine the presence of ENT infections were begun in January 1971. Since illness does determine DOCCUR (see the role of EARPAIN in tables 4 and 5), a simultaneous equation bias in the production function estimates is therefore a danger. To try to remove this bias, the maximum likelihood estimates in Table 2 are based on a predicted value of DOCCUR as the independent variable, where the exogenous determinants of DOCCUR are the nonillness independent variables (prices, income, non-health-related child characteristics, parent attitudes) of the DOCCUR demand equation.[20]

Six of the eight DOCCUR coefficients are positive, as expected, but only two are significantly different from zero. There are two possible reasons for the insignificant effects of DOCCUR. First, for many ENT infections the physician can provide little in the way of direct and effective treatment. For most viral infections, for example, the physician's role is to monitor the disease and to minimize the long-run dangers rather than to "cure" the present illness. But second, in cases wherein physicians can offer effective care, particularly by prescribing antibiotics, patients may often receive this care by phone rather than through an office visit. The parents describe the symptoms and the doctor calls the pharmacy. This format for care is most likely to be used by patients with private physicians in which a "trusting" doctor-parent relationship has been established. Indeed, we notice that curative visits are never significant for the private provider subsamples.

DOCCUR is significant and quite important for children using public providers. Why? First, when doctors and drugs can help, children using public providers must generally go for an office visit to receive their prescription. Because public clinic physicians rarely know the parents personally, the phone cannot be used for a substitute office visit. Second, and perhaps more important, in the many instances in which the physician cannot provide an effective treatment for the present ENT incident, the curative visit may still be a useful preventive encounter. The causes and dangers of the child's present illness are explained to the parent, who also can be taught to look for warning signals and to administer future preventive measures. The parent and the child learn by the *example* of the present illness. Thus curative visits in the past can be an important source of present preventive practices, thereby having a significant positive impact on NOSICK.

Preventive doctor visits—check-ups—have a significant positive effect on health for children only with college-educated mothers using private providers. This seems reasonable since the check-up visit with a private physician often is a lesson in child health practices as well. Because college-educated mothers are more likely to ask questions and to understand the answers, the impact on children's health should be greater for this group. The significant but *negative* sign for preventive visits in the eighth grade-public sample is a bit of a puzzle. Rather than argue that public clinics are a depository of infectious diseases (thus the more you visit, the lower the likelihood of health), the cause of this perverse sign is more likely statistical. Our model is probably not well specified for this subsample. Specifically, for these children COLDHIST is not an adequate control for the presence of chronic, perhaps allergic, ENT infections. COLDHIST is defined by *the parents' response* to the question, "Does your child have three or more colds a year?" For each of the other three subsamples, about 35 per cent of the children were described by their parents as having a history of colds. The corresponding figure for the eighth grade-public sample was 25 per cent, suggesting a possible under-reporting of children with potentially chronic ENT problems. If this is so, and if clinic doctors have encouraged the mothers of these children to come in for regular check-ups, then the negative sign can be explained.

Parents' time per child is significant, positive, and quantitatively important only for children from the eighth grade-public sample. There are reasons, however, to believe that the coefficients on PARTIME/N may be biased downward. Parents' time per child is an "input" not only for the provision of children's physical health but for other child attributes as well, especially sense of self and intellectual development. As these other facets of child development are likely to be produced jointly with health, any production function of health that omits these "joint products" from the specification will likely lead to biased input coefficient estimates. The difference between the estimated and the true input coefficients defines the bias and can be measured by $\beta_{EST} - \beta_{TRUE} = \partial, \xi$, where ∂ is the coefficient of the omitted variable (self-worth, IQ) regressed on the included variables (PARTIME/N in this instance) and ξ is the coefficient of the omitted variable regressed on the dependent variable (NOSICK, NOEARINF). As parents' time per child is likely to be positively related to self-worth and IQ, ∂ will be positive. If we treat child development as a truly joint production process, then over most ranges of the "outputs" the output attributes will be inversely related to one another, *given parental inputs.* Thus ξ will be negative.[21] If these arguments are valid, then $\beta_{\text{TRUE}} > \beta_{\text{EST}}$ for PARTIME/N; the estimates in Table 2 are biased toward zero.[22]

Do the ENT health care technologies described in Table 2 differ across the four education-provider subsamples and, if so, is there a pattern to these differences? Table 3 summarizes our estimates of this technology for overall ENT health. Mean effects of the three health care inputs (β_{it}) are equal to the coefficients from NOSICK, whereas estimates of the variances of their effects ($\sigma^2_{v_{it}}$) are set equal to the squared value of the coefficients' standard errors after normalizing standard error estimates for a common sample size ($n = 200$). Formal tests for the equality of the β_{it}'s and of the $\sigma^2_{v_{it}}$'s can be offered, assuming that the underlying distribution of our parameter estimates is normal. However, the asymptotic properties of the "instrumental variable" logit estimator used to derive β_{it} are not known, so such formal tests for equality of coefficients are probably misplaced.[23]

A casual inspection of the parameter estimates in Table 3 does suggest that children from different mother education-provider subsamples are exposed to different health care technologies. And there appears to be a pattern to these technological differences. The simple correlations of mother's years of schooling with each child's assigned (by membership in a subsample) values of β_{it} and $\sigma^2_{v_{it}}$ show a positive relationship of parental education to β_{it} for DOCPRV (0.85) and negative relationships between education and β_{it} for PARTIME/N(-0.74), β_{it} for DOCCUR (-0.59), and for all $\sigma^2_{v_{it}}$'s (-0.72 for $\sigma^2_{v_{it}}$ for PARTIME/N; -0.44 for DOCPRV; -0.86 for DOCCUR). Comparing the high school-public provider and the high school-private provider subsamples, the children using public providers can expect higher average effects from curative doctor

TABLE 3 The Logit Technology for Children's ENT Health

| | Health Care Inputs | | | | | |
| | PARTIME/N | | DOCPRV | | DOCCUR | |
Sample	β_i	$\sigma^2_{v_i}$	β_i	$\sigma^2_{v_i}$	β_i	$\sigma^2_{v_i}$
Eighth grade–public	3.59	1.84	−1.23	.20	4.37	5.15
High school–public	−.01	.31	.01	.07	1.46	1.86
High school–private	.11	.39	.04	.14	−.32	2.44
College–private	−.45	.20	.47	.10	.45	.36

visits and a lower variance but lower average effects with lower variances for preventive visits.[24]

This pattern of effects of parental education on the ENT technology does not lend strong support to our original hypothesis of a positive relationship between parental education and the effectiveness of health care inputs. Only for preventive visits (DOCPRV) do we see a clear dominance favoring the health technology "available" to children with more highly educated mothers—the average effect rises and the variance falls as education rises.

As mother's education rises, parental time per child has a smaller average impact on health, but the variance or uncertainty of that impact declines as well. But because of the likely bias in our estimate of the PARTIME/N coefficient, this conclusion must be considered tentative at best. Although our earlier arguments have pointed toward a downward bias in estimates of the PARTIME/N coefficient, it may also be true that this bias is greatest for the subsamples with more highly educated mothers. This will be true *if* the impact of a given amount of parents' time on child IQ and sense of self-worth rises as parental education rises. There is some evidence that this is so.[25] If the marginal impact of parents' time on IQ and self-worth (as measured by $\partial > 0$) rises as mother's education rises, and if the tradeoff of child health and IQ or self-worth (measured as $\xi < 0$) does not fall in absolute value as education rises, then our measure of downward bias in β_{it}, $\partial\xi$, will be larger in absolute value for children in the more highly educated mother subsample. The results above may therefore underestimate the true, perhaps positive, relationship between parental education and the average health effectiveness of time with children.

The apparent dominance of public over private providers in Washington, D.C. (discussed above) may explain, in part, the negative correlation between mother's education and the average effect of DOCCUR. Because the lower-educated mothers almost always use public providers (which increases β for this sample) and college-educated mothers always use private providers, we are not able to identify the separate education and provider influences on the family's health technology for these two groups. If the measured positive effect of public providers dominates the (assumed) positive effect of education, then the negative correlations between β_{DOCCUR} and mother's education will result.

Although the evidence here does not force us to reject our original hypothesis that education can improve the health technology, neither does it give it strong support. Overall, the results are more suggestive than conclusive. Although health care services do appear on balance to have a positive effect on children's ENT health, the observed outcomes for any particular child are quite uncertain. The estimates in Table 3 are best interpreted not as a true measure of the best ENT care technology but rather as selected families' perceptions of their received technology. Such an interpretation will still be sufficient for testing the effects of an uncertain technology on the demand for health care commodities. The results are reported in Part B below.

B.

Tables 4 and 5 summarize the results from estimating the demand model for working and nonworking mothers, respectively.

The estimation procedure in all cases was ordinary least squares, which, because each demand equation in the model specifies an identical vector of independent variables, also provides maximum likelihood estimates with our assumed error structure.[26] Given the four assumptions outlined at the beginning of Section 3—the assumed exogeneity of health insurance coverage, family provider of physician services, mother's work status, and number of children—ordinary least squares rather than a two-staged least squares procedure will be justified.[27]

Estimated equations (1a), (2a), and (3a) (Table 4) correspond to a *linearization* of the "equilibrium" specification for working mothers defined by (10)–(12). FULINC is positively related to preventive and curative doctor visits (normal goods) but *negatively* (and significantly) related to parents' time with children. As expected, an increase in FULFEE reduces doctor visits and also reduces parents' time with children. WIFWAGE, the "price" of parents' time with children, is *positively* related to PARTIME and negatively related to doctor visits.

If taken at face value, the results from Equation (1a) suggest that for working mothers "time with children" is an inferior good with respect to income changes and a Giffen good with respect to changes in the price of time, WIFWAGE. There is an alternative and perhaps more plausible explanation for these results. For employed women in our sample with relatively high-paying jobs, the labor market does not permit them to work as many hours as they wish at their current wage. Women who are constrained to work fewer hours than they prefer value market time more highly than time in home activities. Thus, for women in high-paying occupations, children doctor visits that often require time off from

TABLE 4 Working Mothers' Demand for Health Care Activities (n = 880)

Independent Variables	PARTIME			DOCPRV			DOCCUR		
	(1a)	(1b)	(1c)	(2a)	(2b)	(2c)	(3a)	(3b)	(3c)
INC	—	-.0094[a] (.0053)	—	—	.0196[b] (.0084)	—	—	.017 (.014)	—
FULINC	-.00011[b] (.000005)	—	-.0000094[a] (.0000055)	.000020[b] (.000008)	—	.000015 (.000009)[a]	.000017 (.000015)	—	.000019 (.000014)
FULFEE	-.0047[b] (.0021)	—	—	-.0099[b] (.0032)	—	—	-.012[b] (.005)	—	—
DOCFEE	—	-.0046[b] (.0021)	-.0043[b] (.0021)	—	-.0099[b] (.0033)	-.0097[b] (.0035)	—	-.011[b] (.006)	-.0091[a] (.0057)
TIMWAGE	—	—	-.013 (.012)	—	—	-.010 (.019)	—	—	-.0474 (.032)
WIFWAGE	.063[b] (.031)	—	.067[b] (.033)	-.072 (.048)	—	-.046 (.054)	-.068 (.081)	—	-.028 (.089)
TIMCOST	—	-.00058 (.00057)	—	—	-.00029 (.00091)	—	—	-.0018 (.0015)	—
MEANPART	—	—	.19[b] (.10)	—	—	—	—	—	—
VARPART	—	—	-.054[a] (.032)	—	—	—	—	—	—
MEANDOCP	—	—	—	—	—	.395[b] (.165)	—	—	—
VARDOCP	—	—	—	—	—	-.67 (.91)	—	—	—
MEANDOCC	—	—	—	—	—	—	—	—	-.034 (.056)

Variable									
COLLEGE	.14[a] (.08)	.14[a] (.08)	—	.24[b] (.13)	.25[a] (.12)	—	.3[a] (.21)	.39[b] (.20)	-.052 (.048)
HSPRV	.13[a] (.08)	.11 (.07)	—	.041 (.11)	.055 (.11)	—	.7 (.20)	.18 (.19)	—
HSPUB	-.0073 (.07)	-.011 (.07)	—	.11 (.11)	.11 (.11)	—	.10 (.18)	.12 (.18)	—
EARPAIN	—	—	—	—	—	—	.77[b] (.16)	.75[b] (.16)	.75[b] (.16)
COLDHIST	.047 (.037)	.049 (.036)	.049 (.036)	.18[b] (.058)	.17[b] (.06)	.17[b] (.06)	.40[b] (.10)	.41[b] (.09)	.41[b] (.09)
AGE	-.0079 (.0054)	-.0081 (.0055)	-.0081 (.0054)	-.086[b] (.008)	-.086[b] (.008)	-.073[b] (.008)	-.086[b] (.015)	-.073[b] (.014)	-.073[b] (.014)
MALE	-.018 (.033)	-.018 (.034)	-.019 (.033)	.05 (.05)	.056 (.053)	.057 (.054)	-.025 (.089)	-.029 (.088)	-.027 (.089)
N	-.019 (.015)	-.019 (.015)	-.019 (.015)	-.0026 (.023)	-.0041 (.023)	-.0038 (.025)	-.084[b] (.039)	-.084[b] (.039)	-.084[b] (.039)
DOCFAITH	.039 (.038)	.032 (.037)	.032 (.038)	-.14[b] (.059)	-.14[b] (.06)	-.122[b] (.062)	.081 (.099)	.076 (.098)	.11 (.10)
PARHEAL	.0046 (.046)	.012 (.045)	.016 (.047)	.144[b] (.072)	.14[b] (.07)	.15[b] (.075)	.044 (.12)	.04 (.12)	.11 (.12)
FUTURE	-.0013 (.034)	.0069 (.034)	.0076 (.025)	.085[b] (.054)	.074 (.054)	.061 (.058)	.025 (.09)	.029 (.09)	.044 (.093)
BLACK	-.12 (.09)	-.12 (.09)	-.15[a] (.09)	.011 (.14)	.005 (.11)	-.033 (.158)	.05 (.24)	.071 (.24)	-.021 (.244)
RELIGION	.067[a] (.039)	.066[a] (.039)	.063[a] (.041)	-.014 (.062)	-.012 (.062)	-.029 (.066)	.021 (.11)	.022 (.10)	.08 (.10)
MARD	.061 (.045)	.052 (.044)	.095[b] (.046)	.074 (.071)	.074 (.069)	.11 (.075)	-.12 (.12)	-.12 (.12)	-.12 (.12)
$\bar{R}^2$	.04	.04	.04	.19	.18	.14	.12	.11	.12

NOTE: Standard error within parentheses.
[a] Coefficient significantly different from zero at the 0.9 level.
[b] Coefficient significantly different from zero at the 0.95 level.

TABLE 5 Nonworking Mothers' Demand for Health Care Activities ($n = 812$)

Independent Variables	PARTIME (4a)	PARTIME (4b)	DOCPRV (5a)	DOCPRV (5b)	DOCCUR (6a)	DOCCUR (6b)
INC	−.0057 (.0058)	−.0028 (.0055)	.019^b (.010)	.0098 (.011)	.018 (.014)	.019 (.014)
DOCFEE	.0013 (.0024)	.0022 (.0026)	−.0025 (.0043)	−.0011 (.0046)	−.0073 (.0061)	−.0064 (.0066)
TIMCOST	−.0011^b (.00053)	−.0011^b (.00053)	−.0022^b (.00091)	−.0024^b (.0009)	−.0028^b (.0013)	−.0032^b (.0014)
MEANPART	—	−.14 (.11)	—			
VARPART	—	−.062^b (.026)	—			
MEANDOCP				.56^b (.22)		
VARDOCP	—	—		−1.75^b (.81)		
MEANDOCC						−.001 (.05)
VARDOCC	—	—	—	—		−.0085 (.05)
COLLEGE	.16^b (.072)	—	.48^b (.12)	—	.17 (.18)	
HSPRV	.051 (.059)	—	.24^b (.10)	—	.14 (.15)	
HSPUB	.085^a (.052)	—	.29^b (.09)	—	.095 (.13)	
EARPAIN	—	—	—	—	.068 (.14)	.071 (.15)
COLDHIST	.041 (.036)	.042 (.037)	−.00035 (.062)	−.00042 (.007)	.54^b (.09)	.54^b (.09)
AGE	.0056 (.0053)	.0048 (.0047)	−.076^b (.0092)	−.076^b (.0091)	−.053^b (.013)	−.054^b (.014)
MALE	−.016 (.033)	−.021 (.019)	.013 (.057)	.015 (.06)	.097 (.083)	.11 (.08)
N	−.026^b (.013)	−.026^b (.013)	−.0068 (.023)	−.0054 (.031)	−.024 (.033)	−.032 (.033)
DOCFAITH	−.015 (.037)	−.0038 (.038)	−.0021 (.065)	−.024 (.069)	−.0058 (.094)	−.019 (.098)
PARHEAL	.036 (.037)	.025 (.038)	−.059 (.064)	−.035 (.068)	−.057 (.093)	−.017 (.097)

TABLE 5 (Concluded)

Independent Variables	Dependent Variables					
	——PARTIME——		——DOCPRV——		—DOCCUR—	
	(4a)	(4b)	(5a)	(5b)	(6a)	(6b)
FUTURE	$-.12^b$	$-.095^b$	.075	.035	$.26^b$	$.21^b$
	(.036)	(.036)	(.061)	(.065)	(.08)	(.092)
BLACK	$-.11^a$	$-.13^a$	.052	.052	$-.52^b$	$-.52^b$
	(.068)	(.068)	(.11)	(.12)	(.17)	(.17)
RELIGION	$-.011$	$-.0011$	.087	.011	$-.048$	.10
	(.038)	(.037)	(.065)	(.068)	(.095)	(.095)
MARD	.012	.013	19^b	$.23^b$	.062	.073
	(.043)	(.044)	(.075)	(.08)	(.11)	(.11)
$\bar{R}^2$	.04	.03	.15	.09	.11	.11

NOTE: Standard error within parentheses.
[a] Coefficient significantly different from zero at the 0.9 level.
[b] Coefficient significantly different from zero at the 0.95 level.

work are less attractive relative to off-work parent's time as a mechanism for protecting children's health. Therefore as WIF-WAGE rises, time with children is substituted for doctor visits. Indeed, WIFWAGE *as a cross-price effect* (i.e., with FULFEE included) is negatively related to DOCPRV (almost significant at the 0.9 level) and DOCCUR in equations (2a) and (3a).

This "rationed" working-mother model was tested directly in (1b), (2b), and (3b). On the criterion of minimizing the sum of squared residuals, the "equilibrium" model performed slightly better than the "rationed" model—1a(207.2) vs. 1b(207.8), 2a(513.2) vs. 2b(517.1), 3a(1434) vs. 3b(1438)—but the explanatory power of the two models for the whole sample is nearly identical. Equations (1c), (2c), and (3c) split FULFEE into its two components, DOCFEE and the product TIMCOST*WIFWAGE = TIMWAGE. If the "equilibrium" model is the correct specification, then the coefficients on DOCFEE and TIMWAGE should be nearly equal and equal to the coefficient on FULFEE. Only in the DOCPRV equation does this appear to hold. In the PARTIME and DOCCUR equations the coefficient on TIMWAGE is two to five times larger than the coefficient on DOCFEE.

On balance, then, the rationed working-hours model is probably closer to the truth, particularly for working mothers with higher wages. Unfortunately, our wage data are based on broad occupational grouping and do not give us enough variation to split the sample and test for this structural break directly. However, a "compromise" model was tested that included INC, DOCFEE, TIMCOST, and WIFWAGE, each as explanatory variables. The coefficient estimates for INC, DOCFEE, and TIMCOST were identical to those presented in (1b), (2b), and (3b), and the WIFWAGE coefficients were similar to the estimates in (1a), (2a), and (3a). The price and income results appear quite robust across all working-mother specifications.

Equations (1ab), (2ab), and (3ab) give a first test of the hypothesis that health care technologies influence health care consumption. Here education-provider dummy variables for each of our four subsamples were used in the demand equations. The eighth grade-public dummy was excluded to avoid singularity. The children in the college-private subsample (COLLEGE) receive significantly more of each health care input than do children in the high school-private (HSPRV), high school-public (HSPUB), or eighth grade-public subsamples. As the other likely effects of mother's education on health care consumption are accounted for in our model through WIFWAGE, N, and labor force participation, the education-provider dummy variables may be detecting consumption differences attributable to perceived differences in the family's health care technology. If so, and if the pattern of the ENT technology with respect to mother's education is as described in Table 3, then mothers are risk averse with respect to their children's health, preferring the low mean-low variance inputs to the high mean-high variance activities.

Equations (1c), (2c), and (3c) provide one direct test of the mean-variance hypotheses. From Table 3, the expected effects and the variance of the effects of the health care activities from each subsample for the NOSICK equation were assigned to each child according to his subsample membership. The only exception was that negative mean effects were assigned a value of zero under the assumption that mothers do not really believe doctors' or parents' time is detrimental to their children's health.

The coefficient estimates imply that changes in the uncertain health care technology do appear to affect consumption decisions in intuitively reasonable ways. An increase in the average health effectiveness of parents' time (MEANPART) increases the time working mothers spend with their children, whereas an increase in the uncertainty of those effects (VARPART) reduces time spent with children.[28] Both effects are significant. An increase in the effectiveness of preventive visits increases DOCPRV, whereas an increase in variance tends to reduce DOCPRV, but this last result is not statistically significant. DOCCUR appears unaffected by health care technology, suggesting that curative visits may be largely motivated by a desire for parental reassurance and comfort ("Have I done all that's possible?") rather than direct child health effects. From our previous results in (3ab), it appears that college-educated mothers are more sensitive to this reassurance motive.

The remainder of the results in Table 4 are straightforward and need no extensive interpretation. The health history of the child (EARPAIN, COLDHIST) influences the decision to seek care in the expected way. Older children (AGE) get less attention and less doctor care, as do children from larger families (N). There is no sign of sexual discrimination (MALE) by the working mother in her care for children. Religious mothers spend more time with their children; working black mothers spend slightly less time with their children. Healthy parents (PARHEAL) and future-oriented (FUTURE) parents tend to use preventive care more, whereas mothers with faith in the curative power of doctors (DOCFAITH) use preventive care less.

The pattern of the results for the nonworking-mother sample (Table 5) are generally similar to those for working mothers. We do, however, lose the inferior-good quality of parents' time with children. The coefficient on INC in the PARTIME equation is negative, but not significantly different from zero. DOCPRV and DOCCUR are normal goods. Changes in doctor fees (DOCFEE) have no appreciable effect on health care consumption, but changes in time costs per doctor visit are quite important. Higher doctor visit time costs reduce *all* health care activities, doctor visits as well as parents' time with children.

The effects of health care technology on health care consumption are basically similar to those observed for working mothers, except that the mean effect of parents' time on health is no longer a significant positive stimulus to PARTIME. DOCCUR is again immune to changes in the technology, suggesting that parental reassurance may be the key motivation for curative visits for nonemployed mothers as well as for working mothers.

In Table 6 are the elasticities (at the means) of the health care activities with respect to prices, income, technology, and the number of children in the family. Price elasticities (FULFEE, DOCFEE, TIMWAGE, WIFWAGE) rarely exceed 0.15 in absolute value, supporting previous results on the price insensitivity of health care demands.[29] Variation in the TIMCOST of doctor visits is one of the strongest determinants of utilization, particularly for

TABLE 6 Health Care Consumption Elasticities

Independent Variables	Dependent Variables					
	Working-Mother Sample			Nonworking-Mother Sample		
	PARTIME	DOCPRV	DOCCUR	PARTIME	DOCPRV	DOCCUR
INC	-.046	.243	.205	~0	.168	.152, .161
FULINC	-.12, -.10	.559, .419	.461, .516	—	—	—
FULFEE	-.022	-.116	-.137	—	—	—
DOCFEE	-.016, -.015	-.086, -.085	-.092, -.076	~0	~0	-.037, ~0
TIMWAGE	-.017	~0[a]	-.147	—	—	—
WIFWAGE	.099, .106	-.295, ~0	~0	—	—	—
TIMCOST	-.016	~0	-.119	-.032	-.170, -.186	-.208, -.237
MEANPART	.012	—	—	-.007	—	—
VARPART	-.032	.454	—	-.041	—	—
MEANDOCP	—	~0	—	—	.069	—
VARDOCP	—	—	—	—	-.265	—
MEANDOCC	—	—	~0	—	—	~0
VARDOCC	—	—	-.12	-.043	~0	~0
N	-.025	~0	-.270			

[a] If the t statistic for the variable is <1, the elasticity is defined ~0

nonworking mothers. Here the elasticities range from −0.17 for DOCPRV to −0.23 for DOCCUR.

The estimates of income elasticities show that the inferior-good influence of income on parents' time with children is only a mild one. For the working-mother sample, a 10 per cent rise in income leads to at most a 1 per cent fall in parents' time. There is no adverse effect of income on PARTIME for the nonworking-mother sample.

Estimates of the elasticity of doctor visits with respect to income center at 0.16 for the housewife sample and range from 0.2 to 0.56 in the working-mother sample, depending on the model specification—FULINC yielding the higher estimates. The results for FULINC appear to be biased upward, however, because of the assumption regarding working hours needed to define the variable. The true income elasticity is probably closer to 0.25.[30]

The sensitivity of DOCCUR and PARTIME to changes in the health care technology is slight, but the utilization of preventive visits (DOCPRV) does seem rather responsive to alterations in the perceived technology.

Finally, children in larger families have less time with parents, but the actual amount lost is very small. For the working-mother sample, however, there is a significant reduction in curative doctor visits as N increases.

5. TOWARD A PUBLIC POLICY FOR CHILDREN'S HEALTH

ENT infections are one of the most prevalent of childhood diseases. In addition to the discomfort for the child, parental anxiety, and lost days from school and work that such diseases generate, there are possible long-run implications to ENT illness as well. Left untreated, ear infections can lead to permanent hearing loss and/or damage to the child's central nervous system. Chronic ENT disease may mean poor school performance, poor adult health, and losses in future earnings.[31] If one of our health care objectives is to reduce the prevalence of this class of diseases, what policy instruments will work? Our empirical analysis of the family's provision of children's health provides some initial insight into this question. Table 7 lists the expected elasticities of a child's ENT health with respect to three prominently mentioned sets of policy instruments: (1) exogenous income and/or wage subsidies, (2) health insurance, and (3) the availability of care.

TABLE 7 The Elasticities of ENT Health with Respect to Economic Policy Instruments

		Target Population					
		Eighth Grade		High School		College	
Policy	Instrument	Working Mother	Nonworking Mother	Working	Nonworking	Working	Nonworking
Income	INC	.03	.02	.017	.013	.02	.014
	WIFWAGE	.016	—	*	—	*	—
Health insurance	DOCFEE	−.027	−.006	−.007	−.003	−.007	−.002
Access to care	TIMCOST	−.023	−.048	−.01	−.017	−.005	−.013

* See text.

The results are based on the elasticities in Table 6 and on calculated elasticities from Table 2 for the NOSICK and NOEARINF equations. For an upper estimate of the effectiveness of policy on children's ENT health, the higher of the two input elasticities from NOSICK and NOEARINF was used. A zero rather than a negative elasticity was assigned to DOCPRV in the eighth grade-public health equation and to PARTIME/N for the college-private health equation. The only elasticities that are substantially different from zero are 0.16 with respect to PARTIME/N and 0.17 with respect to DOCCUR for the eighth grade-public subsample, 0.082 with respect to DOCCUR for the high school-public subsample, and 0.045 with respect to DOCPRV and 0.041 with respect to DOCCUR for the college-private subsample. The elasticities in Table 7 are based on the sum of policy-induced changes in the use of health care inputs (PARTIME, DOCCUR, DOCPRV) times these average effects of inputs on health.[32] The results are disaggregated by the mother's educational level and work status.

Exogenous income transfers (INC) have a consistently positive effect on children's health, primarily through the inducement to buy more medical inputs. The effects of changes in the mother's wage is unclear. Children whose employed mothers have low levels of education are stimulated by the increase in WIFWAGE to substitute parents' time for less effective doctor visits. The net effect is an increase in the child's chances for ENT health. A similar conclusion probably holds for the employed mother, high school, and college subsamples as well, but a likely downward bias in our estimate of the effects of parent's time obscures this result.

A fall in the out-of-pocket costs of physician visits or in the time cost of such visits also has a positive net effect on a child's health prognosis. Such changes prompt an increase in use of physician services without inducing a sufficiently strong offsetting reduction in home care.

Although the effects of these policy changes on ENT health move in the expected direction, what is perhaps surprising is how small the average policy impact appears to be. Any sizable improvements in ENT health prospects resulting from these economic policy instruments will prove exceedingly costly. To increase the probability of NOSICK from 0.9 to 0.91—a 1 per cent improvement—may require an increase in income equal to about 50 per cent of husband's earnings (the main element in "exogenous" income) or a 25–50 per cent reduction in TIMCOST. A reduction in doctor fees appears no more effective. A 100 per cent reduction in out-of-pocket costs (from $6 to $0), as with universal coverage national health insurance, will increase the probability of no ENT infections for a child from about 0.9 to 0.91–0.93. And each of these calculations assumes no offsetting rise in TIMCOST or fall in quality of care, both of which may arise when increased aggregate demand hits the ambulatory care supply constraint. Whether these health gains can justify such costly policy measures remains to be seen.

The more effective policy strategies may be to improve medical technology and parental health knowledge or to alter the patterns of adult-child interactions. Improvements in medical technology or the health effectiveness of parents' time with children not only yield direct health payoffs through the attribute production function but also appear to induce an increased utilization of the more effective inputs. The net effect may be quite sizable. From our production and demand models, for example, a 10 per cent increase in the average health effectiveness of parents' time or doctor visits will lead to a 4 per cent increase in the probability of NOSICK for children whose mothers have an eighth grade education or less. For children in the higher mother-education subsamples a 1–2 per cent increase in probability of NOSICK may result. In addition, for children in the eighth grade sample, family planning or quality day care may be a useful policy for improving a present child's health prospect. Reducing the number of children under twelve (N) by half can lead to a 2 per cent increase in the probability of NOSICK.[33] The reduction in N increases parents' time with each child as well as the likelihood that a child, once sick, will be given curative care. These two effects have a significant pro-health impact for children in the lower-education subsample.

The point of presenting these numbers is not that they constitute a true basis for a children's health policy, but rather to argue that we should think seriously about analyzing policy alternatives that move beyond the usual income and price instruments of the economic model. At least for one important class of childhood diseases, improvements in health will not come easily. Efforts to influence the family's health performance through the economic parameters of price and income will yield only marginal improvements in children's ENT health. Changes in medical technology, parent health knowledge, and the patterns of adult-child interaction *may* be the more promising policy directions.

National health insurance may still be our protector against the financial risks of major illness, but it is not likely to be the cure for our children's runny noses.

DATA APPENDIX: VARIABLE DEFINITIONS

The variables are defined below and their means (variances) are given for each of the relevant subsamples.

Subsample Key

Eighth grade-public: 8GPUB   High school-public: HSPUB
High school-private: HSPRV   College-private: COLPRV
Working mothers: WM   Nonworking mothers: NWM

Variablo List

AGE: Age of the child in years.

8GPUB	HSPUB	HSPRV	COLPRV	WM	NWM
7.28	6.84	6.96	7.07	7.38	6.56
(11.07)	(10.27)	(9.14)	(10.65)	(9.80)	(10.24)

BLACK: 1 if child is black, 0 otherwise.

WM	NWM
.96	.93
(.03)	(.07)

COLDHIST: 1 if the child has three or more colds a year as reported by parents, 0 otherwise.

8GPUB	HSPUB	HSPRV	COLPRV	WM	NWM
.25	.34	.36	.35	.34	.32
(.20)	(.21)	(.23)	(.23)	(.22)	(.21)

DOCCUR: Number of visits to the doctor within the last six months for ENT diseases as reported by the parents.

8GPUB	HSPUB	HSPRV	COLPRV	WM	NWM
.65	.63	.73	.96	.72	.72
(1.01)	(1.36)	(1.81)	(2.58)	(1.85)	(1.54)

DOCFAITH: 1 if parents agree with "Doctors can cure most serious diseases"; 0 otherwise.

WM	NWM
.72	.73
(.19)	(.19)

DOCFEE: Average out-of-pocket costs for doctor visits as reported by parents.

WM	NWM
5.99	3.63
(64.80)	(53.29)

DOCPRV: Number of doctor check-ups for the child per year as reported by the parents.

8GPUB	HSPUB	HSPRV	COLPRV	WM	NWM
.42	.66	.69	.99	.70	.69
(.56)	(.79)	(.72)	(.74)	(.72)	(.77)

EARPAIN: 1 if child has complained to parents in last two weeks of loss of hearing, dizziness, earaches, plugged ears; 0 otherwise.

WM	NWM
.083	.098
(.07)	(.09)

EARSCAR: 1 if either left or right ear shows scarring of tympanic membrane, 0 otherwise.

8GPUB	HSPUB	HSPRV	COLPRV
.04	.026	.025	.018
(.04)	(.034)	(.024)	(.029)

FUTURE: 1 if parents disagree with "Nowadays, a person has to live pretty much for today and let tomorrow take care of itself"; 0 otherwise.

WM	NWM
.51	.41
(.25)	(.24)

INC: Annual family income in 000's.

WM	NWM
8.69	6.11
(19.27)	(17.22)

INCPC: Annual family income per member of family in 000's.

8GPUB	HSPUB	HSPRV	COLPRV
.87	1.11	1.84	2.55
(.71)	(.62)	(1.04)	(1.39)

MALE: 1 if child is a male, 0 otherwise.

WM	NWM
.51	.51
(.25)	(.25)

MARD: 1 if mother currently married, 0 otherwise.

WM	NWM
.63	.58
(.23)	(.25)

N: Number of children in the family between the ages of 6 months and 12 years.

WM	NWM
2.40	3.03
(1.38)	(1.77)

NOSICK: 1 if child has no diagnosed ENT disease at time of medical survey, 0 otherwise.

8GPUB	HSPUB	HSPRV	COLPRV
.93	.90	.93	.89
(.062)	(.09)	(.06)	(.09)

NOEARINF: 1 if child has no diagnosed symptoms of ear infection (tympanic membrane *not* red or amber/yellow), 0 otherwise.

8GPUB	HSPUB	HSPRV	COLPRV
.96	.93	.97	.94
(.042)	(.059)	(.025)	(.058)

PARHEAL: 1 if mother considers her health good or excellent, 0 otherwise.

WM	NWM
.84	.68
(.14)	(.21)

PARTIME: Amount of time parents spend with all children per day in play or conversation. Based on response to the question "Do you usually play or converse with your children: (1) every day, (2) every other day, (3) once or twice a week, (4) twice a month, (5) once a month or less." Answers were scaled assuming each daily contact with all children was about two hours.

WM	NWM
1.79	1.82
(.25)	(.23)

PARTIME/N: Total estimated time divided by number of children between 6 months and 12 years.

8GPUB	HSPUB	HSPRV	COLPRV
.72	.75	.92	1.09
(.26)	(.25)	(.31)	(.34)

RELIGION: 1 if parents attend religious services once or more a week, 0 otherwise.

WM	NWM
.26	.30
(.18)	(.21)

TIMCOST: The average travel plus average waiting time per child visit to the doctor in minutes.

WM	NWM
47.93	53.37
(880.90)	(1024)

WIFWAGE: Estimated hourly wage of working mothers based on mother's occupation and Washington, D.C., *Area Wage Survey* data.

WM
2.81
(1.32)

NOTES

1. Based on an estimated 20,000 practicing pediatricians earning an average income of $40,000 yearly. The public budget figures include spending at the federal, state, and local level on maternal and child health services and school health. *Statistical Abstract of the United States*, 1973, pp. 68, 71.
2. We concentrate on physical healthiness both in the theoretical and empirical portions of this study simply because the "economic model" is not well-suited for handling the discrete "taste changes" that are likely to accompany changes in mental health.
3. See also Michael Grossman, *The Demand for Health: A Theoretical and Empirical Investigation* (New York: National Bureau of Economic Research, Occasional Paper No. 119, 1972), and Charles Phelps, *Demand for Health*

Insurance: A Theoretical and Empirical Investigation, R-1054-OEO, The Rand Corporation, July 1973.

4. This approach differs from the work of Grossman, *The Demand for Health*, wherein subjective indices are used to specify the individual's healthiness—for example, individual judgments of own health as poor, fair, good, excellent. Grossman is sensitive to the limitations these subjective indices place on his conclusions. Although conclusions about the statistical significance and relative importance of variables can often be made in models involving ordinal dependent variables (see Sanford Labovitz, "The Assignment of Numbers to Rank Order Categories," *American Sociological Review* (June 1970), conclusions about measured marginal impacts are not valid. To correctly specify and estimate a "health production function" requires cardinal, not ordinal, measures of output.

5. This is the approach to health care uncertainty used in all previous work. See, for example, Phelps, *Demand for Health Insurance*.

6. One attractive specification of the attribute technology is to specify (1) as Cobb-Doublas where (1a) incorporates the random effect of $\tilde{u}$ as a shift parameter, $e^{\tilde{u}}$, and $\tilde{v}$ as an additive random term attached to the coefficients on x_i. When $\tilde{u}$ and $\tilde{v}$ are normally distributed, health care attributes, A_t, will be lognormally distributed. For a full development of this case, see Robert Inman, "Health-Care Demand When Outcomes Are Uncertain," mimeo., University of Pennsylvania, 1974.

7. The demand specification above assumes that the consumer's health insurance coverage is exogenously set, either through employment or publicly provided coverage. The recent work of Charles Phelps, *Demand for Health Insurance*; and Isaac Ehrlich and Gary Becker, "Market Insurance, Self-Insurance and Self-Protection," *Journal of Political Economy* (July–August 1972), has led to the development of models in which health care demand and insurance coverage are jointly determined. Our model fits easily into their framework and extends their analysis by allowing for the uncertain effects of health care (self-protection) activities. In the more general model, the consumer's allocation problem can be split into two sequential decisions. At the start of each period, the consumer decides on the level of health insurance coverage, knowing the market prices of x and y, his income I, μ, σ_u^2, β, σ_v^2, A_0, and the market-determined price of health insurance. The demand specifications in (3) above are conditional on the extent of health insurance coverage, especially the coinsurance rate that reduces the gross market prices for health services to the net price, p_x, which is used in (3). Substituting $\phi_i(\cdot)$ into the consumer's utility function $U[x, y, A(x)]$ and optimizing over the insurance parameters allows us to specify preferred insurance coverage (see Phelps, *The Demand for Health Insurance*). Once coverage is set, the consumer buys care according to (3). This extension of our model argues that the price of insurance should be included in the demand equations for health-related goods and services.

8. Of course, if we sufficiently restrict the specification of (1a), and (2), predictions about the demand effects of changes in μ, σ_u^2, β, and σ_v^2 do emerge. See, for example, S. Turnovsky, "A Model of Consumer Behavior under Conditions of Uncertainty in Supply," *International Economic Review* (February 1971), and Walter Oi, "The Economics of Product Safety," *The Bell Journal of Economics and Management Science* (Spring 1973). Turnovsky assumes a quadratic specification for $U(\cdot)$ in (2), whereas Oi assumes a perfect insurance market for commodity failures (in our case, sickness) or a "far-sighted" consumer making many purchases of the good with the uncertain

effect. Neither specification seems particularly attractive for our problem. In another paper, "Health Care Demand When Outcomes Are Uncertain" (mimeo.), University of Pennsylvania, 1974, I develop the demand specifications for a constant relative risk-aversion utility function with lognormally distributed health attributes. There I show that in the three-good cares (preventive care, curative care, and y) with a single health attribute, consumers who are sufficiently risk averse with respect to health (the Pratt-Arrow measure of relative risk aversion exceeding 1) will increase their use of preventive or curative care as the expected marginal health impact for the good increases $(d\beta_{it} > 0)$ or as the uncertainty of the marginal health impact declines $(d\sigma^2_{v_{it}} < 0)$. Section 4 presents some tentative evidence to support this prediction in the case of children's health.

9. The emphasis here on the consumption benefits of child health care does not preclude the notion that health care can be a means to a further end—say, good school performance. However, the model does ignore the human capital formation motive for child health care allocations. See, for example, Michael Grossman, "The Correlation between Health and Schooling," National Bureau of Economic Research, Working Paper No. 22, December 1973; and Marc Nerlove, "Household and Economy, Toward a New Theory of Population and Economic Growth," *Journal of Political Economy*, Part II (March–April 1974). I provide some tentative evidence on the choice between the two models in Section 4. See the discussion of the variable FUTURE below, and the results in tables 4 and 5 for this variable.

10. The survey was conducted as part of the National Academy of Sciences, Institute of Medicine, study entitled "Contrasts in Health Status: An Analysis of Contrasting Forms of Medical Care Delivery." The survey involved a detailed questionnaire of family health attitudes, economic status, and utilization of health care facilities within six months prior to the date of the interview. Interviews were conducted from December 1970 to April 1971. There were 1,435 families in the study's final sample. Children between the ages of 6 months and 12 years in the sample families were then given a detailed ENT clinical examination and those over 3 years were given sight and hearing examinations as well. Approximately 2,600 children were examined by the survey's panel of physicians. My working sample based on complete data for all variables used in this study came to 1,692 children.

11. An earlier version of this paper also examined nose infections, but Lee Benham correctly pointed out that because of the very low prevalence rate and often small sample sizes, these results were virtually useless.

12. For a biological model generating a logit specification for (1,0) health attributes, see J. Truett, J. Cornfield, and W. Kannel, "A Multivariate Analysis of Risk of Coronary Care," *Journal of Chronic Disease* (April 1967).

13. See David Kessner and D. McEldowney, "The Epidemiology of Otitis Media," in K. S. Gerwin and A. Glorig (editors), *Otitis Media: Proceedings of the National Conference* (Springfield, Illinois: Charles C. Thomas, 1972).

14. Parents' time per day per child in play or conversation is based on the parents' response to the question, "Do you usually play or converse with your children: (1) every day, (2) every other day, (3) once or twice a week, (4) twice a month, (5) once a month or less?" Answers were then scaled into an estimate of total parents' time (PARTIME) with all children by assuming that each daily contact with all children consumed about two hours. Recent work by Arleen Leibowitz, "Education and Home Production," *American Economic Review* (May 1974), finds that parents do spend, on average, about two hours per day on the

physical and educational care of their children. Leibowitz also finds that the amount of time per contact is *not* significantly related to parents' educational levels. This fact is relevant, since our production model will be estimated for subsamples based on mothers' educational levels.

15. See L. Pratt *et al.*, "Physicians' Views on the Level of Medical Information among Patients," in W. Scott and E. Volkhaut (editors), *Medical Care: Readings in the Sociology of Medical Institutions* (New York: John Wiley, 1966); and R. Duff and A. Hollingshead, *Sickness and Society* (New York: Harper and Row, 1968). Also, J. Samora *et al.*, "Knowledge about Specific Diseases in Four Selected Samples," *Journal of Health and Human Behavior* (Fall 1952); S. S. Kegeles *et al.*, "Survey of Beliefs about Cancer Detection and Taking Papanicoloan Tests," *Public Health Reports*, No. 80, September 1965; and D. Rosenblatt and E. Suchman, "The Under-utilization of Medical Care Service by Blue Collarites," in *Blue Collar World* (Englewood Cliffs, New Jersey: Prentice-Hall, 1954), have found that lower socioeconomic families have less accurate information about the causes and characteristics of many diseases than higher socioeconomic families.

16. TIMCOST equals the average travel and waiting time for the child for doctor visits over the six months prior to the family interview. If the child did not go to the doctor during this period, TIMCOST was calculated as the average travel plus waiting time of his or her siblings' visits.

17. WIFWAGE is approximated by the average hourly earnings for the occupational class in which the mother is employed. Exact wage data were not available. Occupational wage information was obtained from the *Area Wage Survey*, 1970, Bureau of Labor Statistics, Washington, D.C.

18. DOCFEE equals the average out-of-pocket costs of the child's physician visits during the six months prior to the family interview. If the child did not go to the doctor during this period, DOCFEE was set equal to the average out-of-pocket costs for the child's siblings' visits. Defining DOCFEE as an average of out-of-pocket costs sidesteps the errors-in-variables problems that arise because of the common physician practice of "two-part" pricing—charging a high initial price for each "work-up" visit and then low to zero prices for all follow-up visits.

19. Theil's work on "models with random coefficients" offers a richer econometric specification of our model, closer to the spirit of the work in Section 2. See Henri Theil, *Principles of Econometrics* (New York: John Wiley, 1971), pp. 622–627. In the framework above, uncertainty about health effects arises only because of inadequate inference on the part of the consumer of a true, "certain" health effect, β. Actually, of course, β is rarely known exactly even by health professionals with large samples. Theil's specification allows the variance of β to remain, even as sample size increases. For testing of our demand model, the extension into Theil's "models with random coefficients" is probably not worth the added effort. But in an analysis of health attribute production functions, it is an extension that should be seriously considered.

20. Comparing the results in Table 2 with my initial estimates of the DOCCUR coefficient shows a significant downward bias in the DOCCUR coefficient when this "instrumental variables" procedure was not employed. The estimates of the other coefficients in the model are nearly identical between the two estimating procedures. However, the asymptotic properties of this instrumental variables procedure for the logit model are not known, and the reader should treat these parameter estimates with suitable caution.

21. The coefficient ξ is in effect the slope of the "production possibility frontier"

for child attributes. Given a level of family inputs, more of one attribute may mean less of another.

22. An argument similar to the one just presented for the bias in the PARTIME/N coefficients can be developed for the income per capita variable as well. If parental income is positively related to child IQ and self-worth, as one might expect ($\delta > 0$), then from the model above, the estimated coefficients on INCPC will be biased toward zero. As with the bias to parents' time effects, I know of no evidence that will permit us to judge the seriousness of this underestimation.

The arguments here are not likely to apply to the doctor visit inputs or to past health states since the direct relationship of these variables to IQ or self-worth are likely to be negligible ($\delta \sim 0$).

23. If the parameter estimates, $\tilde{\beta}_{it}$, are normally distributed as $N(\beta_{it}, \sigma^2_{v_{it}})$, then statistical tests for the equality of means and variances across subsamples for each health care input can be made. For a test of equality of variances, the test statistic is the ratio of variance estimates that is distributed as F with parameters $(n - 1, n - 1)$, where $n = 200$. The null hypothesis of equal $\sigma^2_{v_{it}}$'s is rejected for all comparisons made by pairs at the 0.9 level and for all but three at the 0.99 level. For a test of equality of means ($= \beta$'s) of two normal populations with known but different variances, the test statistic is $Z^2 = (\beta_0 - \beta_1)^2 / (\sigma^2_0/n + \sigma^2_1/n)$, which is distributed as χ^2 with one degree of freedom. The null hypothesis of equal mean effect was rejected for all pairwise comparisons at the 0.9 level except for the comparison of β_{it} for DOCPRV for the high school-public and the high school-private subsamples.

Yet even if one accepts the normality assumption for β_{it}, the formal tests for equality of the PARTIME/N coefficients and their variances are biased in an unknown direction because of the bias in our estimates of PARTIME/N. Although we can say with some confidence that β_{it} for PARTIME/N is biased downward, no conclusions about the direction of bias in its standard error can be made. Thus $\sigma^2_{v_{it}}$ is biased away from the true variance in an unknown direction and the formal tests above for PARTIME/N are therefore biased in an unknown direction. Caution should be the keyword here.

24. The pattern is identical for the coefficients and variance estimates from the NOEARINF equation.

25. See, for example, Arleen Leibowitz, "Home Investments in Children," *Journal of Political Economy* (March–April 1972), Part II; and Jerome Kagan and H. A. Moss, "Parental Correlates of Child's IQ and Height," *Child Development* (September 1959).

26. See Arnold Zellner, "An Efficient Method of Estimating Seemingly Unrelated Regressions and Tests for Aggregation Bias," *American Statistical Association Journal* (June 1962).

27. The fact that our analysis is restricted to the provision of ENT health for children makes the first three assumptions less troublesome than they might be for an adult health study or a study of "major" (e.g., crippling) child diseases. Family health coverage is largely exogenous (publicly provided or part of the employee contract) for our sample. For those families buying supplemental insurance, it is unlikely that this coverage will be motivated by a child's ENT diseases.

The choice of the provider—and subsequently the provider's location, which helps define TIMCOST—is also likely to be independent of a child's ENT health. The possible exceptions are children with chronic ENT problems, but they appear to be few in our sample. Acton's simultaneous equation estimate of the role of outpatient visits as a determinant of travel distance is negative, as expected, but not significant. However, in Acton's work distance is a significant (negative) determinant of outpatient visits, a result similar to the one obtained here. See Jan Acton, "Demand for Health Care When Time Prices Vary More Than Money Prices," R-1189-OEO/NYC, The Rand Corporation, May 1973.

The mother's work status is also independent of the family's provision for ENT health. The correlations of mother's work status (1 if works, 0 otherwise) with DOCCUR, PARTIME, DOCPRV, EARPAIN, and COLDHIST never exceed 0.03.

The fourth assumption that assumes the exogeneity of family size is counter to recent household models that argue that number (N) and "quality" of children (of which ENT health is a part) are jointly determined. An alternative view of the parents' decision to have and care for children is to treat the decisions as a sequential process of decision, learning, and decision subject to the constraint that we cannot freely destroy the fruits of prior labor. In such a model, parents decide to have a child and once it is born care for that child as they see fit. The child is a blessing or a burden relative to prior expectations. If a blessing ("quality" greater than expected), they decide to have another. Once born, the parents care for both children as best they choose. Again they compare expected "joy" to received "joy" and decide to have another child or stop the process. It is clear that the fertility-child "quality" model being suggested here is recursive and allows us to identify the true effects on the provision of children's health. Unfortunately, our data base is not sufficiently rich to allow enough degrees of over-identification so that N might be made endogenous and permit us to test these alternative models of the fertility/child-raising process.

28. The fact that our estimates of the mean effect and the variance of this effect are biased for PARTIME/N will not alter our conclusions if the degree of bias is nearly constant across the four subsamples. I have argued earlier, however, that the degree of bias may be systematically related to mother's education. If so, the mother's education should be included in (1c) along with MEANPART and VARPART. But multicollinearity between these variables prevents us from drawing any inferences about the effects of technology in this case. The results in (1c) must therefore be treated as tentative, limited by the proviso that the bias in MEANPART and VARPART is not systematically related to parental education.

29. See, for example, J. P. Newhouse and Charles E. Phelps, "New Estimates of Price and Income Elasticities of Medical Care Services," in this volume.

30. To check for this bias, I reestimated equations (1a), (2a), and (3a), specifying preferred hours worked (t_w) to be a linear function of WIFWAGE. Substituting $t_w = \alpha + \delta$ WIFWAGE into the definition of FULINC [=INC + $(T - t_w)$*WIFWAGE] and this new specification of FULINC into our demand model yielded reduced-form equations in prices, technology, tastes and INC, WIFWAGE, and WIFWAGE^2. Estimating these equations gave "corrected" utilization elasticities with respect to income of about 0.25, suggesting that the true elasticities lie nearer the lower end of the original range.

31. For an interesting study relating childhood health to schooling and adult earnings, see Michael Grossman, "The Correlation between Health and Schooling," National Bureau of Economic Research, Working Paper No. 22, December 1973.

32. The use of the elasticities based on mean health effect, β_{it}, without regard to the

standard errors of these estimates implicitly assumes that society should be
risk neutral when allocating resources to children's health. For arguments to
justify this assumption, see Kenneth Arrow and Robert Lind, "Uncertainty and
the Evaluation of Public Investment Decisions," *American Economic Review*
(June 1970).

33. For a summary of other studies that find that smaller families mean healthier
children, see Joel D. Wray, "Population Pressure on Families: Family Size and
Child Spacing," in National Academy of Sciences, *Rapid Population Growth*
(Baltimore: Johns Hopkins Press, 1971).

6 ‖ COMMENTS

Lee Benham
Washington University

Inman raises two important questions in this paper: (1) How do physician
visits and parents' time spent with children affect children's health? and
(2) How responsive are parents to the health benefits their children receive
from these two inputs? To provide answers to these questions, he develops
and estimates a production function for children's health and a demand
function for health inputs. I will comment on each of these in turn.

In the production function for children's health, health status is measured by
three dummy variables indicating whether the child had an ear, nose, or throat
infection; an inner ear infection; or a cold. Approximately 10 per cent of the
children in the sample had one or more of these illnesses; less than 3 per cent
had a cold. The combination of the relatively small sample sizes and the small
proportion of ill children raises serious questions about the reliability of the
production function estimates. As an extreme case, Table 2 indicates an
eighth grade sample size of 136. According to the overall sample characteristics, approximately 4 children in that group had colds. The dependent
(dummy) variable therefore has a value of 1 in approximately 132 cases and
zero in the other 4. It is difficult to have confidence in production function
estimates based on such small numbers.

Even if the sample size is accepted as adequate for estimating the
systematic association between children's health status and the inputs
examined, the results in Table 2 provide only very weak support for the view
that children's health status is positively associated with inputs of physician
visits and parents' time. Of the 36 estimates of input coefficients reported, 22
are positive and 14 negative. Furthermore, these estimates are rarely significantly different from zero. I am not persuaded that productivity benefits from
these inputs have been shown.

The demand function includes the usual price and income components plus variables obtained from the production function concerning the mean and the variance of the effect of parents' time and physician visits on children's health. Inman's approach is clever. It provides a method of investigating the response of parents to the benefits and uncertainties of inputs to improve their children's health. As these inputs become more effective, the demand should increase, *ceteris paribus*. As the variance of the effects increases, however, the demand should decline if consumers are risk averse. The problem here, however, is that the measures of health benefits used in the demand equation are taken from the production function estimates. If there are no benefits from physician visits or parents' time, or if the production function estimates are not reliable because of sample size, the coefficient estimates for the health productivity variables in the demand equation will not be meaningful. Thus I do not believe that the estimated coefficients of the variables representing the mean and variance of productivity of parents' time and physician visits shown in Table 4 are reliable indicators of parents' demands for these services.

There is a further problem in the demand equation. Several variables that contain both wage (price) and income components are included simultaneously. Consider the composition of the variables included in equations (1a), (2a), and (3a) in Table 4. WIFWAGE is the estimated hourly wage of the mother based on the earnings of women with the same occupation in the Washington, D.C., area. The average occupational wage rate surely includes a large permanent income component, and the coefficient of this variable will in part measure the impact of income on the demand for parents' time and physician visits. FULINC is a measure of full family income that includes the wife's occupational wage times a fixed number of hours per year plus other family income. FULFEE includes wife's wage multiplied by the time cost of visiting a physician plus the physician's fee. In addition, three dummy variables are entered for parents' years of schooling. These variables are also proxies for permanent income. Since several measures of income and wage rates are included simultaneously as independent variables, the interpretation of the individual coefficients is not obvious. This is perhaps why some of the results appear curious when given a straightforward interpretation. For example, Inman writes, "WIFWAGE, the 'price' of parents' time with children, is *positively* related to PARTIME (parents' time with children) and negatively related to doctor visits. These results suggest that for working mothers time with children is an inferior good with respect to income changes and a Giffen good with respect to changes in WIFWAGE!" Economists have been seeking a Giffen good for a long time. Before we conclude that the quest has ended, additional analysis will be necessary to obtain more precise measures of the income and substitution effects.

The problems discussed above are primarily attributable to data deficiencies and should not detract from Inman's contribution in raising some important issues. He has been clever in developing a model that examines both the productivity of inputs on health status and the effects of productivity and uncertainty on the demand for inputs. It is time that we knew more about these questions, and Inman has given us a good start.

David S. Salkever
The Johns Hopkins University

There are a number of aspects of Inman's analysis that deserve comment. Let me first offer a more general commendation. Although the health of children has attracted little attention from economists, it is clearly a major area of current public policy concern. Although the government health care initiatives of the 1960s diminished social-class differences in the receipt of medical care among adults, their impact on children's medical care was modest at best. The ramifications of poor health status and underconsumption of care among children in lower social classes are probably very significant; Grossman's recent work (1973) suggests that the formation of "health capital" in childhood has very significant effects on the accumulation of several forms of human capital in later life. We are indebted to Inman, as well as Grossman, for bringing the issue to our attention in a forceful and interesting way.

As for the empirical analysis, let me first point out that Inman's production function estimates are not exactly encouraging. Leaving aside the few coefficients with significant and correct signs, his results generally suggest that both parental and professional inputs to the medical care production process have little or no impact on the ENT health of children and that the same is true of the "material environment" (INCPC). But if this is the case, what weapons have we in the war against ENT disease? Are we really as helpless as these results imply? Perhaps because I have been brainwashed by the medical profession and the social epidemiologists, I am reluctant to accept this conclusion and therefore am inclined to search for other explanations of these results.

One possible explanation concerns the way Inman has divided his sample. By estimating separate equations for samples defined by educational level, he seems to have substantially limited the range of variation of a number of variables within each equation. For example, data in his appendix suggest systematic variations across samples in per capita income and parental time inputs that are large relative to within-sample standard errors. This homogeneity within samples may be an important explanation for the consistently insignificant findings.

Another explanation, and the one that I regard as most important, relates to Inman's choice of dependent variables. These are 0-1 dummies indicating the presence or absence of colds or ear infections. By and large, these illnesses probably tend to be mild and short-lived even if untreated. The importance of their prevalence as a measure of health status is not readily apparent. But what is most significant is the resistance of these infections (particularly viral infections) to prevention or amelioration by medical care of either the professional or parental variety. Therefore, zero marginal products for medical care inputs are generally what we would expect.

It could, however, be argued that an alternative interpretation of Inman's dependent variables is more appropriate. Given the natural history of most ENT infections, variations in their prevalence rates at any point in time are largely determined by variations in incidence rates; and variations in incidence rates are probably associated with more fundamental differences in physical health that determine susceptibility to infection. Inman's dependent variables could therefore be viewed as proxies for these more fundamental differences. Should we not then be surprised at the result that the "material environment" and parental and professional care have no appreciable effects on these differences?

Again the answer is no, but for a different reason. The differences in physical health that determine susceptibility must certainly be highly correlated with recent health history. But if his dependent variable is a proxy for these differences, Inman's inclusion of independent variables describing recent health history leads me to expect the insignificance of other independent variables. This same point could be made by an unfair analogy. If we obtained data from a cross-section of firms and ran a regression in which today's capital stock was the dependent variable and the two independent variables were yesterday's capital stock and something else, we would hardly be shocked to find that only the coefficient for yesterday's capital stock was significant.

One other possible explanation of the production function results should at least be mentioned. In their more extensive study of the data used by Inman, Kessner, *et al*. (1974) concluded that the medical services provided to children suffering from ear infections were of poor or at best mediocre quality. If there is a relationship between this quality rating and the efficacy of care provided, then Inman's findings are attributable, at least in part, to the failures of individual physicians rather than the limitations of medical science.

In summary, I am not sanguine about curing our children's runny noses, but I would not conclude from Inman's results that health policy can do little to affect the ENT health of children. There is, after all, considerable evidence—from the National Health Examination Survey and elsewhere—that variations exist among income and educational groups in the more serious consequences of ear infection, such as scarring of the eardrum and resultant hearing loss. (Differences in Inman's sample means for EARSCAR bear this out.) I strongly suspect that these variations are attributable to differences in medical care, parental care, and the "material environment" and that policies relating to these variables would indeed pay off in terms of better ENT health. The problem for now is to build on the work considered here to obtain more reliable quantitative estimates of policy effects.

Turning to Inman's estimated demand functions, I shall only offer several brief comments. First, it is interesting that in the doctor-visit equations for the working-mothers sample, the cross-price effects (i.e., the wage coefficients) are negative. A possible explanation is that the time cost of medical services includes time at home in following the doctor's orders as well as travel and waiting time.

Second, the use of out-of-pocket cost as a price measure poses problems because it does not take account of differing insurance coverage. That is, insured persons may purchase more services per doctor visit than uninsured persons or they may frequent higher-quality providers, and their out-of-pocket costs may be the same or higher. Clearly, they face a lower price than uninsured persons, although the out-of-pocket cost measure of price will understate this difference.

Third, I am uneasy with the parental time demand equations for several reasons. The reported means and standard deviations of the parental time variable indicate very little variability. I suspect that this is not true in reality but that Inman's measure is simply too crude to pick up much of the variability that in fact exists. Also, since this variable measures total time input, only a small part of which will be health-related, it is surprising to find significant cross-effects for the time and money prices of medical care. This is rather like finding that the demand for television sets is significantly related to the price of tickets to a baseball game. Finally, I am not wholly convinced by Inman's argument that parental time inputs and the number of children are not simultaneously determined. Even if parents do not formulate multiperiod maximization problems, they may have rather stable preferences for the manner (including time inputs) in which they raise their children, and they will take these into account in deciding how many children to have.

I have thus far avoided discussing Inman's theoretical framework. But with national health insurance so much in the air, I suppose it is imperative that one's comments achieve universal coverage. For the sake of completeness, then, I offer the following two observations.

First, Inman has skillfully expanded on previous work by explicitly introducing uncertainty into his demand model. However, this may be a mixed blessing. Although it adds realism, it also complicates empirical implementation. Given our current difficulties in simply getting reasonable estimates for production function coefficients, one cannot help but feel a little nervous about demand functions that include the *variances* of these coefficients as independent variables.

Second, Inman's logit production functions differ from previous work in that past health status enters multiplicatively. In the past, this variable has been added to a health-increment production function to obtain current health status. The difficulty with Inman's multiplicative specification is that it results in marginal products for medical care that decrease as past health status decreases. The sicker you are, the less the doctor can do for you. Although there may be some instances in which this is true, as a generalization it is not very appealing. It also seems to suggest that illness reduces the demand for medical care, a result that is certainly counter-intuitive.

I would like to conclude with a more general observation, a comment on my comments. A number of the criticisms I have raised about the empirical work in this paper relate directly to deficiencies in data. Although Inman's analysis is interesting and well executed, it is obviously constrained by these deficiencies. And it is just as obvious that further progress in this important area of economic research will depend on the relaxation of data constraints. I believe the best way to ensure this progress is to become actively involved in designing and generating more useful bodies of data.

REFERENCES

1. Grossman, M., "The Correlation between Health and Schooling," National Bureau of Economic Research, Working Paper No. 22, 1973.
2. Kessner, D. M., C. K. Snow, and J. Singer, *Assessment of Medical Care for Children* (Washington, D.C.: Institute of Medicine, National Academy of Sciences, 1974).

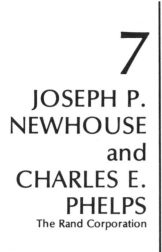

7

JOSEPH P. NEWHOUSE and CHARLES E. PHELPS
The Rand Corporation

New Estimates of Price and Income Elasticities of Medical Care Services

1. INTRODUCTION

In an earlier paper (Newhouse and Phelps, 1974a) we presented preliminary estimates of the price and income elasticities for various medical care services, including hospital length of stay, hospital room and board price, physician visits, and physician price. The theory on which these estimates were based was derived from the work of Grossman (1972) and one of the authors (Phelps, 1973). The estimates were made from data collected in the 1963 Center for Health Administration Studies Survey (Andersen and Anderson, 1967). Our sample was limited to heads who were employed, because these individuals were assumed to have well-defined values of time. In this paper we extend our earlier work, using the same data source. The extension includes reestimating

The authors gratefully acknowledge the help of Ronald Andersen in making the data used in this study available to them and helpful comments and computation assistance by David Weinschrott and Sharon Yamasaki.

The research reported herein was performed in part pursuant to a grant from the Office of Economic Opportunity, Washington, D.C. This project was also supported in part by Grant No. HS-00840-01 from the National Center for Health Services Research and Development. The opinions and conclusions expressed herein are solely those of the authors, and should not be construed as representing the opinions or policy of any agency of the United States government.

the earlier equations on a larger, more diverse sample, plus estimating the determinants of use or nonuse of medical services.

We first briefly recapitulate the specification we are using. We then consider the question of estimating a value of time for those not employed in order to include such individuals in our sample. Unfortunately, computational problems have prevented us from estimating the value of time in an appropriate fashion, and therefore our estimates of demand curves based on the larger sample that includes individuals not employed must be treated as preliminary. But the estimates based on the larger sample are consistent with and support our estimates using the smaller sample of employed heads.

In the earlier paper our estimates of demand were conditional on some use of the medical care system—for example, length of stay in a hospital, conditional on admission. In this paper we consider, in addition, the question of use or nonuse of hospital and office services. Thus, we estimate an admissions equation for hospital services and its analogue for physician services. Some theoretical complications of estimating these demand curves are discussed and estimates of the price elasticity are presented. With these estimates we are in a position to compute the elasticity of medical care expenditure with respect to price and income. In an appendix we present revised estimates based on the smaller sample used in our earlier paper. These estimates correct some computational errors; the revisions moderately affect the earlier estimates.

2. THE MODEL

This section reviews the specification used in Newhouse and Phelps (1974a); this will also be the basic specification used in this paper. Our specification is a generalization of Michael Grossman's investment model (Grossman, 1972). The significant generalizations include: (1) disaggregation of medical services, so that medical services are not considered a homogeneous commodity; (2) treatment of insurance as endogenous; (3) permitting price to vary among providers and treating the price of the provider selected as endogenous. For a more complete discussion the reader is referred to the earlier paper (Newhouse and Phelps, 1974a). We begin with the dependent variables and then turn to the explanatory variables.

The Dependent Variables

In this paper we explain variation in hospital admissions, hospital length of stay conditional on admission, and hospital room and board price per day conditional on admission. We do not explain variation in hospital ancillary services, so our estimates do not include all components of hospital expenditure.[1] The importance of this omission can be seen by disaggregating hospital expenditure. Hospital expenditure is the product of patient days and price per day. Patient days is the product of the admission rate, whose determinants are discussed in Section 3, and length of stay, whose determinants are discussed in Section 4. Price per day is a weighted average of the room and board price and ancillary services in price per day, with the shares of room and board price and ancillary services in total price per day as weights. These shares each equal approximately one-half (Health Insurance Association of America, 1968). In Section 4, we also explore determinants of the room and board price. To derive estimates of the responsiveness of total hospital expenditure to exogenous variables, one must make an assumption about the responsiveness of ancillary services; we assume that they respond the same way that room and board price does.

We also explain use of the ambulatory services with a similar set of equations (use of any ambulatory visits, number of visits conditional on positive visits, and price per visit conditional on positive visits). Unlike the case of hospital services, our estimates of price per visit include ancillary services received per visit.

In this and in the earlier paper, hospital length of stay (nonobstetrical days) is weighted by the average price across the sample for the type of accommodation (one, two, and three or more bed medical or surgical accommodations); the room and board price equation is estimated as a deviation from the average price for the type of accommodation used. Similarly, physician visits are weighted by the average price across the sample for the type of provider seen (general practitioner or specialist); the physician visit price equation is a deviation from the average price across the sample, given the type of provider used. The rationale for this disaggregation is that variation in average price across type of accommodation or type of provider is assumed to reflect productivity differences. Multiplication of physical units by the average price is therefore assumed to convert utilization to efficiency units. Variation of price holding provider type constant is assumed to reflect amenities, shorter queues, or incomplete search. Our estimates of expenditure elasticities, presented at the end of the paper, are invariant to this disaggregation.

Own-Price

In the length of stay and physician visit equations, this variable represents the price paid for a marginal unit (net of insurance benefits) measured in dollars. The theory underlying either an investment model (Grossman, 1972) or a consumption model (Grossman, 1972; Phelps, 1973) specifies marginal price in the first-order conditions; excluding the Giffen good case, a negative sign is expected. However, the theory assumes that price per unit is constant, and this assumption is violated if a deductible is present in the policy; price per unit then falls with expenditure. In this case, the true price of the price the consumer acts on when below the deductible is less than the observable price, because a unit of consumption raises the probability of later exceeding the deductible (Keeler, Newhouse, and Phelps, 1974). Because the true marginal price cannot be observed, we have excluded individuals with deductibles in their policies, except where otherwise noted. There are other examples of variation in unit price as total expenditure varies (such as an upper limit); however, we do not regard these as empirically important.[2]

Because sicker individuals tend to purchase better insurance (Phelps, 1973), net price is treated as an endogenous variable. Our excluded exogenous variables are size of work group (an instrument for insurance price) and nine occupation dummy variables.[3]

In the equations explaining deviation from the average price, the own-price variable is the coinsurance rate at the margin. In the case of hospital policies it was necessary to account for the policies that pay up to a certain dollar amount per day and nothing thereafter; in this case, the dollar amount of the limit was entered if the policy was of that type (zero otherwise). In addition, we entered a dummy variable that took the value of 1 if the policy did not have a dollar limit so that the intercept could also adjust for this type of policy. These variables are all endogenous. In the price equations (but not the utilization equations) we have excluded individuals who sought care for which there was no charge made by the provider, either for reasons of charity or professional courtesy. This amounted to some 10 to 15 per cent of the sample. Such individuals were of necessity excluded because there is no gross price variable for them.

Because we use the actual marginal price (the marginal coinsurance rate times the gross price) in the length of stay and visit equations, and because the gross price is a function of the coinsurance rate, we cannot simply add the estimated "utilization" and "price" elasticities to derive an expenditure elasticity with respect to coinsurance. To do so would involve some amount of double counting. In order to derive the elasticity of expenditure with regard to coinsurance, we have reestimated the length of stay and visit equations with just the coinsurance rates as the own-price and cross-price variables and have used the resulting elasticity of utilization with respect to coinsurance in our concluding section.

In the admission equation and use-nonuse of office visits equation, we do not use marginal price but, rather, coinsurance rates as explanatory variables. The rationale for this approach is explained in Section 4. Also, the hospital coinsurance rate is a weighted average of the room and board coinsurance rate and the inpatient physician coinsurance rate. (See Section 4.)

Cross-Price

In the length of stay and visit equations, the cross-price is specified as the net price paid for a marginal unit, measured in dollars. It is the physician office visit price in the length of stay equation and the hospital room and board price in the physician visit equation. The predicted sign is ambiguous, depending on whether the good is a complement or substitute. As in the case of own-price, to estimate an expenditure elasticity we have reestimated the length of stay and visit equations using only the coinsurance rate.

In the use-nonuse equations the cross-price is specified as the coinsurance rate, for reasons explained in Section 4.

Wage Rate

This is measured in dollars per week (averaged over the year), because a week is the shortest time period available in the 1963 data. Thus, we assume that labor force adjustments occur through reallocation of weeks worked per year rather than hours worked per week if the wage rate changes. The expected sign of the wage rate (summing its effect over all medical services) is positive in the investment model; the variable has no predicted sign in the consumption model.

Two complications arise when testing this concept empirically. If the health status variables do not adequately control for health status, there will be a downward bias in the measured effect of income, because poor health is often associated with negative transitory income. The second complication concerns sick leave and disability insurance provisions about which we have no data. To the extent that such provisions improve with wage income, the measured effect of income is positively biased.[4] The net effect of these two complications on our estimates cannot be known with certainty; we feel that they are likely to be roughly offsetting.

Nonwage Income

This is measured in dollars per year. There should be no relationship between nonwage income and demand in the investment model, and a positive relationship in the consumption model. The hypothesis of no relationship is difficult to test because the theoretical prediction relates to a lifetime, one-period model, and nonwage income in any single year may be only weakly related to the present value of all nonwage income flows. If the error in measuring the theoretical construct is random, both the coefficient and the t statistic are inconsistent toward zero (Cooper and Newhouse, 1971).

Family Size

This is the number of individuals in the family unit, which is defined as the group of related individuals living together. Family size is expected to have a negative effect if nonwage income has a positive effect, although it may also have an effect if nonwage income has no effect (Grossman, 1972). If neither family size nor nonwage income is significant, support for the investment model is strengthened.

Education

Education is measured by the highest grade completed. The effect is expected to be negative in the investment model (Grossman, 1972); the consumption model yields no simple prediction on the sign.

Age

Age is measured in years; the effect on consumption is expected to be positive if the depreciation rate rises with age. If depreciation rates are fully captured in health status variables, age should have no effect.

Sex and Race

These are dummy variables that take the value of 1 for females and nonwhites. They are included to standardize for possible underlying differences between the sexes in demand for care and differences in access (especially travel costs) that may confront persons of different races.

Self-Perceived Health Status and Disability Days

These are included as a measure of health stock. As self-perceived health status decreases and disability days rise, demand is expected to rise. Because disability days may be endogenous, we estimated equations with it omitted, and our results did not change.[5]

Beds-Population and Physician-Population Ratios

These ratios refer to the medical resources in the county of residence and are included to account for the stochastic nature of medical demand. The greater community supply is relative to community demand, the smaller proportion of the time will facilities be overfull. Although we have measures of community supply, we have no measure of community demand. Because of the likely positive covariance between community supply and demand, the coefficient of the supply variable is biased toward zero as a gauge of the behavior we seek to measure.

Notice that the problem of simultaneity that exists when equations are estimated from aggregate data is not necessarily present in these data on the demand of individuals. In particular, it will not exist if the error term for the individual is distributed independent of geography (that is, the omitted variables and measurement error are independent of geography).

Region

Four regional dummies are included in the price equations to standardize for differences in nominal prices among regions. The Pacific region is the omitted region.

Rural Place of Residence

This dummy takes the value of 1 if the place of residence is rural and is intended to standardize for differences in travel time and other demographic characteristics between rural and urban areas.

Functional Form, Estimators, and Data Summary

We have entered the variables in a simple linear form. For some variables (price, nonwage income) we have tested a quadratic form; this has not resulted in any improvement. We present estimates using both two-stage least squares (TSLS) and ordinary least squares (OLS).[6] Summary statistics are presented in Appendix 1, Table 1.

3. DEMAND FOR CARE FROM INDIVIDUALS WHO ARE NOT EMPLOYED

Adding individuals who are not employed to our sample has two helpful effects. First, it considerably increases the size of the sample available for estimation, thereby improving the precision of our estimates. Second, the employed population greatly underrepresents individuals who are not prime-age males. If there are interactions between sex (and age) and price elasticities, estimates that do not account for such interactions could be quite inaccurate. But if there are few non-prime-age males in the sample, it is difficult to test for interactions.

The major problem to be solved before individuals who are not employed can be included is estimating an opportunity cost of time for them. For those who are employed, we have followed the conventional practice of assuming that a wage rate (dollars per week in our case) measured this opportunity cost.[7] Obviously, for individuals who are not employed, a wage rate is not available.

The most significant work on estimating the value of time for nonemployed individuals has been done by James Heckman (1974). (See also Gronau, 1973a, 1973b.) Heckman postulated an offered wage function for housewives:

(1) $w = f$ (education, experience) $+ e$

and a wage-asking function:

(2) $w^* = f$ (hours, number of children under 6, spouses' wage, education, net assets) $+ u$

Furthermore, for women free to choose their working hours

(3) hours $\cdot (w\text{-}w^*) = 0$

If $w > w^*$ when hours equal 0, then the woman will work positive hours until $w^* = w$. If $w \leqslant w^*$ when hours equal 0, the woman will not work (that is, hours are 0). It is the wage-asking equation that is relevant for our purposes, because it yields the value the nonworking woman places on her time.

Heckman estimates equations (1) and (2) with a simultaneous equation version of tobit (Tobin, 1958), allowing the covariance of u and e to be non-zero.[8] The estimator is a nonlinear estimator, and Heckman uses a maximum likelihood routine.

We attempted to use Heckman's procedure, but computational difficulties arose.[9] We therefore resorted to a procedure known to be biased—estimating a wage for those in the labor force and using the resulting equation to estimate values of time for those not in the labor force by setting weeks worked equal to zero. Thus, we estimate (2) using OLS separately for men and women in the labor force and then apply the resulting equations to those not in the labor force, setting the weeks variable to zero to obtain a value of time.[10]

A priori, one cannot say whether this procedure is biased up or down; this reflects ignorance of whether the person does not work because w is "low" (for some reason the person is not suited to the labor force) or because w^* is "high" (the person is very productive at nonmarket work). The direction of bias, if any, in our estimate of w^* will depend on which reason predominates. Based on the work of Gronau (1973a), there is some reason to believe that the bias introduced is substantial and varies with demographic characteristics, such as age, education, and race. Therefore, if the w^* estimated by OLS is applied to the nonworking subsample and used in a demand equation, the coefficient of w^* will be biased toward zero, and the coefficients of the demographic characteristics will also be biased. It is not necessarily the case, however, that the price elasticity is biased. Our estimates using the subsample of employed heads suggest that any bias in the price elasticity is likely to be small.

To estimate w^* we used the specification described in (2) (substituting weeks for hours because that was the measure of labor supply in the 1963 survey) and added two health variables (self-perceived health status and disability days), dummy variables for "don't know" or "not applicable" responses, and used nonwage income rather than net assets. The resulting estimates are shown in Appendix 1, Table 2.[11] Because these equations are used merely to produce an estimated wage and because the procedure is known to contain biases, the results of these auxiliary equations are not discussed.

4. HOSPITAL ADMISSIONS AND USE OR NONUSE OF PHYSICIAN

Hospital Admissions

A major theoretical question to be faced in estimating an equation predicting the probability of admission to a hospital is the specification of the price variable. The issue arises because there is typically some uncertainty about the out-of-pocket price the consumer will have to pay when the physician and the patient contemplate admission to the hospital. The problem may be formulated as follows. Assume that there is a distribution of possible out-of-pocket expenditures resulting from an admission. Assume that the parameters of this distribution depend on the health stock loss and insurance policy of the consumer, so that the distribution can be written as $f(x;L,I)$ where f is a density function of expenditures measured in terms of other goods x that can be bought after paying for medical care. The density function is conditional on the health stock loss L and the insurance policy I. There is also some probability distribution of final health status H after the hospital stay, because neither the physician nor the consumer knows what the outcome of the hospital stay will be. Let this distribution (the benefit) have a density function $g(H;L)$; this function is also conditional on the health stock loss.

The admission decision is discrete; the patient is either admitted or not admitted. Under standard assumptions concerning behavior under uncertainty, the physician and the patient choose admission if the expected utility is positive. That is, the patient is hospitalized if

(4) $$V = \int U(x,H;L)\, g(H;L)\, dH - \int U(x,H;L)\, f(x;L,I)\, dx > 0$$

where U is a utility function in other goods, x, and health status, H; utility is conditional on the loss. In this expression the first term is the expected benefit, conditional on the loss, and the second term is the expected cost, in terms of utility lost from foregoing consumption of other goods, conditional on the loss and the insurance plan.

The change this formulation makes from the standard model is that uncertainty about price is explicitly introduced. The uncertainty occurs because the consumer is not given a price per unit and asked how many units he wants, but rather an uncertain price for an entire stay (depending on length, tests ordered, etc.) and asked whether he wants exactly one unit (one admission). Deriving the theoretical properties of introducing uncertainty about the price is not important for the purpose of this paper; we point out, however, that for risk-averse consumers the introduction of uncertainty decreases the probability of admission (relative to the certainty case at the same expected price).[12]

What is significant for present purposes about the above model is that demand for admissions is a function of the expected benefits from hospitalization and the expected out-of-pocket expenditure (and perhaps higher moments of the distributions as well). Neither of these values is observable, but they are functions of the health stock loss and the insurance policy. Our basic strategy is to take advantage of this dependence and enter variables that approximate health stock loss and key parameters of the insurance policy. Because policymaking interest centers around the response to insurance, this deviation from the theoretical model loses little, if anything. However, measurement of the health stock loss and the insurance variable is not straightforward.

Health stock loss is not directly observable, yet it is obvious that both the expected benefits and expected costs are typically greater for someone with a severe or life-threatening illness than for a minor illness. It would be a heroic assumption to assume that the variation in L causes no change in V (i.e., that $\partial V/\partial L = 0$). If one is not willing to make this assumption, variation in L will in general affect the probability of hospitalization. Indeed, health stock loss may well be the most important variable in explaining admissions. It is therefore necessary to approximate L, and we have included a general measure of self-perceived health status for this purpose.

This is obviously an imperfect measure, but should serve as a reasonable first approximation. Moreover, the errors in measuring the effect of health stock loss are likely to be random and therefore should not cause estimates of the effect of insurance to be inconsistent.

The difficulties in measuring the insurance variable are largely caused by the presence of deductibles.[13] This can be seen by writing down the expression for expected out-of-pocket price, a natural variable to use in explaining demand:

(5) $$E(f(x)) = \int_0^D xh(x)dx + C \cdot \int_D^\infty xh(x)dx$$

where $h(x)$ is the distribution of gross expenditure (assumed given for the moment) and C and D are the coinsurance rate and the deductible, respectively. If the deductible is zero, the first term is obviously zero, so that the expected out-of-pocket costs are proportional to the coinsurance rate. But if the deductible is positive, the expected out-of-pocket price is clearly not proportional to the coinsurance rate.[14] Therefore we estimate the responsiveness of hospital admissions to the coinsurance rate among those who have no deductibles in their policies.[15]

Additionally, in the admissions and use of physician equation we have used the coinsurance rate and not the expected price as an explanatory variable. This is done for two reasons. First, it is difficult to define an expected price for the 92 per cent of the sample who were not admitted to a hospital. Second, if the expenditure distribution $h(x)$ were invariant with respect to C, the result of estimating the response of admissions to C would be equivalent to estimating the response of admissions to expected out-of-pocket price. Unfortunately, the assumption that $h(x)$ is independent of C is unwarranted; the results presented in Section 5 of this paper show that length of stay and choice of hospital respond to C. This means that estimates of the responsiveness of admissions to the expected out-of-pocket price will *overestimate* the responsiveness to changes in C, because a reduction in the coinsurance rate (which would, *ceteris paribus*, reduce out-of-pocket payments) also introduces a partially offsetting rise in total expenditures with a consequent rise in expected out-of-pocket price (except in the limiting case of full insurance).[16] However, policymaking interest centers around the responsiveness to insurance parameters because that is what policy controls. Therefore, the overall response to coinsurance (rather than the *ceteris paribus* response to expected price) is an important value to derive. To find the responsiveness of demand to expected price, it is necessary to add estimates of the responsiveness of the expenditure distribution to estimates of the response to coinsurance.

The results of estimating an equation in which the explanatory variable is the coinsurance rate are presented in Table 1. For these purposes the coinsurance rate is a weighted average of the coinsurance rates for hospital and inpatient physician expenditures, with budget shares as weights (i.e., the hospital coinsurance rate was weighted by hospital expenditure as a fraction of hospital plus inpatient physician expenditures).[17] The coinsurance rate is considered exogenous in these results. Use of an instrumental variable estimate of the coinsurance led to estimates of the own-price elasticity that were further from zero; as a result, we do not present them.[18] The results shown in Table 1 have been generated from a logit regression. This procedure estimates the probability of admission, P, as a function of a vector of explanatory variables X; the function is:

(6) $\qquad P = 1/(1 + e^{-\beta x})$

The advantage of this procedure relative to a simple least squares estimation is that it constrains the probability to lie between zero and one, thereby incorporating the prior information that this must be true. This function is obviously nonlinear in β; we have used a maximum likelihood routine to estimate β.[19]

For dummy variables (sex, the health status variables, the rural variable, and race) Table 1 shows the difference in P if the variable assumes the value of 1 (continuous variables at their means, other dummy variables at zero); for continuous variables we show the elasticity at the mean of all variables.[20]

The results in Table 1 show a substantial response to both own-coinsurance and cross-coinsurance; the elasticity at the mean for hospital room and board coinsurance is -0.17 (asymptotic $Z = 2.99$) and for physician office visit coinsurance is -0.57 (asymptotic $Z = 4.82$). Hospital and physician services therefore appear to be strongly complementary, although there are so few individuals with insurance for physician services that it is hard to place a great deal of weight on this conclusion. Self-perceived health status is very important; with it included, age is not significant at conventional levels. Nonwhites are around 3.6 percentage points less likely to be admitted to a hospital. Joint tests on the supply variables indicate that they are not significant at the mean.

TABLE 1 Hospital Admissions[a]

Variable	Coefficient	Asymptotic Z Statistic (absolute value)	Elasticity for Continuous Variables; Change in Probability for Dummy Variables[b]
Hospital room and board rate coinsurance	−.34	2.99	−.17
Physician office visit coinsurance	−.71	4.82	−.57
Sex	−.054	.45	−.005
Age	.0006	.19	.018
Wage income	.00002	.66	.023
Nonwage income	.00007	2.87	.037
Health status good	.76	5.56	.069
Health status fair	1.39	7.73	.20
Health status poor	2.40	10.74	.66
Family size	−.014	.45	−.058
Education	−.019	1.82	−.10
Rural dummy	−.030	.22	−.036
Physician-population	.0028	.53	−.28
(Physician-population)^2	−.000042	.97	—
Bed-population	−.10	1.26	.41
(Bed-population)^2	.020	2.69	—
Race	−.63	3.16	−.036
Estimated value of time	.0013	.75	.037
Constant	−2.18	5.02	—

Chi-square of estimate (18 d.f.) = 228.78 ($p < 0.01$)

[a] $n = 4,522$. The sample is arrived at by excluding: (a) 2,760 individuals whose policies were not verified; (b) 38 individuals who have more than three insurance policies; this exclusion was for computational reasons; (c) 7 individuals with wages higher than $500 per week in 1963; (d) 8 individuals who exceeded $50 per visit for office visits; (e) 305 individuals with non-zero hospital deductibles; and (f) 247 individuals with non-zero office visit deductibles. Some individuals are excluded for more than one reason. The mean probability of admission is 0.078.

[b] In computing elasticities, all variables are at their means. In computing the change in probability induced by a change in the dummy variable, continuous variables are at their means and dummy variables are set to zero. The elasticity with respect to the supply variables is shown next to the linear term.

Physician Office Visits

We have also estimated a use-nonuse equation for the use of physician office visits; the dependent variable takes the value of 1 if there were any physician office visits. The underlying model is the same as for hospital admissions, but the rationale for estimating a separate "admissions" equation is somewhat different. In the case of hospital admissions, we emphasized the uncertainty surrounding the price of an admission relative to the price of an extra day. This uncertainty is not present to the same degree for office visits. But there is a different rationale for estimating a separate visit equation (rather than an equation that combines individuals with some visits and individuals with no visits in an equation estimated by tobit methods). The decision to seek any care from a physician is almost always made solely by the consumer, with no information supplied by the physician. Further visits may well incorporate information from the physician, and this information may alter the responsiveness to the explanatory variables. In this case, combining information on those having visits with those having none is inappropriate.

In our sample the probability of consulting a physician is 56 per cent—well below the estimate for the National Health Survey of 70 per cent. This difference is probably attributable to differences in definition; the CHAS survey does not include telephone consultations in its definition of visits whereas the National Health Survey does.

The CHAS 1963 sample is not optimal for estimating the responsiveness of demand for ambulatory physician services to price, because 89 per cent of the sample does not carry insurance for physician services. With that caveat we present our results for use-nonuse of the physician in Table 2.

The own-coinsurance and cross-coinsurance elasticities are both negative and highly significant, as in the case of hospital admissions. Health status is of considerable importance, as is race; nonwhites have a lower probability of making any visits. The wage, value of time, and nonwage income variables exhibit a small, though significant, elasticity; family size has a significant and negative effect. Notice that with self-perceived health status in the equation, age has a negative effect on use. A joint test on the supply variables shows that the physician-population ratio is significant at the mean (asymptotic $Z = 1.99$), but the bed-population ratio is not.

TABLE 2 Any Use of Physician Services[a]

Variable	Coefficient	Asymptotic Z Statistic (absolute value)	Elasticity for Continuous Variables; Change in Probability for Dummy Variables[b]
Physician office visit coinsurance	−.28	2.60	−.11
Hospital coinsurance rate	−.27	3.94	−.07
Sex	.47	6.90	−.11
Age	−.011	5.32	−.14
Wage income	.000076	4.77	.044
Nonwage income	.000043	2.34	.013
Health status good	.30	4.19	.07
Health status fair	.86	7.69	.21
Health status poor	1.41	8.41	.33
Family size	−.12	7.15	−.23
Education	−.005	.85	−.013
Rural dummy	.069	.84	—
Physician-population	.0019	.67	.049
(Physician-population)^2	.0000036	.30	—
Bed-population	−.046	.92	.035
(Bed-population)^2	.0063	1.28	—
Race	−1.06	11.45	−.22
Estimated value of time	.0053	4.75	.071
Constant	.76	3.00	—

[a] $n = 4,522$. The sample is the same as in Table 1. The mean probability of a visit is 0.56.
[b] In computing elasticities, all variables are at their means. In computing the change in probability induced by a change in the dummy variable, continuous variables are at their means and dummy variables are set to zero. The elasticity with respect to the supply variables is shown next to the linear term.

5. AMOUNT OF MEDICAL CARE SERVICES DEMANDED, CONDITIONAL ON SOME BEING DEMANDED

In Table 3 we summarize the price and wage elasticities for the amount of medical care services demanded, conditional on some services being demanded. The complete equations can be found in Table 3 of Appendix 1. All own-price elasticities estimated using OLS are small, but all are significantly different from zero. The

TABLE 3 Price and Wage Income Elasticities[a]

	Length of Hospital Stay ($n = 364$)		Physician Office Visits ($n = 2,617$)	
	TSLS	OLS	TSLS	OLS
Hospital coinsurance × room and board price	.08 (.43)	−.062 (1.92)	−.14 (.95)	−.055 (2.95)
M.D. office visit coinsurance × visit price	−.23 (.84)	.003 (.07)	−.073 (.46)	−.081 (4.65)
Wage income per week	.10 (.92)	.038 (.89)	.029 (.60)	.028 (1.88)
Nonwage income (less than $3,000 per year)	−.037 (.95)	−.023 (.77)	−.00008 (.007)	−.004 (.43)

	Room and Board Price ($n = 313$)		Physician Visit Price ($n = 2,346$)	
	TSLS	OLS	TSLS	OLS
Coinsurance rate of service	−.022 (.49)	−.051 (2.50)	−.21 (1.01)	−.15 (3.30)
Wage income per week	.022 (.81)	.010 (.45)	.072 (2.31)	.075 (5.93)
Nonwage income (less than $3,000 per year)	.041 (2.12)	.022 (1.41)	.005 (1.47)	.009 (.94)

[a]The absolute values of t statistics are in parentheses. Elasticities are computed at the mean.

TSLS estimates are also near zero but are uniformly not significant at conventional levels.

Length of Hospital Stay

In the length of hospital stay OLS estimates, the own-price elasticity is −0.062 ($t = 1.92$). In the TSLS results, own-price is insignificant and positive; residual variance is around 30 per cent higher in the TSLS estimates than in the OLS estimates, reflecting the lower efficiency of that estimator. Wage and nonwage income elasticities are small and insignificant.

The full equation is shown in Appendix 1, Table 3. Inspection of the equation reveals that nonwage income higher than $3,000 is positive and significant in the OLS results, although with a small elasticity. This result is consistent with the consumption model, but little should be made of it, because only 5 per cent of the sample has a nonwage income higher than $3,000. A joint test on the supply variables at their means shows them to be insignificant at conventional levels. The effect of race is to increase length of stay, the opposite of the results found in the admissions equations (see Table 1). Although the probability of admission for nonwhites is 3.6 percentage points less than for whites, their length of stay is 2.9 to 3.7 days higher, on average, than for whites. On net, the reduction of admissions more than offsets the increase in length of stay, so that community-rated hospital insurance plans cause some racial redistribution away from nonwhites; the expected number of weighted patient days among nonwhites is some 20 per cent lower than among whites.[21]

In these equations, if a person was employed during 1963, his actual wage rate was entered as an explanatory variable; otherwise, the wage rate variable was zero. If a person was not employed, the estimated time value is entered as a separate variable; this variable takes the value of zero if the individual is employed. Thus, we permit the estimated response to the value of time to differ for the employed and nonemployed, while constraining all other coefficients for the employed and nonemployed to be equal. If the wage and the estimated value of time variables were added together, the estimated coefficients would be constrained to be equal; we leave them separated to test that hypothesis. Although in general we cannot reject the hypothesis that the two coefficients are equal, we have not shown results when we constrained the variables to have the same coefficient because we felt that the wage variable was less subject to measurement error and wanted a separate estimate of it. In any event, the estimates of price elasticity were hardly affected. In the length of stay equations, both the wage and the estimated value of time show elasticities near zero and are not significantly different from zero.

Room and Board Price

The response of hospital price to coinsurance is small, but the elasticity is quite significant in OLS. Based on the OLS result, a change from no coverage to full coverage (other variables at their means) would increase the room and board price by approximately 23 per cent.[22] There is little response to wage or nonwage income. We infer that neither amenities nor time saved from shorter queues are very important in explaining the room and board price, given the type of accommodation. Weighted hospital days is the most significant variable in this equation. A joint test on the physician-population ratio shows it is significant at the 5 per cent level at the mean $(t = 2.2)$; we view this result as reflecting the more specialized (and costly) facilities that exist where physicians are concentrated.[23] The bed-population ratio is not significant at its mean, although its elasticity is negative. The full equation is shown in Table 5 of Appendix 1.

Physician Office Visits

In the physician office visit equation using OLS, the estimated elasticity at the mean is -0.08 $(t = 4.65)$. The TSLS estimate is -0.07 $(t = 0.46)$, so that one cannot determine if the significance of the OLS estimate is due to adverse selection or not. The cross-price elasticity is -0.06 and highly significant in OLS; it is somewhat higher but not significant in TSLS. The negative cross-price elasticities in the admissions and physician office visit equations are consistent with the hypothesis that hospital and office services are complements.[24] The estimated elasticity for wage income is very small, as are the elasticities for nonwage income. Family size is significant and is negative, indicating consumption aspects may play a role in physician utilization. Joint tests on the supply variables indicate that they are very significant, but the elasticities in the vicinity of the mean are very small—.03 for the physician-population ratio and .002 for the bed-population ratio. The negative sign on the coefficient of the (physician-population)² variable supports the hypothesis that additional physicians reduce the fraction of time that demand exceeds capacity. Visits are slightly higher (0.6 visits more) for nonwhites $(t = 1.99$ in OLS), an increase of 10 per cent above visits for whites, but this does not offset the sharply lower probability of nonwhites using any services.

Physician Price

The responsiveness of physician price to coinsurance in OLS and TSLS is -0.15 and -0.20, respectively, although the coefficient is only significant in OLS. Thus, the apparent significance of the result may be attributable to adverse selection. Using the OLS result, an increase from no coverage to full coverage increases the price of the physician selected by 18 per cent.[25] Wage income elasticities are very significant, but small in both TSLS and OLS, whereas nonwage income is not significant. This pattern supports the inference that a higher-priced physician represents less waiting time or less time devoted to search rather than additional amenities. The quantity of physician office visits is significant in OLS but not TSLS; the OLS result supports the hypothesis that people who make more visits search for lower-priced providers.

Separate Equations for Those in and out of the Labor Force

We estimated results for the subsamples with positive wage income and those with estimated values of time separately. In general, the OLS estimates of the important parameters were not very different between the two subsamples, although some of the TSLS parameters did change. We performed the standard Chow test to determine if the two subsamples could be assumed to come from the same population; in some instances we could reject this hypothesis and in others we could not. Because the greatest interest centers in the estimates for the entire population (and for the sake of economy), we have relegated the results for those with positive wage income to Appendix 2 and have not presented the results for the subsample with zero wage income.

Interaction Effects

We reestimated the length of stay and physician visit equations, allowing the price variable to interact with the following variables: health status good or fair; health status poor (these variables permitted testing whether those in worse health are more or less sensitive to price); wage income; nonwage income; and price itself (i.e., a quadratic term). In the length of stay equations, the additional interaction terms were uniformly insignificant. In the physician visit equation, however, two of them (the interactions of price with poor health and nonwage income) were significant in the OLS results; in addition, a joint test on all the interaction terms was significant at the 1 per cent level in the OLS results. Those with poor health have higher price elasticities (further from zero), whereas those with high nonwage incomes exhibit lower elasticities.

The predicted number of visits from this equation for two levels of health status, four coinsurance rates, and three combinations of wage and nonwage income (on an annual basis) is shown in Table 4; the complete equations are shown in Table 4 of Appendix 1. The effect of both interaction terms on responsiveness to co-insurance appears small; visits appear some 10 to 15 per cent higher with full insurance than with no insurance. This estimate of responsiveness does not include the decision on use of the physician at all, nor the effect of insurance on the price per weighted visit. In the next section we attempt to combine these effects.

6. OVERALL ESTIMATES AND CONCLUDING REMARKS

In this section we pull together our elasticity estimates for particular services and attempt to estimate overall coinsurance and wage

TABLE 4   Physician Visits per Person for Various Levels of Insurance, Income, and Health Status

Self-Perceived Health Status Good[a]					
Income		Coinsurance			
Wage	Nonwage	1.0	.5	.25	0
3,000	0	4.75	5.01	5.13	5.26
5,000	300	4.89	5.13	5.25	5.37
10,000	1000	5.25	5.46	5.56	5.66

Self-Perceived Health Status Poor[a]					
Income		Coinsurance			
Wage	Nonwage	1.0	.5	.25	0
3,000	0	8.90	9.56	9.89	10.22
5,000	300	9.04	9.69	10.01	10.34
10,000	1000	9.40	10.01	10.32	10.63

[a] Individual assumed to be white, male, 45 years old, single, with a high school education. Other variables at means, including gross price per visit.

income elasticities at the means of our data for hospital and physician expenditures. The obvious imprecision and omissions in our data make such an exercise hazardous, but the policy importance of the issue justifies even crude calculations.

Our most important problem in making such estimates is that neither the OLS nor the TSLS estimates are ideal; the OLS estimates of insurance elasticities are inconsistent away from zero, if there is advance selection of insurance, but the TSLS estimates are very imprecise and may in fact have larger mean square errors than the OLS estimates. We have solved this problem by accepting the OLS estimates but increasing their standard errors so that a 95 per cent confidence interval would include zero. There may be some upward bias in our estimates as a result; the reader who is not happy with this solution can easily construct similar estimates using the TSLS results.

A second problem is that the results for length of stay and physician visit equations use actual price. A change in the coinsurance rate includes a partially offsetting rise in the gross price, as shown by the price equations, and therefore use of an elasticity with respect to the actual price would be expected to overstate the elasticity with respect to the coinsurance rate. (See also the discussion in Section 4.) We have therefore reestimated the length of stay and visit equations substituting the own- and cross-coinsurance rate for the own- and cross-price. The resulting own-coinsurance elasticities are summarized in Table 5, along with the wage and nonwage income elasticities. The expected bias appears in the length of stay results; however, in the physician office visit equa-

TABLE 5 Estimates of Elasticity if Coinsurance Is Used Rather than Marginal Price[a]

	Length of Hospital Stay		Physician Office Visits	
	TSLS	OLS	TSLS	OLS
Coinsurance elasticity	.10	−.020	−.037	−.16
	(.47)	(.50)	(.07)	(3.29)
Wage income elasticity	.071	.047	.014	.018
	(.71)	(1.08)	(.41)	(1.19)
Nonwage income elasticity[b]	−.030	−.029	−.001	−.005
	(.77)	(.98)	(.12)	(.49)

[a] The t statistics are in parentheses.
[b] Nonwage income less than $3,000.

tion the coinsurance elasticity is further from zero than the marginal price elasticity in Table 3. We attribute this result to sampling error.

The question then arises whether the results in Table 3 or Table 5 should be used; because policy interest primarily attaches to changes in the coinsurance rate *per se*, we have used those in Table 5. This means we add elasticities with respect to only the coinsurance rate to arrive at an overall estimate.

A third problem was lack of information on the response of hospital ancillary services to the coinsurance rate. We have assumed that ancillary services, and therefore price per day, respond to coinsurance in the same fashion as do room and board prices. Modest differences in how ancillary services respond to coinsurance will not substantially affect the results. Finally, we have assumed that the estimates are independent of one another for purposes of calculating standard errors.

The values we used to make our calculations are shown in Table 6; they are taken from figures presented in tables 1, 2, 3, and 5. These estimates yield an elasticity with respect to coinsurance of −0.24 for hospital expenditure; this figure is shown in the line entitled summary. A 95 per cent confidence interval is from −0.05

TABLE 6 Values Used to Estimate Summary Elasticities at Means

	Hospital Services		Physician Services	
	Elasticity	Standard Error	Elasticity	Standard Error
Coinsurance				
Admission or use-nonuse	−.17	.085	−.11	.055
Length of stay or visits	−.020	.040	−.16	.08
Price	−.051	.0255	−.15	.075
Summary	−.24	.097	−.42	.12
Wage income				
Admission or use-nonuse	.023	.034	.044	.0092
Length of stay or visits	.047	.044	.018	.015
Price	.010	.022	.075	.013
Summary	.080	.060	.137	.022
Nonwage income				
Admission or use-nonuse	.037	.013	.013	.0056
Length of stay or visits	−.029	.030	−.005	.010
Price	.022	.016	.009	.0096
Summary	.030	.036	.017	.015

to −0.44. The elasticity with respect to physician services is higher, −0.42. A 95 per cent confidence interval is from −0.18 to −0.66. In appraising this estimate we would reemphasize that very few individuals in our sample had insurance for physician office visits, and therefore these figures should not be taken as a very reliable estimate of the effect of changes in coinsurance.

Table 6 also shows summary estimates of wage and nonwage income elasticities. For hospital services the elasticity is 0.08, with a 95 per cent confidence interval from −0.04 to 0.20, and for physician services the elasticity is 0.137, with a 95 per cent confidence interval from 0.094 to 0.18. For nonwage income the elasticity for hospital services is 0.030, with a 95 per cent confidence interval from −0.041 to 0.101, and for physician services it is 0.017, with a 95 per cent confidence interval from −0.012 to 0.046.

From these services we can obtain an estimate of wage income elasticities for hospital and physician services combined, using the fact that 75 per cent of the expenditures on these two services combined are for hospital services (Cooper and Worthington, 1973). The resulting overall value is 0.094, with a 95 per cent confidence interval from 0.006 to 0.18. Because the confidence interval does not include zero, this test supports Grossman's investment model.

Adding nonwage income elasticities for each service in a similar fashion (using the elasticities for nonwage income less than $3,000) yields a value of 0.027 as the elasticity, with a 95 per cent confidence interval from −0.026 to +0.080. Because the confidence interval does include zero, this result is also consistent with the investment model. But as has been pointed out, nonwage income for one year does not exactly correspond to the nonwage income concept of the model; therefore, we would caution against placing much emphasis on this particular finding.

A weak test of this result is the analogous overall elasticity for the family-size variable. For hospital services, family size is quite insignificant; the elasticity is −0.10, with a confidence interval from 0.173 to −0.383. For physician services, quite the opposite result obtains; the elasticity is −0.37 and highly significant, with a 95 per cent confidence interval from −0.24 to −0.50. This is consistent with a non-zero income effect; however, it is also possible to attribute the result to a complementarity between the health stock of adults in a family and child-rearing activities (Grossman, 1972). Across both hospital and physician services, the imprecision of the results for hospital services dominates; the combined elasticity with respect to family size is −0.17, with a 95 per cent confidence interval from 0.04 to −0.38.

Our estimates of elasticities at the mean with respect to coinsurance are somewhat lower than those in the literature (Feldstein, 1971; Davis-Russell, 1972). However, the data used to construct those estimates contain errors in measuring the price variable, which cause the estimates to be inconsistent, most likely in an upward direction (Newhouse and Phelps, 1974b). Our estimates are somewhat higher than those we have made using insurance premium data (Phelps and Newhouse, 1974). But our insurance premium data come from a substantially lower range of coinsurance, and there is some evidence in those data that elasticity falls with coinsurance.

Nevertheless, we would not exempt the data used in this paper from the charge of errors in measurement. Although they are richer than almost any other existing survey data, they are far from ideal. Insurance coverage is measured at the end of the year, and there is no guarantee that the insurance was in force throughout the year. Ambulatory utilization was measured by recall over the year, a procedure known to contain systematic biases by demographic group (Marquis, Cannell, and Laurent, 1972). Although abstracting the key features of the insurance policy and deriving the price of the marginal unit has involved a very lengthy process, there is variation in insurance policies that we have not measured. For example, some policies might not cover a physical examination or psychiatric procedures, whereas others might. Most important, the TSLS results are almost never significant, so the possibility that all elasticities are in fact zero cannot be dismissed on the basis of these data.

Thus, these estimates are fragile. Moreover, our elasticity estimates as well as those in the literature are really most helpful for appraising the effect of variation in coinsurance. To estimate the effect of varying a deductible is a more difficult problem because the marginal price is not a constant, and these estimates shed little light on the question of the effects of varying a deductible. It is obvious that much remains to be learned about the effect of insurance on consumer behavior.

APPENDIX 1

TABLE 1-1 Summary Data Statistics

	Mean[a]	Standard Deviation[a]	Number of Zeros
Exogenous Variables ($n = 2{,}617$, with positive office visits)			
Nonwage income (0 if > $3,000)	328.08	651.17	1606
Nonwage income (0 if ≤ than $3,000)	322.63	2151.91	2473
Nonwage dummy (1 if nonwage income > $3,000)	0.05	0.22	2473
Wage income/week	31.70	60.97	1828
Value of time	33.82	35.88	789
Disability days	10.10	32.61	1169
Health status good	0.39	0.49	1596
Health status fair	0.13	0.34	2246
Health status poor	0.05	0.21	2473
Married	0.47	0.50	1389
Sex	0.55	0.50	1180
Race	0.086	0.28	2373
Family size	4.10	1.88	0
Age 25-34	0.13	0.33	2296
Age 35-54	0.24	0.43	1996
Age 55-64	0.081	0.27	2398
Age ≥ 65	0.095	0.29	2328
Education 9-11 years	0.16	0.36	2207
Education 12 years	0.19	0.39	2137
Education 13-15 years	0.081	0.27	2415
Education ≥ 16 years	0.059	0.24	2471
Physician-population	113.16	47.98	0
Bed-population	4.22	2.20	151

TABLE 1-1 (concluded)

	Mean[a]	Standard Deviation[a]	Number of Zeros
Endogenous Variables			
Weighted length of stay[b] (n=364)	7.39	7.49	0
Hospital price[b] (n=313)	47.75	26.19	0
Marginal hospital coinsurance rate (n=313)	0.27	0.39	142
Weighted office visits[b] (n=2,617)	4.58	4.76	0
Office visit price[b] (n=2,346)	7.12	6.43	0
Marginal office visit coinsurance rate (n=2,346)	0.85	0.35	236

[a] Means and standard deviations include zero values in wage and nonwage income variables. Means and standard deviations are weighted to be representative of national sample by work-group size and income.
[b] The weights are the normalized average prices for the type of service used (1,2,3 or more bed surgical; 1,2,3 or more bed medical hospital room; general practitioners, specialist, or clinic). For example, if a specialist visit cost $10 and the average physician visit price were $8, the specialist weight was 1.25. The price variable is total expenditure divided by the weighted number of days or visits.

TABLE 1-2 Value of Time Equations—Dependent Variable Wage Income per Week

Explanatory Variable	Males (n = 900) Coefficient (t statistic)	Females (n = 527) Coefficient (t statistic)
Weeks worked	.54	.20
	(2.43)	(1.90)
Spouse's wage	−.17	.06
	(3.18)	(1.78)
Spouse dummy (=1 if no spouse)	−25.68	−2.83
	(2.00)	(.27)
Spouse retired	.69	15.68
	(.02)	(1.49)
Nonwage income	.003	.0008
	(1.47)	(.47)
Dummy = 1 if no nonwage income reported	21.28	9.28
	(1.02)	(.87)
Education	7.10	6.45
	(11.29)	(10.74)
Married	23.38	−9.76
	(2.65)	(1.85)
Disability days	.04	.22
	(.42)	(3.64)
Health status good	−3.19	−3.22
	(.71)	(.85)
Health status fair	−10.67	−12.13
	(1.54)	(2.32)
Health status poor	−19.93	−5.53
	(1.48)	(.55)
Number of children under 6	—	−8.00
		(2.74)
Constant	−.11	−9.71
	(.01)	(1.07)
R^2	.19	.27
Corrected R^2	.18	.25

TABLE 1-3 Utilization Equations

Explanatory Variable Coefficient (t ratio) (n = elasticity)	Dependent Variable = Hospital Length of Stay (n = 364) (weighted by average price of type of room)				Dependent Variable = Physician Office Visits (n = 2,617) (weighted by average price of type of provider)			
	TSLS		OLS		TSLS		OLS	
Hospital coinsurance × price of bed	.05 (.43181)	η = .08	-.04 (-1.9199)	η = -.06	-.05 (-.95249)	η = -.14	-.02 (-2.9520)	η = -.06
M.D. office coinsurance × price	-.51 (-.83824)	η = -.23	.006 (.07482)	η = .003	-.06 (-.46173)	η = -.07	-.07 (-4.6463)	η = -.08
Wage income/week (0 if no wage income)	.02 (.92384)	η = .10	.008 (.88551)	η = .04	.004 (.60444)	η = .03	.004 (1.8787)	η = .03
Estimated value of time (0 if wage income >0)	.02 (.38801)	η = .07	.005 (.38786)	η = .02	.005 (.27144)	η = .03	.002 (.53543)	η = .01
Nonwage income (0 if > $3,000)	-.0007 (-.94810)	η = -.04	-.0004 (-.77462)	η = -.02	-.000001 (-.00666)	η = -.00008	.00006 (-.43262)	η = -.004
Nonwage income if > $3,000	.0005 (1.3529)	η = .04	.0004 (3.0631)	η = .03	.00002 (.16405)	η = .001	.000005 (.08639)	η = .0003
Dummy = 1 if nonwage income > $3,000	-1.83 (-.91436)		-1.80 (-1.0516)		.44 (.76068)		.45 (.86717)	
Education 9-11 years	1.54 (1.3023)		1.03 (1.0310)		.05 (.20275)		.08 (.37187)	
Education 12 years	1.71 (1.3208)		1.33 (1.21171)		a		a	
Education 13-15 years	-2.92 (-1.0926)		-1.6605 (-.87987)		-.1 (-.24149)		-.04 (-.10285)	
Education 16+ years	1.26 (.47202)		.48 (.20978)		-.76 (-1.3402)		-.66 (-1.5546)	

TABLE 1-3 (concluded)

Explanatory Variable Coefficient (t ratio) (n = elasticity)	Dependent Variable = Hospital Length of Stay (n = 364) (weighted by average price of type of room)		Dependent Variable = Physician Office Visits (n = 2,617) (weighted by average price of type of provider)	
	TSLS	OLS	TSLS	OLS
Age 25-34 years	1.20 (.64941)	1.51 (.94820)	-.03 (.06806)	-.08 (-.25135)
Age 35-54 years	2.83 (1.5025)	3.78 (2.5526)	a	a
Age 55-64 years	3.79 (1.6297)	4.61 (2.4101)	.26 (.58305)	.23 (.52337)
Age 65+ years	5.35 (2.9007)	5.46 (3.4259)	.27 (.65321)	.27 (.66649)
Family size	-.07 (-.23526)	-.17 (-.78243)	-.17 (-3.0474)	-.16 (-3.0265)
Sex (=1 if female)	1.60 (1.3919)	.89 (1.1444)	.39 (1.4533)	.42 (2.1834)
Race (=1 if nonwhite)	2.90 (1.6409)	3.66 (2.7842)	.89 (1.7351)	.63 (1.9900)
Disability days	.03 (2.7459)	.03 (4.1484)	.02 (4.4782)	.02 (5.4518)
Health status good	-.23 (-.22586)	-.37 (-.40236)	1.24 (5.6117)	1.22 (6.1537)
Health status fair	2.09 (1.4809)	1.50 (1.3038)	3.24 (8.1745)	3.12 (10.464)

	(1)	(2)	(3)	(4)
Health status poor	.68 (.38235)	.21 (.14528)	5.71 (9.2735)	5.50 (11.125)
M.D.s per 100,000 population ratio	.03 (.75588) $\eta = .45$	.01 (.32379) $\eta = .16$	.02 (1.5452) $\eta = 38$	.02 (2.3820) $\eta = .48$
(M.D.s per 100,000 population ratio)²	-.0002 (-1.0369) $\eta = -.35$	-.00009 (-.62583) $\eta = -.17$	-.00006 (-1.5550) $\eta = .003$	-.00007 (-2.0187) $\eta = -.22$
Beds per 1,000 population ratio	-.25 (-.42985) $\eta = -.15$	-.13 (-.25356) $\eta = -.08$	-.26 (-1.8271) $\eta = -.24$	-.30 (-2.3165) $\eta = -.28$
(Beds per 1,000 population ratio)²	.05 (.80308) $\eta = .16$	.04 (.92660) $\eta = .15$	.02 (1.8739) $\eta = .005$	.03 (2.2566) $\eta = .14$
Married	-.07 (-.04842)	-.73 (-.67247)	.37 (1.2801)	.35 (1.3241)
Constant term	1.77 (.43692)	3.45 (1.4644)	3.80 (3.1519)	3.39 (5.8703)
R^2	—	.28	—	.16
Corrected R^2	—	.23	—	.15
Dhrymes F	3.09	—	10.47	—
(d.f.)	(27,7)	—	(25,9)	—
t ratio adjustment factor	.87	—	.76	—
F	—	4.92	—	19.65
(d.f.)	—	(27,336)	—	(25,2591)

[a] Included in category immediately preceding.

TABLE 1-4 Physician Visit Equations with Interactions

	Dependent Variable = Physician Office Visits; n = 2,617 (weighted by average price of type of provider)		
	TSLS	OLS	
Physician coinsurance × price of visit	.48 (.35) η = .56	-.06 (-1.65)	η = -.05
Hospital coinsurance × price of bed	.04 (.22) η = .12	-.02 (-2.32)	η = -.07
Wage or estimated value of time	.03 (.93) η = .37	.004 (1.67)	η = .06
Nonwage income (0 if >$3,000)	-.001 (-.84) η = -.09	-.0001 (-.93)	η = -.01
Nonwage income if > $3,000	-.0002 (-.21) η = -.01	-.00002 (-.35)	η = -.001
Dummy = 1 if nonwage income >$3,000	-6.54 (-1.12)	.10 (.19)	
Education 9-12 years	.35 (.29)	.05 (.23)	
Education 13-15 years	-.81 (-.52)	-.09 (-.26)	
Education 16+ years	-.62 (-.45)	-.67 (-1.59)	
Age 25-54 years	-2.02 (-1.01)	-.02 (-.07)	
Age 55-64 years	-1.48 (-.83)	.26 (.62)	
Age 65+ years	-1.03 (-.77)	.24 (.58)	

	Column 1		Column 2	
Family size	−.23 (−1.51)		−.16 (−3.03)	
Sex	−.36 (−.42)		.4 (2.11)	
Race	−.21 (−.11)		.66 (2.09)	
Number of disability days	.02 (2.24)		.02 (5.46)	
Health status good	5.06 (.83)		1.32 (5.20)	
Health status fair	6.96 (1.18)		3.23 (9.59)	
Health status poor	38.05 (1.62)		6.28 (9.72)	
Physician-population	.02 (.78)	$\eta = .42$	.02 (2.36)	$\eta = .47$
(Physician-population)^2	−.00008 (−.97)	$\eta = -.26$	−.00007 (−1.98)	$\eta = -.22$
Bed-population	−.31 (−.98)	$\eta = -.29$	−.30 (−2.35)	$\eta = -.28$
(Bed-population)^2	.04 (1.16)	$\eta = .18$	.03 (2.28)	$\eta = .14$
Married	1.14 (1.23)		.39 (1.47)	
(Physician coinsurance × price of visit)^2	.02 (.66)		−.0002 (−.17)	
Net price × health status good or fair	−.78 (−.66)		−.02 (−.64)	
Net price × health status poor	−5.89 (−1.43)		−.15 (−2.09)	

TABLE 1-4 (concluded)

	Dependent Variable = Physician Office Visits; $n = 2,617$ (weighted by average price of type of provider)	
	TSLS	OLS
Net price × nonwage income	.0002	.00002
	(.77)	(2.59)
Net price × wage income or estimated value of time	−.004	−.000007
	(−.82)	(−.06)
Constant	1.62	3.28
	(.26)	(5.53)
R^2	—	.16
Corrected R^2	—	.15
Dhrymes F	17.47	—
(d.f.)	(29,5)	—
t ratio adjustment factor	2.19	—
F	—	17.25
(d.f.)	—	(29,2587)

TABLE 1-5 Price of Care Equations

	Hospital Room and Board Price (n = 313)		Physician Office Visit Price (n = 2,346)	
	TSLS	OLS	TSLS	OLS
Room and board coinsurance rate	-4.00 $\eta = -.02$ $(-.49124)$	-9.24 $\eta = -.05$ (-2.5040)		
Number of hospital days	-1.26 $\eta = -.19$ (-2.4169)	-1.54 $\eta = -.26$ (-7.9618)		
Maximum payment per hospital day	1.03 (1.6102)	$.04$ $(.19714)$		
Dummy (=1 if no limit on $/day)	-35.71 (-1.4987)	3.81 $(.58805)$		
Physician office visit co-insurance			-1.73 $\eta = -.21$ (-1.0125)	-1.27 $\eta = -.15$ (-3.3033)
Number of physician office visits			$.09$ $\eta = .06$ (1.2043)	$-.09$ $\eta = -.06$ (-3.4615)
Wage income/week (0 if no wage income)	$.03$ $\eta = .02$ $(.81409)$	$.01$ $\eta = .01$ $(.45336)$	$.01$ $\eta = .07$ (5.3895)	$.02$ $\eta = .07$ (5.9284)
Estimated value of time (0 if wage income >0)	$.03$ $\eta = .02$ $(.56632)$	$.02$ $\eta = .01$ $(.39000)$	$.01$ $\eta = .04$ (1.4437)	$.01$ $\eta = .04$ (1.6210)
Nonwage income (0 if > $3,000)	$.005$ $\eta = .04$ (2.1218)	$.003$ $\eta = .02$ (1.4139)	$.0001$ $\eta = .005$ $(.4655)$	$.0002$ $\eta = .009$ $(.9387)$
Nonwage income if > $3,000	$.0004$ $\eta = .005$ $(.54128)$	$.0006$ $\eta = .007$ (1.0793)	$.0001$ $\eta = .005$ $(.3869)$	$.00004$ $\eta = .002$ $(.4420)$
Dummy = 1 if nonwage income >$3,000	-10.483 (-1.4544)	-10.138 (-1.6120)	$-.45$ $(-.1071)$	$.9181$ (1.1695)
Education 9-11 years	5.16 (1.1852)	4.99 (1.3386)	$.56$ (1.4491)	$.45$ (1.1850)

TABLE 1-5 (concluded)

	Hospital Room and Board Price (n = 313)		Physician Office Visit Price (n = 2,346)	
	TSLS	OLS	TSLS	OLS
Education 12 years	5.91 (1.2626)	.84 (.24023)	.32 (.7611)	.25 (.6768)
Education 13-15 years	1.37 (.19276)	-4.64 (-.82013)	1.73 (3.4881)	1.68 (3.6613)
Education 16+ years	4.27 (.63200)	3.30 (.59941)	.83 (1.5753)	.62 (1.3327)
Family size	.27 (.29659)	-.05 (-.07058)	-.14 (-1.6133)	-.20 (-2.7072)
Race	10.786 (1.4946)	6.91 (1.1949)	.67 (1.2531)	.79 (1.6161)
Region: Northeast	-6.62 (-1.1395)	-6.12 (-1.2408)	-2.3 (-4.5711)	-2.17 (-4.7685)
Region: North Central	1.50 (.24536)	-2.71 (-.56037)	-.72 (-1.2368)	-.85 (-1.9059)
Region: South	-5.72 (-1.0498)	-6.36 (-1.3395)	-.24 (-.4604)	-.34 (-.7541)

Region: Mountain	-3.59		-2.3		.93		.77	
	(-.35944)		(-.26700)		(1.0508)		(1.0272)	
M.D.s per 100,000 population ratio	.27	$\eta = .61$	.2	$\eta = .45$	.0009	$\eta = .01$	.006	$\eta = .09$
	(1.6535)		(1.4582)		(.0685)		(.4553)	
(M.D.s per 100,000 population ratio)^2	-.0005	$\eta = .16$	-.0003	$\eta = .28$	.0001	$\tau = .19$	.0001	$\eta = .14$
	(-.77473)		(-.48873)		(1.5656)		(1.2592)	
Beds per 1,000 population ratio	.81	$\eta = .08$	.03	$\eta = -.002$	.30	$r = .18$	.22	$\eta = .13$
	(.36104)		(.01302)		(1.5239)		(1.1543)	
(Beds per 1,000 population ratio)^2	-.22	$\eta = -.12$	-.08	$\eta = -.09$	-.03	$r = -.009$	-.02	$\eta = -.007$
	(-1.0121)		(-.45284)		(-1.5126)		(-1.1579)	
Constant term	28.155		46.424		5.99		6.72	
	(1.7698)		(4.4359)		(3.3595)		(6.8796)	
R^2	—		.31		—		.09	
Corrected R^2	—		.25		—		.08	
Dhrymes F	3.07		—		1.71		—	
(d.f.)	(23,17)		—		(21,18)		—	
t ratio adjustment factor	1.08		—		.43		—	
F	—		5.61		—		10.48	
(d.f.)	—		(23,289)		—		(21,2324)	

APPENDIX 2

Recalculating Elasticities for Family Unit Heads

In our earlier paper (Newhouse and Phelps, 1974a) we presented results based on heads of households who had been hospitalized or who used a physician. It later came to our attention that the data included a number of heads who had no wage income during the year. Our algorithm had assigned these individuals a zero wage and hence a zero value of time, obviously an error. Therefore, we reestimated these equations using the subset of heads with positive wage income. In these revised estimates we excluded individuals with deductibles in their policies for reasons explained in the text; these individuals were included in the earlier results. We also excluded from the price equations individuals who had obtained care for which no charge had been made, which we had not done in our earlier estimates. The results are sufficiently changed from those in the earlier paper to warrant some discussion. In general, the elasticities estimated using TSLS are near zero and not significantly different from zero; the elasticities estimated using OLS are rather small, but generally significant. We first consider hospital admissions, then length of hospital stay, and then physician office visits (nonsurgical). We did not estimate a use-nonuse of physicians equation for the subsample of employed heads.

Hospital Admissions

The results (Table 2-1) show that the admissions response to coinsurance among heads is very similar to the full sample; the estimated elasticity is -0.21. Wage income is quite significant and has an elasticity of 0.29, higher than in the full sample, whereas nonwage income has practically no effect (elasticity of 0.04) and is not significant at conventional levels. This finding tends to support Grossman's investment model, although errors in measuring the appropriate value of nonwage income make a strong conclusion about its true value unjustified. However, the weakness of the family-size effect also supports the investment model, and this result is less easily attributed to errors in measurement. These results must, however, be added with the results for length of stay and hospital price to obtain an overall test of the investment model, as is done in the text for the full sample.

Hospital beds in the county of residence were entered in linear form in this table; unlike the full sample they exert a moderately

TABLE 2-1 LOGIT Estimation of Nonobstetrical Admission Equation: No Positive Deductibles, Non-Zero Wage Income[a]

Variable	Elasticity at Mean for Continuous Variables; Change in Probability for Dummy Variables	Absolute Value of Asymptotic Normal Variable (significance level in parentheses)
Hospital coinsurance rate	−0.21	2.19 (.03)
Office visit coinsurance rate	−0.40	2.26 (.02)
Sex (1 if female)	0.016	1.56 (.12)
Age	0.22	0.81 (.42)
Wage rate	0.29	2.16 (.03)
Nonwage income	0.036	1.25 (.26)
Health status good (1 if good)	0.050	3.59 (.01)
Health status fair (1 if fair)	0.074	3.62 (.01)
Health status poor (1 if poor)	0.30	6.44 (.01)
Family size	−0.054	0.29 (.77)
Education	−0.41	1.29 (.20)
Rural area dummy (1 if rural area)	−0.007	0.76 (.45)
Physician-population	−0.24	1.01 (.81)
Hospital bed-population	0.35	2.04 (.04)
Race (1 if nonwhite)	−0.022	2.29 (.02)
Constant	−2.33	—

Chi-square of estimate (15 d.f.) = 83.6, significant at 0.01

[a] $n = 1{,}579$. This is the sample remaining after excluding from the original sample of 7,803 individuals: (a) 2,760 individuals whose policies are not verified; (b) 38 individuals with more than three policies; this exclusion was for computational convenience; (c) 3,244 individuals with zero wage income or wage income in excess of $500 per week (1963 prices); and (d) 305 individuals with positive hospital or medical deductibles. Some individuals are excluded for more than one reason. The mean probability of admission is 0.077.

strong and statistically significant effect on hospital admissions. We would expect this effect to be even more pronounced had we included variables measuring community demand, as explained above. Even as it stands, the result supports the notion that there is nonprice rationing of hospital services (see also Rafferty, 1971). This discrepancy from the full sample may be attributable to the difference in functional form; we are continuing to explore this question.

The health status dummy variables are the most important determinants of admissions, as in the full sample. (Excellent health status is the omitted value.) Controlling for health status, age does not have a significant effect.[1]

Education has the negative effect predicted by the investment model but the effect is not statistically significant at conventional levels. The rural dummy variable is not significant.

In the results presented in Table 2-1 we excluded individuals whose insurance policy contained a deductible. In order to take account of variation in a deductible, as well as a coinsurance rate, we have entered an expected total price variable directly. We are not very confident about the results, however, because of the difficulties of estimating the expected price. For those who did not go to the hospital, we assumed that the mean gross price of those who went was what was expected and applied the insurance policy they had to this expenditure. For those who did go to the hospital, we made two alternative assumptions: (1) that the expected expenditure was the actual realized expenditure, and (2) that the expected gross expenditure was the mean gross expenditure. We then applied the insurance policy to determine the expected net expenditure. The former is probably the more realistic assumption, because the physician and the individual usually have some information about diagnosis when the patient is being admitted. For this reason, the elasticity with respect to actual price could be expected to be greater (in absolute value) than that estimated using the mean price; those individuals who expected a low price would tend to be admitted more readily, and vice versa. There is a second reason why use of the actual price could be expected to result in a greater elasticity than the mean price. The mean price is approximately proportional to the coinsurance rate in this sample (it is exactly proportional for the 88 per cent of the observations with no deductible); as argued in the text, use of the coinsurance rate results in a lower elasticity estimate than use of actual price because a change in the coinsurance rate introduced a partially offsetting change in expenditure.[2]

The results from these two alternative assumptions are shown in Table 2-2. As expected, the elasticity using actual expenditure is much higher than that using the mean price (0.67 vs. 0.16). This elasticity with respect to expected price compares with an elasticity of approximately 0.2 with respect to the coinsurance rate.

The other results in Table 2-2 are similar to those in Table 2-1, with the following exceptions: (1) The nonwage income coefficient is significant when using actual expenditure (asymptotic Z equals 2.26), but the elasticity is still very small (0.07); (2) The education coefficient has become significant at a 5 per cent level when using

TABLE 2-2 LOGIT Estimation of Admission Equation; Positive Deductibles Included[a]

Variable	Elasticity at Mean for Continuous Variables; Change in Probability for Dummy Variables		Absolute Value of Asymptotic Normal Variable (significance level in parentheses)	
	Actual Expenditure	Mean Expenditure	Actual Expenditure	Mean Expenditure
Expected price	−.67	−.16	5.99 (.01)	1.69 (.09)
Physician office visit coinsurance	−.36	−.46	2.00 (.04)	2.57 (.01)
Sex	.011	.011	1.56 (.12)	1.29 (.20)
Age	.25	.26	0.88 (.38)	0.97 (.33)
Wage rate	.26	.28	1.92 (.05)	2.10 (.03)
Nonwage income	.064	.040	2.26 (.02)	1.40 (.16)
Health status good	.032	.045	3.36 (.01)	3.60 (.01)
Health status fair	.052	.069	3.63 (.01)	3.76 (.01)
Health status poor	.25	.28	6.59 (.01)	6.52 (.01)
Family size	−.086	−.084	0.43 (.67)	0.44 (.66)
Education	−.66	−.48	2.02 (.04)	1.52 (.13)
Rural area dummy	−.002	−.004	0.36 (.72)	0.52 (.60)
Physician-population	−.16	−.15	0.68 (.43)	0.66 (.51)
Hospital bed-population	.25	.28	1.42 (.15)	1.58 (.11)
Race	−.011	−.019	1.53 (.12)	2.20 (.03)
Constant	−1.92	−2.38		

Chi-square of estimate using actual expenditure (15 d.f.) = 125.02, $p<.0001$; using mean expenditure (15 d.f.) of 82.77, $p<0.01$.

[a] $n = 1,761$. The sample is the same as for Table 1 plus 182 individuals with positive deductibles who satisfied the other restrictions.

actual expenditure; (3) The size of the elasticities and the asymptotic normal statistics drop somewhat for the hospital bed-population ratio. The values are, however, sufficiently similar to those in Table 2-1 to support the conclusions drawn there.

The results of estimating length of stay, visit, and price equations are summarized in Table 2-3 and shown in detail in tables 2-4 and 2-5.

Length of Hospital Stay

The own-price elasticities at the mean for length of hospital stay are estimated to be −0.29 using TSLS and −0.13 using OLS, somewhat

TABLE 2-3 Own-Price, Cross-Price, and Wage Income Elasticities, Heads Only[a]

	Length of Hospital Stay (n = 76)		Physician Office Visit (n = 563)	
	TSLS	OLS	TSLS	OLS
Hospital coinsurance × price of bed	−.29	−.13	−.10	−.12
	(1.89)	(1.28)	(1.08)	(3.04)
M.D. office coinsurance × price	.20	−.09	−.03	−.10
	(1.14)	(.79)	(.21)	(2.70)
Wage income-week	−.35	−.15	.07	.08
	(1.46)	(.53)	(.93)	(.99)

	Room and Board Price (n = 57)		Physician Price (n = 517)	
	TSLS	OLS	TSLS	OLS
Coinsurance rate	−.04	−.03	.26	−.25
	(.66)	(.56)	(.56)	(2.25)
Price per day limit in $	.08	−.0004	—	—
	(.77)	(.006)	—	—
Wage	−.08	−.07	.14	.13
	(.33)	(.32)	(1.31)	(1.61)

[a] The absolute value of t statistics are in parentheses. For TSLS, the t statistics are the Dhrymes alternative t statistics (Dhrymes, 1969). We arrived at the sample used to estimate these equations as follows. There were 2,376 heads; of these, 788 had insurance that was not verified and 13 had more than three insurance policies. This latter group was excluded for computational reasons. This left 1,566 heads. This subsample of 1,566 of the national probability sample whose insurance was verified is not representative by work-group size and income of the entire population. Therefore, we weighted the sample along these dimensions to be representative of the national population. To obtain the sample of 76 for the length of stay equation we applied the following restrictions to the 1,566 sample (the numbers in parentheses are the number of 1,566 that the restriction excluded): zero wages or wages greater than $500 per week (1963 dollars) (475); no hospital days or hospital days exceeding 40 days (1,443); physician office visit price higher than $50 per visit (1); positive deductible in the hospital policy (92); expenses exceeding upper limit of policy (3). Some individuals were excluded for more than one reason. The physician visit equation started with the same 1,566 heads, which were reduced to 563 by the following restrictions; zero wages or wages greater than $500 per week (1963 dollars) (475); physician office visit price higher than $50 per visit (1); no physician visits or physician visits exceeding 30 (717); positive deductible in insurance policy applying to physician visits (67). The numbers are reduced for the price equation by the number of individuals who received care for which no charge was made.

TABLE 2-4 Utilization of Heads

Explanatory Variable Coefficient (t ratio) (elasticity)	Dependent Variable = Length of Hospital Stay n = 76; Heads Only (weighted by average price of type of room)				Dependent Variable = Physician Office Visits n = 563; Heads Only (weighted by average price of type of provider)			
	Eq. (1) TSLS		Eq. (2) OLS		Eq. (3) TSLS		Eq. (4) OLS	
Hospital coinsurance × price of bed	-.25 (-1.89)	$\eta = -.29$	-.11 (-1.28)	$\eta = -.13$	-.038 (-1.08)	$\eta = -.10$	-.046 (-3.04)	$\eta = -.12$
M.D. office coinsurance × price	.54 (1.14)	$\eta = .20$	-.25 (-.79)	$\eta = -.09$	-.024 (-.21)	$\eta = -.03$	-.083 (-2.70)	$\eta = -.10$
Wage income-week	-.024 (-1.46)	$\eta = -.35$	-.010 (-.53)	$\eta = -.15$	.003 (.93)	$\eta = .07$	.003 (.99)	$\eta = .08$
Nonwage income	-.001 (-.87)	$\eta = -.05$	-.0017 (-.95)	$\eta = -.08$	.0003 (.98)	$\eta = .02$	.0002 (.64)	$\eta = .01$
Nonwage income if > $3,000	.001 (-.54)	$\eta = -.02$	-.00037 (-.12)	$\eta = -.008$	.0015 (3.42)	$\eta = .07$	.0015 (2.40)	$\eta = .07$
Dummy = 1 if nonwage income > $3,000	1.77 (.17)		.22 (.01)		-5.93 (-2.43)		-5.89 (-1.75)	
Education 9-11 years	1.58 (.92)		1.86 (.73)		-1.00 (-2.01)		-.97 (-1.50)	
Education 12 years	-1.16 (-.58)		.68 (.24)		-.25 (-.60)		-.26 (-.43)	
Education 13-15 years	2.69 (.87)		.13 (.03)		-.09 (-.16)		.008 (.01)	
Education 16+ years	.21 (.09)		1.09 (.31)		-1.12 (-2.08)		-1.05 (-1.44)	

TABLE 2-4 (concluded)

Explanatory Variable Coefficient (t ratio) (elasticity)	Dependent Variable = Length of Hospital Stay n = 76; Heads Only (weighted by average price of type of room)		Dependent Variable = Physician Office Visits n = 563; Heads Only (weighted by average price of type of provider)	
	Eq. (1) TSLS	Eq. (2) OLS	Eq. (3) TSLS	Eq. (4) OLS
Age 25-34	2.57	4.49	-1.96	-2.04
	(.65)	(.75)	(-2.55)	(1.89)
Age 35-54	7.19	8.08	-2.04	-2.02
	(1.85)	(1.34)	(-2.78)	(-1.93)
Age 55-64	13.64	15.00	-1.58	-1.58
	(3.00)	(2.28)	(-1.96)	(-1.38)
Age 65+	9.25	14.08	-1.60	-1.56
	(1.84)	(2.06)	(-1.70)	(-1.18)
Family size	-.097	-.33	-.10	-.11
	(-.21)	(-.48)	(-.96)	(-.72)
Sex	-8.29	-6.75	1.89	1.90
(=1 if female)	(-2.98)	(1.63)	(2.57)	(1.86)
Race	3.28	1.72	1.79	1.90
(=1 if nonwhite)	(1.58)	(.57)	(3.34)	(2.70)
Disability days	.063	.058	.028	.028
	(5.09)	(3.17)	(6.01)	(4.21)

	(1)	(2)	(3)	(4)
Health status good	-.39 (-.18)	1.21 (.41)	1.38 (4.10)	1.36 (2.88)
Health status fair	-2.47 (-1.03)	-.54 (-.16)	3.48 (7.64)	3.47 (5.36)
Health status poor	-5.00 (-1.82)	-2.34 (-.61)	6.70 (8.16)	6.66 (5.72)
M.D.'s/100,000	-.028 (-1.86), $\eta = -.35$	-.23 (-1.09), $\eta = -.29$	.007 (1.64), $\eta = .17$	.008 (1.65), $\eta = .18$
Beds/1,000	.48 (1.71), $\eta = .26$	.28 (.72), $\eta = .15$	-.05 (-.63), $\eta = -.04$	-.03 (-.34), $\eta = -.03$
Married	-6.12 (-2.10)	-2.95 (-.75)	1.35 (1.94)	1.42 (1.45)
Constant term	10.03 (1.69)	4.84 (.64)	3.30 (2.38)	4.04 (2.80)
R^2	.45	.45	—	.23
Corrected R^2	.20	.20		.20
Dhrymes F	4.29	—	12.46	—
(d.f.)	(24,8)	—	(24,8)	—
t ratio adjustment factor	1.70	—	1.43	—
F	—	1.76	—	6.89
(d.f.)	—	(24,51)	—	(24,538)

TABLE 2-5 Price of Care Equations, Heads Only[a]

	Hospital Room and Board Price (n = 57)				Physician Office Visit Price (n = 517)			
	TSLS		OLS		TSLS		OLS	
Room and board coinsurance rate	-11.23 (-.66)	$\eta = -.04$	-8.28 (-.56)	$\eta = -.03$	—		—	
Number of hospital days	-.72 (-1.15)	$\eta = -.13$	-1.09 (-2.40)	$\eta = -.19$	—		—	
Maximum payment per hospital day	.50 (.77)		-.003 (-.006)		—		—	
Dummy (=1 if no limit on $/day)	42.31 (1.23)		17.07 (.84)		—		—	
Physician office visit coinsurance	—		—		2.68 (.56)	$\eta = .26$	-2.49 (-2.25)	$\eta = -.25$
Number of physician office visits	—		—		.17 (.76)	$\eta = .10$	-.18 (-2.49)	$\eta = -.11$
Wage income	-.030 (-.33)	$\eta = -.08$	.023 (.32)	$\eta = .07$	.01 (1.31)	$\eta = .14$	.009 (1.61)	$\eta = .13$
Nonwage income (0 if >$3,000)	.008 (1.16)	$\eta = .07$	.006 (1.06)	$\eta = .06$	.0002 (.28)	$\eta = .008$	.0002 (.31)	$\eta = .007$
Nonwage income > $3,000	.013 (1.09)	$\eta = .07$	.008 (.70)	$\eta = .04$	-.002 (-1.19)	$\eta = -.05$	-.001 (-.93)	$\eta = -.03$
Dummy = 1 if nonwage income >$3,000	-47.21 (-.75)		-20.78 (-.36)		10.36 (1.24)		6.10 (.98)	
Education 9-11 years	-4.49 (-.40)		-1.33 (-.13)		.88 (.60)		.61 (.54)	
Education 12 years	-5.08 (-.48)		-4.93 (-.49)		1.41 (.94)		.70 (.63)	

Education 13-15 years	-34.88 (-1.71)	-29.75 (-1.61)	4.49 (2.55)	3.87 (2.92)
Education 16 + years	-8.20 (-.52)	-6.37 (-.44)	1.41 (.79)	.47 (.35)
Family size	.75 (.29)	.29 (.12)	.06 (.20)	.004 (.02)
Northeast	-22.40 (-1.53)	-22.40 (-1.62)	-3.10 (-1.64)	-2.11 (-1.63)
North Central	-29.59 (-1.99)	-27.63 (-1.99)	-2.61 (-1.19)	-.98 (-.76)
South	-38.62 (-2.12)	-35.62 (-2.15)	-2.00 (-.97)	-.53 (-.40)
Mountain	-31.77 (-1.22)	-23.80 (-1.01)	-2.35 (-.71)	-.03 (-.01)
Physician-population	-.01 (-.11) $\eta = -.03$	-.001 (-.008) $\eta = -.002$	.04 (2.82) $\eta = .50$	.04 (4.21) $\eta = .57$
Beds-population	1.20 (.73) $\eta = .13$	1.11 (.71) $\eta = .12$	.22 (.84) $\eta = .11$	.17 (.84) $\eta = .09$
Constant	73.93 (3.06)	72.82 (3.21)	-.58 (-.13)	4.70 (2.22)
R^2	—	.41	—	.12
Corrected R^2	—	.11	—	.09
Dhrymes F	1.17	—	2.13	—
(d.f.)	(19,18)	—	(17,20)	—
t ratio adjustment factor	.99	—	.80	—
F	1.37	1.37	—	4.13
(d.f.)	(19,37)	(19,37)	—	(17,499)

a Excluding those who received care for which no charge was made.

larger than the full sample. OLS should be biased away from the TSLS result (Newhouse and Phelps, 1974b), yet the TSLS result is larger in absolute value; consequently, we feel that the TSLS result is likely to be too high, though how much too high is difficult to say. The cross-price elasticity changes signs between the two estimators and is not significantly different from zero.

Wage income elasticities are negative but are not significant at conventional levels. The negative wage income elasticity by itself does not contradict Grossman's investment model because that model applies to all medical expenditure rather than to any particular component of medical expenditure. Moreover, in the full sample wage elasticities become positive, as shown in Table 1-3. The negative sign on wage income may also indicate a downward bias because of the decline in income associated with sickness. Non-wage income elasticities are not significant.

As for demographic variables, length of stay increases with age, is shorter for females, and shorter for married individuals. This is consistent with the effect of these variables taken one at a time in the data gathered by the National Health Survey (Gordon, 1973). There is no relationship apparent with education nor with self-perceived health status; evidently, self-perceived health status is too crude to measure differences in health status among the hospitalized population.

Room and Board Price

The elasticity of room and board price with respect to the coinsurance rate is near zero and not significant in both OLS and TSLS. This is a marked change from our earlier paper. Wage income elasticities are also not significantly different from zero, nor are nonwage income elasticities. As in the case of the full sample, we infer that neither amenities nor time saved from shorter queues are very important in explaining the deviation of the room and board price, given the type of accommodation. Weighted hospital days are negatively related to the price; those who are in the hospital longer tend to use cheaper hospitals, given the type of accommodation.

Physician Visits

It is difficult to estimate demand for physician services from these data because 85 per cent of this sample had no insurance for physician services.[3] As a result, there is relatively little price variation. The elasticities using TSLS are small and not significantly different from zero; the OLS elasticities (own-price and cross-price) are around −0.1 and quite significant. Because both price and insurance are endogenous, one could argue that there is a bias away from zero in the OLS results. However, other work we have done persuades us that this elasticity is at least as high as −0.1 (Phelps and Newhouse, 1972; Newhouse, Phelps, and Schwartz, 1974). Wage income elasticities are small and not significant; nonwage income is also not significant except for the 5 per cent of the sample whose nonwage income is higher than $3,000, in which case the elasticity is 0.07, and quite significant in both OLS and TSLS. Health status variables are the most closely related to visits; visits steadily increase as self-perceived health status worsens and also increase with disability days. Additional physicians show a weak positive relationship to visits, but beds show none. Non-whites and females make more visits.

Physician Price

The physician visit price appears quite responsive to coinsurance using the OLS estimate; the elasticity is −0.25 and significant. The TSLS result is of the wrong sign. An increase in insurance from no coverage to full coverage increases the price per (weighted) visit by about 30 per cent. Those who visit the physician more frequently seek out lower-priced physicians; the elasticity with respect to the number of visits is −0.11 (OLS). Wage income has a positive effect that borders on significance at usual levels (the effect is very significant if non-heads are included), whereas nonwage income has no effect. We interpret this to mean that a higher-priced physician means less time spent in search or in a queue, and not additional amenities. The physician-population ratio bears a very strong and positive relationship to price. We have not attempted to treat this variable as endogenous, and therefore its interpretation must remain ambiguous.

NOTES

1. Ancillary services frequently have different insurance provisions. Work is now in progress to estimate their responsiveness to price.
2. We have, however, excluded from the sample all individuals who have exceeded an upper limit, on the grounds that we could only imperfectly control for health stock loss. This excluded a negligible number of individuals. See note to Table 1.

3. The nine are professional, managerial, sales, foreman, agriculture-mining-construction, manufacturing, finance, public administration, and entertainment.
4. We are indebted to Karen Davis for this point.
5. We did not feel we had a sufficient degree of overidentification to treat disability days as endogenous.
6. Because our data come from a multistage probability sample (around seventy-five primary sampling units), the estimated standard errors are biased downward. The amount of bias depends on the size of covariances within the primary sampling units. On the basis of unpublished analyses of utilization data within New York City census tracts, we would guess that these covariances are sufficiently small so as to create negligible bias in the estimated standard errors.
7. This is a heroic assumption; it assumes that individuals who are paid by salary are similar to those paid a wage, as are those who are self-employed. Sick leave provisions are ignored, as is the possibility that one's opportunity cost of time may fall if one is sick. Nonpecuniary aspects of work are assumed to be a constant proportion of the money wage. Despite these problems, the simple wage rate seems to predict some phenomena reasonably well (most particularly use or nonuse of the medical care system and physician price).
8. Michael Grossman has pointed out to us that hours of work at any stage in the life cycle should depend on the rate of interest relative to the rate of time preference. This implies that age should be in Equation (2), and that if it were, (2) might become underidentified, because age is strongly related to experience. The problem can be solved by specifying other variables (such as industry mix in the area) in (1); because Heckman's procedure failed computationally (see text), we have not pursued this issue.
9. The estimator converged to different values depending on the starting point.
10. We also attempted to use the following method for estimating the reservation wage: Let $H = a(w - w^*) + e_H$, where H = hours, w and w^* are as defined in (1) and (2), and e_H is an error term. Let $w^* = bX + e_r$, where X is the vector of variables described in the text. Substituting, $H = aw + cX + e$, where $c = -ab$ and $e = e_H - ae_r$. Therefore, b can be estimated as $-c/a$ and w^* estimated as bX. When we followed this procedure, the results were unsatisfactory. Using an OLS estimator to estimate a and c, many of the predicted reservation wages were negative. Using a tobit estimator, a different problem arose; the standard deviation of the estimated reservation wages seemed unreasonably high (it was six times the standard deviation of w). We therefore resorted to the procedure described in the text, one known to be biased, but nevertheless producing estimates that appeared to have less mean square error. We are exploring alternative estimates of time value.
11. The total number of individuals in the sample for the equation is larger than in the utilization equations because individuals with deductibles in their policies have not been excluded.
12. The proof follows the standard proofs of the level of investment in any risky asset. The asset with the certain return is preferable.
13. Throughout this discussion we ignore the presence of upper limits. We have excluded the 0.2 per cent of individuals in our sample who exceeded an upper limit and have assumed that the behavior of the remainder was not affected by the presence of an upper limit. Because the probability of exceeding an upper limit is slight, this assumption should have little effect on our estimates (Keeler, Newhouse, and Phelps, 1974).

14. Nor is it in general proportional to the deductible. This is easily seen by differentiating (5) with respect to D:

$$\frac{dE\,(f(x))}{dD} = (1-C)\,Dh\,(D)$$

This is proportional to D only if $h\,(D)$ is constant or, equivalently, if $h'(D)$ is zero, which will be true only in the special case of local maximums and minimums or a uniform distribution of expected expenditure. As a result, if the responsiveness to expected price is linear, responsiveness of demand to a deductible is some nonlinear function.

15. Suppose that higher moments of $f(x)$ as well as the first moment are relevant in explaining demand; policies with no deductibles are more convenient for estimation in this case also. If D is zero, the nth moment is homogeneous of degree n.

16. Partially offsetting, on the assumption that the elasticity is less than 1, as appears reasonable from our estimates in Section 5.

17. This procedure can lead to biased estimates if the services tend to be covered at different rates and one is used without the other (Newhouse and Phelps, 1974b). However, these two services are covered at nearly identical rates (roughly 0.3), and the quantities of services consumed are probably roughly in proportion.

18. Using the instrumental variable estimate of C, the elasticity at the mean for the specification used in Table 2 was on the order of -0.4; asymptotic normal statistics were slightly in excess of 1.

19. The program uses a Fletcher-Powell minimization algorithm.

20. Differentiating (4), one can compute that the elasticity at the mean is $(1-\bar{P})\beta x$.

21. This result can be approximated by assuming that whites have the mean admission rate and length of stay (0.078 and 7.39 days, respectively), whereas nonwhites are similar to whites except for the racial dummy variable effect. The conclusion ignores effects of race on the price per weighted day, if any; however, race is not significantly different from zero in price equation presented next.

22. $0.23 = 9.24/40.97$. The 9.24 is the coefficient in the OLS room and board price equation; the 40.97 value is the predicted room and board price at a coinsurance rate of 1.

23. Both this equation and the physician visit price equation were run without the physician-population and bed-population ratios to guard against a simultaneous equation problem. The estimated coefficients were virtually unchanged.

24. There is a positive but essentially zero (and insignificant) cross-price coefficient in the OLS length of stay equations.

25. $0.18 = 1.27/6.93$. The 1.27 figure is the coefficient in the price equation; 6.93 is the predicted price selected by an individual with no insurance (other variables at their means).

NOTES TO APPENDIX 2

1. Age and education are not entered in interval form in the logit equations in order to minimize computational costs.

2. This may not be true of a change in a deductible. All those hospitalized in our

sample exceeded the deductible in their policies. A small change in the deductible, therefore, would not affect the marginal conditions.
3. This may explain the near zero cross-price elasticity in estimating cross-price in the length of stay equation.

REFERENCES

Andersen, R., and O.W. Anderson, *A Decade of Health Services* (Chicago: University of Chicago Press, 1967).

Cooper, Richard V., and Joseph P. Newhouse, "Further Results on the Errors-in-the-Variables Problem," P–4715, The Rand Corporation, October 1971.

Davis, K., and L.B. Russell, "The Substitution of Hospital Outpatient Care for Inpatient Care," *Review of Economics and Statistics*, 54 (May 1972), pp. 109–120.

Dhrymes, Phoebus J., "Alternative Asymptotic Tests of Significance and Related Aspects of 2SLS and 2SLS Estimated Parameters," *Review of Economic Studies*, 36 (April 1969), pp. 213–226.

Feldstein, Martin S., "Hospital Cost Inflation: A Study of Nonprofit Price Dynamics," *American Economic Review*, 61 (September 1971), pp. 853–872.

Gordon, Evelyn W., "Average Length of Stay in Short-Stay Hospitals: Demographic Factors," Vital and Health Statistics Series 13, Number 13, DHEW Publication No. (HSM) 73-1764 (Washington, D.C.: Government Printing Office, 1973).

Gronau, Reuben, "The Intrafamily Allocation of Time," *American Economic Review*, 63 (September 1973), pp. 643–651.

———, "The Measurement of Output of the Nonmarket Sector: The Evaluation of Housewives' Time," in Milton Moss (editor), *The Measurement of Economic and Social Performance* (New York: National Bureau of Economic Research, 1973).

Grossman, Michael, *The Demand for Health* (New York: National Bureau of Economic Research, Occasional Paper No. 119, 1972).

Health Insurance Association of America, "A Comparison of Group Medical Care Insurance Benefits to Charges," New York, 1968.

Heckman, James, "Shadow Prices, Market Wages, and Labor Supply," *Econometrica*, 42 (July 1974).

Keeler, Emmet B., Joseph P. Newhouse, and Charles E. Phelps, "Deductibles and the Demand for Medical Services: The Theory of a Consumer Facing a Variable Price Schedule under Uncertainty," R-1514-OEO/NC, The Rand Corporation (1974).

Marquis, Kent H., Charles F. Cannell, and Andre Laurant, "Reporting Health Events in Household Interviews," *Vital and Health Statistics*, Series 2, No. 45, DHEW Publication No. (HSM) 72-1028 (Washington, D.C.: Government Printing Office, 1972).

Newhouse, Joseph P., and Charles E. Phelps, "Price and Income Elasticities for Medical Care Services," in Mark Perlman (editor), *The Economics of Health and Medical Care* (London: Macmillan, 1974a).

———, "On Having Your Cake and Eating It Too: An Analysis of Estimated Effects of Insurance on Demand for Medical Care," R-1149-NC, The Rand Corporation, April 1974b.

_____, and William B. Schwartz, "Policy Options and the Impact of National Health Insurance," *New England Journal of Medicine*, 290 (June 13, 1974), pp. 1345–1359.

Phelps, Charles E., "The Demand for Health Insurance: A Theoretical and Empirical Investigation," R-1054-OEO, The Rand Corporation, July 1973.

_____, and Joseph P. Newhouse, "Effects of Coinsurance on Demand for Physician Services," R-976-OEO, The Rand Corporation, June 1972. An abridged version of this paper was published as "Effects of Coinsurance: A Multivariate Analysis," *Social Security Bulletin*, 35 (1972), pp. 20–29.

_____, "Coinsurance, The Price of Time, and the Demand for Medical Services," *Review of Economics and Statistics*, 56 (August 1974).

Rafferty, John A., "Patterns of Hospital Use: An Analysis of Short-Run Variations," *Journal of Political Economy*, 79 (1971), pp. 154–165.

Tobin, James, "Estimation of Relationships for Limited Dependent Variables," *Econometrica*, 16 (January 1958), pp. 24–36.

7 ‖ COMMENTS

Paul B. Ginsburg
Michigan State University

Newhouse and Phelps have made a valuable contribution to the literature on econometric analysis of the demand for medical care. Their work is careful and detailed. They pay ample attention both to rigorous use of economic theory to derive hypotheses and to the relevance of the specification to major policy considerations. Although by no means the first econometric study of this topic, it is distinctive in a number of important ways. First, data on individuals are used instead of data on families or data aggregated by state. Compared to aggregate data, Newhouse and Phelps' data have the advantage of avoiding general aggregation problems (discussed by Theil and others), and provide superior opportunities for accurately specifying price. However, with data on individuals, a change in the price faced by a single individual should have different effects from an across-the-board change for all individuals in an area as community norms of health care change. National health insurance may approximate the latter model (change in utilization through norms) more closely.

A second distinct aspect of this work is specification of a particularly accurate marginal coinsurance rate. This is accomplished through information on the benefit structure of individual insurance policies and by eliminating individuals with deductibles from the sample. Other studies have used the average coinsurance rate to calculate net price. This method is theoretically defective because deductibles cause net price to be underestimated for low expenditures and overestimated for high expenditures, which causes an upward bias in price elasticity estimates. Another problem with the average rate is that it is a function of the dependent variable, giving rise to a bias in the opposite direction. Unfortunately, the overall direction of bias is not clear. A third difference from other studies is treatment of insurance as endogenous. Sicker people allegedly buy more extensive insurance coverage. Although this is not a problem for studies using aggregate data, adverse selection among individuals could give rise to an upward bias in price elasticity estimates. TSLS estimation is used here. Exogenous variables in the insurance equation that are excluded from the demand for care equation are size of the employee group and a series of occupational dummies. A fourth difference from other studies is the inclusion of health status variables in the demand equations. Their inclusion substantially improves the fit in many equations and avoids potential specification bias resulting from their omission. A fifth distinct aspect of this study is estimation of equations for price paid. The authors see differences from the mean in price paid to reflect variation in amenities, queuing, and degree of search. Finally, Grossman's model of the demand for health care as a human capital investment decision is used as the theoretical basis for this work. Although the theory does not suggest inclusion of any new variables, some ambiguity with respect to predicted signs is removed. Wage rate, nonwage income, education, and family size are the principal variables affected.

The elasticity of expenditures with respect to price are estimated to be -0.33 for hospital care and -0.22 for physician services. These estimates, particularly the physician estimates, are lower than those reported by other researchers. (The equations are linear, so elasticity is evaluated at the mean. It should be pointed out that mean coinsurance rates are 0.27 for hospital care and 0.85 for physician services.)

A number of aspects of these results warrant detailed discussion. First, TSLS estimates were uniformly poor. Elasticities were often insignificant, and if not, they tended to be higher than OLS estimates, contrary to a priori expectations. Certain implications can be drawn from this result. Adverse selection probably is not so quantitatively important as had been thought, which is plausible considering the large proportion of insurance that is purchased by employers. In fact, the sick may have less insurance rather than more, for they tend to be unemployed or employed by companies without health insurance benefits, thus facing a higher loading charge. In empirical analysis of aggregate data, Frech has found adverse selection to be quantitatively small.

Another implication of these results is that the TSLS estimation is not very efficient in this context. Since other researchers are unlikely to be able to estimate a superior demand for insurance equation to obtain an instrument for insurance coverage, treating insurance as endogenous is not a fruitful endeavor.

A highly interesting series of results are the negative cross-elasticities obtained, implying that hospital and physician services are complements.

These findings run counter to the usual notion of absence of coverage of physician services causing outpatient services to be performed on an inpatient basis. Although this may be the case, this effect is apparently swamped by other cross-price relationships.

Estimating interactions between the price variables on the one hand and income and health status on the other did not turn up any significant interactions. This result is contrary to a general expectation that price elasticities might be higher for low-income individuals and lower for individuals who are ill. However, the authors do not consider their evidence as a firm indication that such interactions do not exist.

Although I am generally enthusiastic about both the competence of the analysis and the usefulness of the results, I have a few criticisms worth mentioning. The authors have been rather ruthless in cutting down their sample in the interest of avoiding errors in the independent variables. For example, all persons other than heads of households were eliminated because of difficulties in establishing a value for their time. (They later were put back.) Those with insurance policies with deductibles were dropped because of difficulties in assigning them a marginal coinsurance rate. For the same reason, those individuals exceeding the limit of their policy were dropped.

Although the reasons for reducing the sample are valid, the costs of doing so are not discussed. By focusing only on heads of households, a large part of the population with potentially different behavior is ignored, reducing substantially the efficiency in estimation. Apparently, as seen in the later results, price elasticities for heads were not different, but the increase in standard errors from reducing the sample was large.

Dropping those individuals with deductibles and limits may cause the estimates to be inconsistent. It is rational for those with high price elasticities for medical care to purchase insurance with large deductibles if their premium depends on use (as in the case of a group of similar individuals). Excluding those choosing deductibles could affect the estimates, although the bias in this sample is limited by the small number of individuals who have deductible provisions in their policies. To maintain consistency, it might be desirable to also drop all of those approaching the limits of their policy as the marginal coinsurance rate is exceeded by the implicit rate that those individuals face. It may be best not to eliminate either group, but to attempt to impute implicit coinsurance rates to all. Although this will be quite a challenge, the preponderance of deductibles in recent proposals for national health insurance makes such an analysis highly relevant.

The equations using price paid as dependent variables are potentially very valuable and are much easier to estimate with data on individuals than with aggregated data. The efficiency of estimation could be improved if the average price in the respondent's community was used instead of the average price over the entire sample. Three regional dummy variables do not do an adequate job of reflecting varying degrees of local monopoly power, differences in wage levels and construction costs, and price differences caused by immobilities of medical resources. Consequently, a great deal of variation in the deviation from average prices is attributable to factors other than amenities, queuing, and search activity—the factors that the deviations are supposed to reflect. Since sampling is concentrated in a limited number of primary sampling units, there may be enough data to obtain prices from the sample for each area. If not, outside price data should be brought in.

Because of the unique position of the physician as an agent for the patient as well as provider of health care, and the evidence that health care markets tend to stay out of equilibrium for long periods of time, supply variables have been included in most economists' estimates of the demand for health care. When individual observations are used, however, variables reflecting demand for care in the community should be included along with the supply variables. For instance, an area may have a large number of hospital beds per capita, but if the population is old and has extensive insurance coverage, the survey respondent may be facing a market in which there is excess demand rather than excess supply. Thus, omitting community demand variables risks losing some of the information that the supply variables are intended to provide.

The authors use type of accomodation to adjust hospital length of stay for productivity in health care. This variable strikes me more as a reflection of amenities than productivity in delivering health care. To the extent that productivity is not adjusted for in the length of stay equation, there should be a downward bias in the price elasticity estimate. However, productivity will wind up in the price of care equation, giving an upward bias to price elasticity in that equation. The net effect when price elasticity of expenditures is computed should be zero. The problem does not affect the physician service equation so severely, because the price differences between G.P.'s and specialists are much better indicators of productivity difference.

Since this study clearly adds to our knowledge about medical care demand, it is appropriate to ask where we should go from here. There are a number of directions that I can see. One, which is suggested by Newhouse and Phelps, is studying the demand for ancillary services in the hospital. Feldstein's calculations of changes in hospital costs over time show that increases in inputs per patient day are a significant cause of cost inflation. In his theory, this increase is predominantly demand-determined. This makes the study of demand for ancillary services particularly important.

Use of health status variables is an endeavor of great potential. Although Newhouse and Phelps characterize their variables as crude, they contribute to the explanatory power of a number of equations. The usefulness of health status variables is pointed out by some of the results that Karen Davis presented in her paper at this conference. With health status variables included, utilization was a positive function of income. With the variables omitted, the relationship was U-shaped.

Finally, more work on the interactions between price and health status, income, age, and other variables is desirable. National health insurance is often advocated not only to correct alleged market failure in private health insurance, but also to subsidize medical care for certain groups such as the poor and the sick to increase their use. All plans involve a tradeoff between welfare losses from financing the plan and moral hazard on the one hand and the benefits of increased utilization by target groups on the other. Detailed price elasticity information is needed to both assess and design public financing plans with these considerations in mind.

Harold S. Luft
Stanford University

This most recent paper by Newhouse and Phelps is important for two reasons, one positive and one negative. On the positive side, it demonstrates the usefulness of microdata sets and the potential for much more detailed analysis of the demand for medical care services. On the negative side, we should be wary of too much concentration on the question of demand and remember that the market for medical care has unique characteristics that require much more study of the supply conditions.

The use of micro survey data by Newhouse and Phelps has several real advantages. They are able to move beyond data based on geographical aggregates for which we have little knowledge of the underlying distributions and for which mean values may be inappropriate. A primary example of the improvement afforded by microdata is the very detailed description of insurance coverage available in the NORC data. This allows the coinsurance and deductible provisions in the policies to be separated and a demand function to be estimated in which the price is truly the marginal price and not an implicit average price based on gross and net expenditures. These microdata also allow the specific decisions concerning the marginal unit of care to be more clearly identified. In addition, the use of a household survey allows data on individual health status to be incorporated. Newhouse and Phelps were also able to include some estimates of geographically based variables, such as the supply of physicians and beds per capita for the counties from which the sample was drawn.

There are, however, a number of problems and cautions that are raised by the use of microdata. The need for using the appropriate sample for each equation and the problem of missing data can lead to widely varying numbers of observations. For instance, the final hospital elasticity results are composed of estimates for length of stay (364 observations), admissions (1,579 observations), and price (313 observations). Other related regressions are based on samples ranging from 76 to 4,536. Although even the smallest of these samples is reasonably large for aggregate series, one must be careful that a variable does not represent only a very small number of observations that may, in the particular sample used, be aberrant. For instance, based on the proportions found in the total sample, only 7 of the 76 people are black and only 4 of 76 have nonwage incomes in excess of $3,000.

When working with aggregate data, ignorance usually leads us to assume that all variables are equally reliable or unreliable. (Discussion of the effects of errors in measurement can usually be traced to coefficients that appear with the "wrong" sign or magnitude.) Concern about the measurement of variables is probably more important for microdata sets in which errors are less likely to average out in aggregation, and the mere number of observations makes looking at the residuals a particularly painful task. In fact, one of the reasons for the Newhouse-Phelps paper was to correct an error in the algorithm that generated the wage variable in their original paper.

Finally, there are some statistical problems that should be recognized. The NORC sample is clustered; this invalidates the assumptions of independence of observations and leads to standard error estimates that are biased downward.[1] This bias should be considered when reporting the results. The clustering also implies that the data for some variables, such as the physician-population ratios, are based on the number of clusters in the sample, not the number of persons.

On the negative side, and more important than the use of microdata, is the use of such data in the context of a very traditional market framework. There are a number of characteristics of the medical care sector that should cause us to focus at least some of our attention on the behavior of the physician rather than solely on the rational consumer making choices among a number of commodities. The pathbreaking article by Kenneth Arrow on "Uncertainty and the Welfare Economics of Medical Care" clearly indicated the importance of uncertainty and the asymmetry of information in medical care.[2] In a recent review of the econometric literature, Martin Feldstein argues persuasively that it is inappropriate to either ignore the physician or assume that utilization is determined solely by the physician.[3] Instead, he proposes that future research consider the physician to be an agent for the consumer and then examine the behavior of the physician when this relationship is not perfect.

Newhouse and Phelps should continue their analysis with this model and further disaggregate the decision process. For instance, the total utilization of hospital care is appropriately broken down into the decision to admit, the length of stay, and the level of services consumed. The admission equation should utilize the expected net price of the episode, including *all* hospital services, (not just the room charge) *and* the net price of physicians' services in the hospital. To test the impact of physicians on the demand curve, it may be appropriate to include a measure of the marginal profit to the physician resulting from the admission decision. (Under fee-for-service, this will be positive and related to gross physician charges; under prepaid plans the marginal profit is zero or negative. It is also likely to vary substantially for surgical and medical procedures.)

After the decision to undergo hospitalization, it is important to examine the determinants of the "intensity of services" or the cost per patient day. Again, net price to the patient and marginal profit to the decision makers are often thought to be completely based on technical considerations and are probably those in which the patient is least competent.[4] Intensity is often a function of the availability of special services in the hospital and standard practices in the area. For instance, costs per day in the West are consistently higher than in the East, but this is probably because of shorter lengths of stay. Long-run availability of services and practice patterns should also be investigated.

The final hospitalization decisions concern the length of stay. For the marginal day in the hospital, the net price of hospital services will be based primarily on the room charge and coinsurance rate; there are generally few ancillary services. The physician is also likely to gain little relative to an additional office visit, and especially little relative to major surgical fees. (The hospital, however, tends to make money on the marginal day and may exert informal pressures on the physician.)

When examining the utilization of physician visits it is important to distinguish four types: (1) those required for employment, insurance, etc.; (2)"purely preventive"—patient initiated; (3) response to symptoms—patient initiated; and (4) physician-suggested follow-up with patient compliance. The first type is relatively uninteresting although it may account for a substantial fraction of the visits of certain population subgroups. Even the purely preventive visit may not be completely patient initiated because the physician can alter the consumer's perception of the benefits of such care. For instance, the proportion of women who think that yearly Pap smears are necessary is probably not independent of the supply of gynecologists in the area. It is, however, in the area of preventive care that Grossman's investment model is probably most applicable.[5] There is also some question about whether preventive visits should be considered in the investment or the consumption category. Education is consistently one of the most important predictors of check-ups but there is little medical evidence to support the value of such visits.

Physician visits in response to symptoms may be viewed in part as investments, but they are largely "consumption" services to reduce pain and anxiety. Net price, search, and time costs are probably of primary importance, but other factors influencing symptom recognition and choice of the type of provider should also be investigated. Finally, physician-suggested follow-up visits comprise a substantial fraction of total visits and are probably the group of visits most subject to provider influence. This influence occurs not just through the statement that the patient should return for a follow-up. This suggestion can be made with varying degrees of force and, in the absence of other specialized information, is likely to shift the location of the demand curve.

The Newhouse-Phelps paper is a valuable contribution; these comments are intended to suggest that further research needs to be done with microdata and with still more disaggregated, and perhaps more realistic, models of the medical care market.

NOTES

1. For estimates of the magnitude of this bias see Leslie Kish and Martin Frankel, "Balanced Replications for Standard Errors," *Journal of the American Statistical Association,* 65 (September 1970), pp. 1071–1094.

2. *American Economic Review,* 53 (December 1963), pp. 941–973.
3. "Economic Studies of Health Economics," in M. Intriligator (editor), Frontiers of Quantitative Economics, II (Amsterdam: North-Holland Publishing Company, 1974).
4. The potential consumer may be willing to pay a substantial premium beyond actuarial value so that he or she is sure to face a very low price (coinsurance rate) when decisions must be made that directly affect his or her health. Moral hazard may be a positive good for the consumer.
5. The testing of such a model is very difficult. For instance, positive coefficients for wage income are predicted by the model and are found by Newhouse and Phelps. One might predict the same findings on the basis of the sliding scale of fees that is more closely related to what the physician *thinks* the patient earns than total income including unearned income. The sliding scale has become less important in the last ten years, so that a comparison of the Newhouse-Phelps results and more recent data should help to answer this question. See Michael Grossman, "On the Concept of Health Capital and the Demand for Health," *Journal of Political Economy,* 80, 2 (March–April 1972), pp. 223–255.

8

FRANK A. SLOAN
University of Florida

Physician Fee Inflation: Evidence from the Late 1960s

1. INTRODUCTION

The second half of the decade of the 1960s was one of dramatic change in the physicians' services market. The Medicare and Medicaid programs, instituted in 1966, provided coverage for medical services for post-age 65 and poverty groups. Growth of private insurance coverage for outpatient services was also substantial. Per capita out-of-pocket expenditures on physicians' services actually declined during the 1965–1970 period, in spite of a rise in the physician fee index at a rate almost twice the Consumer Price Index and an even greater rate of growth in money expenditures on physicians' services. Whereas patients' out-of-pocket payments to vendors of medical services constituted 63 per cent of total expenditures on physicians' services in 1965, this percentage was down to 40 by 1970.[1] Two previous studies (Feldstein, 1970; Steinwald and Sloan, 1974) report that insurance coverage has a positive impact on physicians' prices.

During this half-decade the physician-population ratio increased by 7 per cent, reflecting an increased domestic medical school output as well as greater immigration of foreign medical school graduates.[2] One would expect that higher ratios would depress physicians' fees, but several studies (Feldstein, 1970; Huang and Koropecky, 1973; and Newhouse, 1970) report that the physician-population ratio has a zero or even a positive impact. Some research on the demand for hospital and medical services suggests that per capita population use of health care services is greater in high physician-population areas and that use is in part a consequence of physician availability (Davis and Russell, 1972; Feldstein, 1971a, 1971b; Fuchs and Kramer, 1972). If an increased stock of physicians causes both higher prices *and* higher utilization, policy-makers may desire to reevaluate current government medical education policy that favors expansion of medical school capacity.

Product price increases often follow factor price increases. Wages of allied health personnel rose substantially during 1965–1970. Unlike the situation in many manufacturing industries, the growth in money wages was not partially offset by productivity gains.[3] Total visits per physician week (an admittedly crude measure of physician productivity) did not rise during this period. Although there is some interyear variation in the visits per week series, no trend is evident.[4]

Many experts maintain that group practice is a better organizational form than solo practice. Judging from the rapid growth in medical groups (8 per cent per year from 1965 to 1969), physicians are increasingly favoring this mode of practice.[5] Given certain aspects of the internal incentive structure of medical groups, Sloan (1974) warns that physicians practicing in groups may charge higher fees, *ceteris paribus.*[6] If this hypothesis is substantiated empirically, policy-makers would certainly want to question the statements of many experts.

This study develops a model of physician fee-setting and tests the model with state cross-sections covering four years, 1967–1970. The 1965–1970 period logically defines an era for this market, immediate pre-Medicare-Medicaid to the year before price controls (1971), but fee data are not available before 1967. The fee data and information on physician characteristics used in this study come from annual surveys of physicians' practices conducted by the American Medical Association. Other data, available from published sources, are described below.

The empirical analysis emphasizes general practitioners for two reasons: First (and more important), the AMA surveys contain approximately twice as many general practitioners as physicians in any other single field. State means for general practitioners merit more confidence that those of other specialties with relatively few observations for the smaller states.[7] Second, public concern about citizens' access to primary medical care of the type provided by GP's is particularly acute. During 1965–1970, fee increases for primary care procedures were higher than those for other procedures often performed by physicians (herniorrhaphy, tonsillectomy, and adenoidectomy).[8]

In Section 2, I develop a model of physician output and price decisions. Section 3 contains empirical results from the physicians' fee analysis. In Section 4 I compare the results of this study with past research and present conclusions and pertinent policy implications. In the appendix I describe the methods used to construct, and the sources of variation in, several insurance and wage variables that are important to this study.

2. MODEL AND VARIABLE SPECIFICATION

Demand Equation

Let the demand schedule for the physician firm be:

$$(1) \quad P = a_0 + a_1Q + a_2AT + a_3INS + a_4DEM + a_5MDPOP$$
$$\pm \text{ or } - \qquad \pm \text{ or } + \qquad \pm \text{ or } -$$
$$+ a_6INC + a_7PO$$
$$+ \qquad +$$

where P is the physician's fee (or an index of fees); Q, the quantity of services demanded; AT, attributes of the physician affecting demand; INS, private and government health insurance coverage of his potential patients; DEM, demographic characteristics of the physician's potential patients; MDPOP, the physician-population ratio in the physician's market area; INC, income of potential patients; and PO, the price of other providers of ambulatory medical services. Signs below the a's indicate whether the expected effect is positive or negative.

Rather than specifying a demand curve for each type of medical or surgical procedure, Equation (1) represents all services. Patients are likely to judge a physician's overall costliness, not his charge for a specific procedure. They cannot select one surgeon for office visits and another for an appendectomy. A certain number of office and hospital visits are complementary with an appendectomy.[9]

Three variables represent physician attributes: board certification, experience, and foreign medical education. Board certification in a specialty (BRD) should have a positive impact on demand.[10] A proxy for experience is LIC10, a variable indicating that the physician has been licensed less than ten years in his current state of practice. This variable is expected to have a negative effect if it primarily accounts for relative inexperience in physician practice and/or for a lack of patient contacts in his present location. But if recently licensed physicians have been the recipients of a much more technically advanced medical education than other physicians, the net impact of this variable on demand may be positive.[11] The professional education of foreign medical school graduates (FMG) may be regarded by some potential patients as technically inferior, implying a negative impact on demand. All three physician attribute variables are expressed as percentages.

Third-party reimbursement enters in several ways. One specification contains three variables: (1) private health insurance expenditures on health care services other than hospital (PRIVH); (2) Medicare Supplemental Medical Insurance Expenditures (MCARE), representing the part of the Medicare program that covers physicians' services; and (3) Medicaid expenditures on physicians' services (MCAID). Each is divided by state population. In a second specification, the percentage of the population with major medical insurance (MMED) is substituted for PRIVH. There is far less private insurance coverage under basic insurance plans for physicians' office visits, and home visits are typically covered under major medical plans once the deductible has been satisfied.[12] The fraction of medical expenditures paid by insurance (K), the sum of PRIVH, MCARE, and MCAID divided by an estimate of expenditures on medical services in the state per capita population, represents insurance in a third specification. As indicated below, the use of K is associated with a minor modification in Equation (1).

Medical care prices may affect the levels of insurance coverage as well as the reverse.[13] To obtain consistent parameter estimates, predicted values from regressions of PRIVH and K on a set of exogenous variables are used in the empirical analysis of fees. A regression for MMED has also been estimated, but an actual rather than a predicted series represents MMED in the fee analysis. The appendix provides details on reimbursement variable construction, results of PRIVH, K, and MMED regressions, as well as justification for using actual rather than predicted values of MMED.

The Medicare variable (MCARE) primarily reflects the proportion of the state's population over age 65 and demographic characteristics of persons in this age group (and thus may be considered a demographic as well as an insurance variable), characteristics of the state's health delivery system, and, finally, Medicare carrier reimbursement policy. An account of the sources of variation in MCARE is provided in the appendix. Available evidence indicates that determinants of MCARE's variation are outside the model developed in this study, and, therefore, it is appropriate to treat MCARE as exogenous in the empirical analysis. Unfortunately, equally strong evidence is not available for MCAID. However, it too is considered exogenous.

Physicians per 10,000 population is expected to have a negative impact on per physician demand. The empirical analysis includes two measures: the number of physicians in the physician's field per 10,000 population (MDPOP1) and the number of physicians in all other fields per 10,000 population (MDPOP2). The use of a single measure does not permit distinguishing among varying degrees of substitutability of physicians' services in different specialty fields. The within-field cross-elasticity of demand should be higher than the between-field cross-elasticity. In fact, physicians in other fields may be sources of referrals, implying that MDPOP2 may have a positive impact on demand for services of physicians in the field included in MDPOP1. But evidence presented in Shortell (1971, p. 5) indicates that general practitioners receive few patients on referral (3 per cent of all new patients).[14] For this reason, and because MDPOP1 and MDPOP2 are highly collinear, MDPOP2 has been excluded from the general practitioner fee regressions.

State per capita income (INC) should generally have a positive impact on demand. One expects that the price of other providers, such as outpatient departments of hospitals and health maintenance organizations, should have a positive effect. Preliminary regressions with the price of other providers of ambulatory services (PO) were not encouraging. Therefore, the variable has been excluded from the regressions presented in this study.[15]

Cost Equation

There are two cost functions for the physician firm. The first reflects non-physician input costs:

$$(2) \quad C_1 = \underset{\pm \text{ or}}{c_{10}} + \underset{+}{c_{11}\text{WAGE}} + \underset{+}{c_{12}\text{RENT}}$$

$$+ (\underset{\pm \text{ or}}{c_{13}} + \underset{+}{c_{14}\text{WAGE}} + \underset{+}{c_{15}\text{RENT}})Q$$

As Equation (2) is specified, both fixed and marginal costs are functionally dependent on factor prices, which are treated as exogenous to the physician (and to the physician services sector as a whole). Measures of the wage rate of nonphysician personnel (WAGE) and of the per unit cost of space (RENT) represent the factor prices. The method used to construct WAGE (expressed in terms of the weekly wage rate for secretarial-clerical personnel) is discussed in the appendix. The largest part of the inter-physician variation in capital costs probably relates to space. Unfortunately, measures of rental rates available for this study are poor. The available unit cost of space measure proved to be highly collinear with other variables in the regressions. All capital costs, actual and/or imputed, constitute only approximately 10 per cent of total practice expenses, certainly far less of the total than the nonphysician labor component. For these reasons, RENT is excluded from the regressions presented in this study.[16]

The principal input to the physician firm is the physician himself. Although there is no transaction between the self-employed physician as buyer and this physician as seller of his own labor, the value he imputes to his own input affects his price and output behavior. The second cost function represents the imputed value of physician effort.

The imputed value of physician's time (C_2) depends on a number of personal and professional factors. Using previous research as a guide, the following personal factors are relevant. As the physician grows older, his personal return to further asset accumulation diminishes. Thus, older physicians are likely to place a higher value on leisure time. Sloan (1975) reports that physician hours of work decline with age. The variable AGE refers to the percentage of physicians by field, state, and year who are aged 55 or over. Judging from Sloan (1973, 1975) physician income from property has a small positive effect on the physician's imputed wage;[17] female physicians with children have higher imputed wages. This is not true of female physicians without children. Unfortunately, data on physicians' property income and children are not available in a form usable for this study.[18] It is possible to distinguish between male and female physicians, but without data on the number of children, a variable indicating the percentage of physicians who are female would serve no useful function.

Although health status would appear to affect the imputed wage a priori, Sloan (1975) failed to find a relationship between health status and physician effort. Thus, the lack of suitable data on physicians' health is not disturbing. Feldstein (1970) hypothesized that physicians will work more when their income falls relative to others in the community. However, the variable to measure this ("reference income") effect is significant in only one out of the nine regressions he presents. Sloan (1974b) also found this variable to be unreliable. Therefore, although data for a relative or reference income variable are available, past research has not been sufficiently encouraging to warrant this variable's inclusion.

Several variables related to the physician as a professional may influence the physician's imputed wage. Clearly, some physicians enjoy the practice of medicine more than others, and these physicians impute a correspondingly lower wage to their effort. Unfortunately, it is difficult to find objective factors associated with a "love of medicine."[19] The board certification variable (BRD), included above as a demand variable, may serve this role, assuming that board-certified physicians derive more pleasure from the practice of medicine than others. If so, the positive demand effect of board certification on physicians' fees may be offset by a negative supply effect on fees.[20]

The second cost function, measuring the physicians' imputed wage, is specified as

(3)
$$C_2 = c_{20} \quad + \quad c_{21}AGE \quad + \quad (c_{22} \quad + \quad c_{23}AGE)Q$$
$$\pm \text{ or } \quad + \qquad\qquad \pm \text{ or } \quad +$$

According to Equation (3), imputed fixed and marginal costs rise with physician age.[21] Because of the aforementioned uncertainty about the use of BRD as a supply variable, it has not been included as part of Equation (3). If it were to be included, it would enter in the same manner as AGE, but it would have a negative rather than a positive effect on C_2. The unavoidable exclusion of property income and female physicians with children is unfortunate.

Output and Price Equations

The model assumes that the physician's objective, given equations (1) through (3), is to maximize profit, defined as his earnings above his imputed wage. Including the imputed wage allows for physician preferences for leisure as well as goods. Empirical evidence to support the profit maximization assumption is given in Steinwald and Sloan (1974).[22]

(4)
$$\pi = P \cdot Q - C_1 - C_2$$

Differentiating π, one obtains the following expressions for optimal quantity and price (Q^* and P^*).

(5) $\quad Q^* = (1/2a_1)(-a_0 - a_2AT - a_3INS - a_4DEM - a_5MDPOP - a_6INC$

$\quad\quad - a_7PO + c_{13} + c_{14}WAGE + c_{15}RENT + c_{22} + c_{23}AGE)$

and

(6) $\quad P^* = (1/2)(a_0 + a_2AT + a_3INS + a_4DEM + a_5MDPOP + a_6INC$

$\quad\quad + a_7PO + c_{13} + c_{14}WAGE + c_{15}RENT + c_{22} + c_{23}AGE)$[23]

If K is the proportion of the fee paid by both private and public third parties, then Equation (1) may be rewritten as $P = a_1Q + bX + KP$, (1)′, where X stands for all exogenous demand variables. KP replaces a_3INS in Equation (1). Letting the sum of the two cost equations be

(7) $\quad C = C_1 + C_2 = d + eQ$

(8) $\quad Q^* = [e(1-K) - bX]/2a_1$

and

(9) $\quad P^* = [e + bX/(1 - K)]/2$

According to Equation (9), each exogenous demand variable is divided by the proportion of the out-of-pocket fee paid by the patient. This specification implies that patients possess perfect knowledge of their insurance coverage before purchasing medical services and hence base utilization decisions on the price *net* of insurance. But if patients gain precise information about their coverage after the fact, equations (5) and (6), which allow a higher utilization response to gross price than to insurance, may provide better explanations of observed behavior than equations (8) and (9).[24] With one modification, equations (6) and (9) provide the basis for the empirical analysis of physicians' fees.

Group Practice

A substantial number of physicians share costs and/or revenues with other physicians.[25] If one could be certain that decisions involving practice price, output levels, and input purchases were made collectively by group members, a model appropriate for the solo practitioner would fit group medical practice equally well. But if these decisions are made by individual physicians within the group, the model must be modified. Sharing costs reduces the incentive to minimize non-physician costs in that the individual physician member bears an increasingly smaller proportion of the financial consequences of his failure to control costs as group size rises. If both revenues and costs are shared, the financial return to individual effort decreases as group size rises. Although an arrangement such as one in which physicians share both revenues and costs equally results in equal reductions in both marginal revenue *and* the marginal cost associated with non-physician inputs, sharing does not reduce the marginal cost associated with individual physician labor, the cost represented by Equation (3). If c_{22} and c_{23} of Equation (3) were zero, output and price given by equations (5) and (6) would be unaffected, but this is very unlikely.[26]

As demonstrated formally in Sloan (1974a), under the assumption of no economies of scale arising from better use of non-physician labor and capital inputs, it is appropriate to multiply both c_{22} and c_{23} by the number of physicians (n) in the group if net income of the practice is divided equally among its physician members. When net income is divided into unequal shares (θ_i, a fraction signifying the share to the ith physician), c_{22} and c_{23} should be multiplied by $1/\theta_i$. Intuitively, smaller shares of net income are greater disincentives to individual effort. Although a price equation containing age/group-size interaction terms would be desirable on conceptual grounds, the sample size limits the number of variables that may usefully be included. Regressions in the empirical section contain two group-size variables entered in a linear, noninteractive fashion (GRP1 = percentage of physicians by field, state, and year practicing in groups of three to ten physicians; GRP2 = percentage of physicians in groups of eleven or more physicians).

Proponents of group practice stress potential economies of scale resulting from more efficient use of non-physician labor and sophisticated capital equipment. Scale economies from these sources may offset disincentives to individual physician effort. Kimbell and Lorant (1973) report increasing returns to scale for small to medium-size groups relative to solo practice and decreasing returns for large groups. Results made available to this author by Kimbell and Lorant indicate maximum efficiency for single-specialty groups with six physicians and a slow decline in the efficiency of single-specialty groups thereafter. Multispecialty groups, which generally include more than ten physicians, appear on the basis of Kimbell and Lorant's work to be inefficient relative to single-specialty groups, which usually have fewer than this number. On the basis of Kimbell and Lorant's research, one would expect GRP1's and GRP2's parameter estimates to be negative and positive, respectively.

Usual Fees Versus Average Revenue

Two types of price variables serve as dependent variables: the fee usually charged by the physician; and average revenue, which is the physician's gross annual revenue divided by an estimate of his total annual visits. The usual fees analyzed correspond to the physician's follow-up office visit, hospital visit, and appendectomy. These procedures are frequently performed by physicians and reflect the physician's mean fee level.

For purposes of empirical analysis of physician fee inflation, however, usual fees have two potential deficiencies. First, if there is price discrimination and/or related behavior (e.g., a collection ratio less than 1), the usual price overstates the physician's average price. If such behavior is unrelated to the fee equation's explanatory variables, this presents no problem. Some experts contend, however, that a major effect of increased third-party reimbursement has been to reduce price discrimination. Judging from data presented in Owens (1973), the dollar value of "free and reduced-fee services" in 1971 was from 1 to 2 per cent of gross billings. Since this percentage is so low, price discrimination is not likely to be an important factor in a 1967–1970 cross-sectional study.

Second, although the AMA requests usual fees for specific procedures in its annual mail questionnaires, some ambiguity from the standpoint of the responding physician undoubtedly remains. For example, it may be customary for some physicians to include routine laboratory services as part of the office visit charge. Instead of raising his fees, physicians may decide to bill separately for laboratory work and hold the usual charge for the office visit constant. To the extent that this type of behavior is unrelated to the independent variables, the only consequence is a relatively poor fit for the regression equation as a whole. But evidence presented in Sloan and Steinwald (1975) suggests that the structure of basic insurance plans does encourage the physician to bill separately for minor tasks that might otherwise be included in office visit, hospital visit, and/or surgical charges.

The average revenue measure overcomes these objections, but it too has deficiencies. First, it does not hold the physician's procedure mix and the number of procedures performed per visit constant. Research by Bailey (1970) indicates that group-practice physicians perform more procedures per visit than their colleagues in solo practice. Lab tests, for example, may be performed by the group physician who owns the necessary equipment. The solo physician may refer the patient to a commercial laboratory for testing. This implies that group-practice coefficients in average revenue equations may be biased upward. Second, there are probably measurement errors in visits, the denominator of the average revenue series. Visit data appear to be particularly difficult to collect by mail questionnaire. Although errors in visits may affect goodness of fit, no potential biases are apparent.

In sum, neither measure is fully appropriate. Analysis of both is likely to be more informative than analysis of either one in isolation. Dependent variables and all monetarily expressed explanatory variables are deflated by a state price index.[27]

3. EMPIRICAL RESULTS

Tables 1 and 2 present fee regressions based on general practitioner, surgeon, and internist data. All regressions are weighted by the square root of state population.

Table 1 Regressions

The performance of the reimbursement variables in the Table 1 regressions is mixed. The private health insurance benefits variable (PRIVH) has a consistently implausible negative sign in preliminary office and hospital visit fee regressions and is therefore excluded from the office and hospital visit fee regressions presented in Table 1. The PRIVH variable includes basic insurance payments, and, as stated above, there is some evidence that basic insurance encourages the physician to submit bills for more narrowly defined procedures. A visit that does not include lab tests and the like is likely to cost less than one that does. This "billing effect" may have introduced a negative bias into the PRIVH parameter estimates. Future surveys should make particular efforts to ensure that physicians' responses to fee questions refer to homogeneous procedures. By contrast, PRIVH is always positive and significant in the average revenue equations, with implied elasticities at the means of the observations of 0.75 (general practitioners) and 1.20 (internists). The average revenue measure does not reflect the billing effect.

Major medical insurance (MMED) demonstrates a greater impact on average revenue than on usual fees. This variable is highly collinear with INC, however, and for this reason one should examine MMED and INC together. Without INC, Regression (1) of

TABLE 1   Price Equations: General Specification[a]

Dependent Variable	INC	PRIVH	MMED	MCARE	MCAID	INS	MDPOP1	MDPOP2	BRD
				General Practitioners					
1. Office	—	—	0.020[c]	0.088[c]	—	—	−0.11	—	—
visit fee	(—)	(—)	(0.005)	(0.014)	(—)	(—)	(0.08)	(—)	(—)
2. Office	0.00095[c]	—	−0.0015	0.069[c]	0.0033	—	−0.22[c]	—	—
visit fee	(0.00017)	(—)	(0.0058)	(0.014)	(0.0076)	(—)	(0.08)	(—)	(—)
3. Office	0.0010[c]	—	—	—	—	0.0098	−0.23[c]	—	—
visit fee	(0.0002)	(—)	(—)	(—)	(—)	(0.0056)	(0.09)	(—)	(—)
4. Hospital	0.0011[c]	—	0.013	0.162[c]	—	—	−0.39[c]	—	—
visit fee	(0.0003)	(—)	(0.010)	(0.025)	(—)	(—)	(0.14)	(—)	(—)
5. Hospital	0.00092[c]	—	0.0036[c]	0.161[c]	0.022	—	−0.36[b]	—	—
visit fee	(0.00030)	(—)	(0.0010)	(0.025)	(0.015)	(—)	(0.15)	(—)	(—)
6. Average	−0.00035	—	0.054	0.436[c]	0.036[c]	—	−1.65[c]	—	—
revenue	(0.00080)	(—)	(0.031)	(0.075)	(0.011)	(—)	(0.44)	(—)	(—)
7. Average	−0.0011	0.25[c]	—	0.50[c]	0.059	—	−1.93[c]	—	—
revenue	(0.0077)	(0.06)	(—)	(0.07)	(0.104)	(—)	(0.44)	(—)	(—)
				Surgeons					
8. Appen-	—	—	0.21	0.84	0.061	—	−29.81[c]	6.67[c]	—
dectomy	(—)	(—)	(0.19)	(0.63)	(0.322)	(—)	(10.11)	(1.25)	(—)
fee									
9. Appen-	−0.014	—	0.49[b]	0.97	−0.076	—	−31.84[c]	7.56[c]	—
dectomy	(0.008)	(—)	(0.24)	(0.64)	(0.331)	(—)	(10.53)	(1.36)	(—)
fee									
				Internists					
10. Average	—	—	0.091[b]	0.78[c]	—	—	−1.94[c]	—	—
revenue	(—)	(—)	(0.042)	(0.10)	(—)	(—)	(0.64)	(—)	(—)
11. Average	−0.0022	0.48[c]	—	0.87[c]	−0.052	—	0.46	−0.40	−0.005
revenue	(0.0014)	(0.12)	(—)	(0.12)	(0.185)	(—)	(1.86)	(0.47)	(0.009)

[a] Standard errors in parentheses.
[b] Indicates 5 per cent significance level (two-tail test).
[c] Indicates 1 per cent significance level (two-tail test).

Table 1, MMED has a significant impact on the general practitioner's office visit fee. The implied elasticity at the means of the observations is small, 0.17. With INC included, Regression (2), MMED's parameter estimate becomes negative with a high standard error. The elasticity associated with INC in all office and hospital visit fee regressions presented in Table 1 is around 0.6. The coefficients of MMED are positive and larger than their standard errors in both hospital visit regressions ([4] and [5]). As before, the implied elasticities are small. Steinwald and Sloan (1974), an empirical analysis of physicians' fees at the level of the individual physician using 1971 data, reports low MMED (defined as in this study) elasticities derived from GP office and hospital visit fee regressions. However, the Steinwald-Sloan

LIC1O	FMG	WAGE	AGE	GRP1	GRP2	Constant	
			General Practitioners				
-0.0006	0.0047	0.048^c	—	—	—	-0.35	$R^2 = 0.52$
(0.0037)	(0.0046)	(0.007)	(—)	(—)	(—)	(0.63)	$F(6,182) = 32.31^c$
—	—	0.038^c	-0.006^b	-0.010^b	0.016	-0.82	$R^2 = 0.61$
(—)	(—)	(0.007)	(0.003)	(0.004)	(0.014)	(0.62)	$F(9,179) = 30.5^c$
-0.0015	0.0014	0.041^c	-0.009^c	-0.009^b	0.021	-1.12	$R^2 = 0.55$
(0.0040)	(0.0052)	(0.007)	(0.003)	(0.004)	(0.016)	(0.67)	$F(9,179) = 24.7^c$
—	—	0.049^c	—	—	—	-2.14^c	$R^2 = 0.54$
(—)	(—)	(0.012)	(—)	(—)	(—)	(1.09)	$F(5,182) = 42.7^c$
—	—	0.049^c	0.035	-0.024	0.026	-1.33	$R^2 = 0.59$
(—)	(—)	(0.012)	(0.048)	(0.000)	(0.026)	(1.09)	$F(9,178) = 27.9^c$
—	—	0.035	0.004	0.047^c	-0.0013	2.43	$R^2 = 0.39$
(—)	(—)	(0.031)	(0.014)	(0.018)	(0.0072)	(3.09)	$F(9,133) = 9.4^c$
-0.0013	-0.0070	0.049	0.010	0.036^b	0.0057	1.32^c	$R^2 = 0.45$
(0.018)	(0.023)	(0.030)	(0.015)	(0.018)	(0.069)	(0.42)	$F(11,131) = 9.7^c$
			Surgeons				
—	—	1.88^c	—	—	—	-35.97	$R^2 = 0.58$
(—)	(—)	(0.25)	(—)	(—)	(—)	(26.5)	$F(6,163) = 32.7^c$
—	—	1.95^c	—	—	—	-14.04	$R^2 = 0.59$
(—)	(—)	(0.26)	(—)	(—)	(—)	(29.3)	$F(9,160) = 25.3^c$
			Internists				
—	—	-0.66	—	0.027	0.010	8.13	$R^2 = 0.35$
(—)	(—)	(0.46)	(—)	(0.024)	(0.020)	(4.60)	$F(8,118) = 7.8^c$
-0.016	0.055	-0.47	0.006	0.043	0.007	8.23	$R^2 = 0.42$
(0.023)	(0.042)	(0.54)	(0.023)	(0.024)	(0.020)	(5.53)	$F(13,113) = 6.4^c$

parameter estimates are significant at the 5 per cent level or better in all instances whereas those in Table 1 are not. The higher precision of the Steinwald-Sloan estimates probably reflects a lower degree of collinearity between the income measure and MMED. The elasticities associated with the MMED coefficients in the Table 1 appendectomy fee equations (based on surgeon data) are also small, 0.1 and less. Major medical insurance has a much greater impact on average revenue. MMED elasticities based on regressions (6) and (10) are 0.48 and 0.52, respectively.[28]

Medicare supplemental insurance benefits per capita population (MCARE) is significant in all but the appendectomy fee equations. If MCARE primarily reflected usual fee levels, it would probably perform better in the office, hospital, and the appendectomy fee

TABLE 2 Price Equations: Effect of the Proportion Covered by Third Parties[a]

Dependent Variable	INCK	MDPOP1K	MDPOP2K	FMGK	LIC10K	1K	WAGE	AGE	GRP1	GRP2	Constant	
1. Office visit fee	0.00055^c	-0.096	—	-0.0037	0.0051	-1.88^c	0.045^c	—	-0.010	0.033	1.66	$R^2 = 0.63$
	(0.00010)	(0.053)	(—)	(0.0030)	(0.0028)	(0.39)	(0.011)	(—)	(0.007)	(0.020)	(1.19)	$F(8,87) = 18.3^c$
2. Hospital visit fee	0.00089^c	-0.127	—	0.0066	-0.0013	-3.37^c	0.043^b	-0.011	-0.020	0.062	4.71^b	$R^2 = 0.61$
	(0.00018)	(0.093)	(—)	(0.0062)	(0.0056)	(0.69)	(0.020)	(0.010)	(0.012)	(0.035)	(2.27)	$F(9,86) = 15.0^c$
3. Lab fee	0.00013	-0.004	-0.018^c	0.0013	-0.0024	-0.49	0.022^c	-0.004	-0.003	0.020	1.13	$R^2 = 0.39$
	(0.00008)	(0.035)	(0.009)	(0.0026)	(0.0021)	(0.27)	(0.008)	(0.004)	(0.004)	(0.014)	(0.86)	$F(10,85) = 5.5^c$
4. Average revenue	0.0018^c	-1.14^c	—	-0.030	0.017	0.005	0.063	—	0.065	0.073	-6.93	$R^2 = 0.34$
	(0.0007)	(0.36)	(—)	(0.021)	(0.017)	(2.46)	(0.060)	(—)	(0.038)	(0.112)	(6.69)	$F(8,63) = 3.99^c$
5. Average revenue	0.0017^c	-1.18^c	0.084	-0.043	0.024	-0.242	0.052	—	0.070	0.021	-5.79	$R^2 = 0.35$
	(0.0007)	(0.36)	(0.080)	(0.024)	(0.018)	(2.47)	(0.061)	(—)	(0.038)	(0.122)	(6.77)	$F(9,62) = 3.67^c$

[a] Standard errors in parentheses.
[b] Indicates 5% significance level (two-tail test).
[c] Indicates 1% significance level (two-tail test).

equations than in the average revenue equations. This clearly is not the case. Elasticities from average revenue equations are far higher (0.6 to 0.75) than are those from the usual fee equations (around 0.1). As explained in the appendix, MCARE reflects the state's demographic characteristics, features of its health care delivery system, and deliberate policies of the Medicare carriers. These exogenous influences have clearly had an impact on physicians' price and output behavior, particularly on average revenue. In some preliminary regressions, the percentage of persons in the state aged 65 and over was substituted for MCARE. That variable performed relatively poorly. Steinwald and Sloan (1974) report similarly inconclusive results using the percentage over age 65 variable in usual fee equations.

The Medicaid (MCAID) variable demonstrates no impact on fees in the Table 1 regressions. Table 1's Regression (3) contains INS, the sum of PRIVH, MCARE, and MCAID. Although almost significant at the 5 per cent level, the associated elasticity is low (0.05). This result principally reflects the poor performance of PRIVH and MCAID, as demonstrated by other regressions.

Coefficients of MDPOP1 are significant in the general practitioner regressions. GP regressions containing both general practitioners per 10,000 population (MDPOP1) and physicians in other fields per 10,000 population (MDPOP2), not reported, have also been estimated. Sums of the coefficients of the two physician variables are negative and significant at the 1 per cent level.[29] The MDPOP1 and MDPOP2 coefficients in the appendectomy fee equations for surgeons are also significant (negatively) individually and as a sum. The physician-population coefficients in the internist regressions are implausible. Elasticities associated with MDPOP1 are generally small (under -0.2), with the exception of general practitioner average revenue, in which they are around unity. The parameter estimates corresponding to board certification (BRD), the newly licensed physician (LIC10), and the foreign medical school graduate (FMG) are unreliable. Similar results have been obtained previously (Steinwald and Sloan, 1974).

Wages affect office, hospital visit, and appendectomy fees in the expected manner; associated elasticities range from 0.66 to 0.92. Although insignificant at conventional levels, the wage parameter estimates in the average revenue equations imply similar elasticities (0.63 to 0.68). The only implausible wage coefficients are in internist average revenue equations. In these, reimbursement dominates the effects of the other variables. Age coefficients (AGE) are often negative and, as a rule, imprecise.

Judging from Kimbell and Lorant (1973), the GRP1 and GRP2 parameter estimates should be negative and positive, respectively. If increased scale does not result in better utilization of aides and equipment, Sloan's assumption (1974a), then both GRP coefficients should be positive and GRP2's should exceed GRP1's coefficient. The GRP signs in Table 1 are too erratic to lend strong support to either view. Moreover, significance tests on the sum of Table 1's GRP coefficients are never significant.

Table 2 Regressions

The equations in Table 2 are based on the alternative specification of insurance. All five regressions are based on general practitioner data. The lab fee regression pertains to urinalysis, a frequently performed laboratory procedure.

As above, the effect of third-party reimbursement on average revenue is much more obvious than on usual fees. From Equation (9), it is evident that

$$(10)^{30} \quad \partial P^*/\partial K = \left[bX/2(1 - K)^2 \right]$$

where X represents all exogenous demand equation variables. Based on (10), the elasticity of average revenue with respect to the proportion paid by third parties, evaluated at the means of the observations, is slightly above unity.[31] The derivative $\partial P^*/\partial K$ corresponding to the usual fee equations is negative at the means of the observations (at which the derivative is evaluated), an implausible result but one that is consistent with the implausible behavior of PRIVH in Table 1's usual fee equations. PRIVH accounts for about three-fourths of total third-party reimbursements, K's numerator.

As shown in the appendix, income's coefficient in the K equation is negative. Therefore, the coefficients of INC overstate the impact of income on both usual fees and average revenues. The following adjustment procedure considers the indirect effect of INC through K on P as well as the INC's direct effect on P. Let $\hat{b}_1$ be the parameter estimate of INC and $\hat{b}_2$, the parameter estimate of other exogenous demand variables interacting with K, and X_1 be the other exogenous (noninsurance) demand variables. Then,

$$(11) \quad \partial \hat{P}^*/\partial INC = \hat{b}_1/2[1 - K(INC)] + \{\hat{b}_1 INC/2[1 - K(INC)]^2\}(\partial K/\partial INC)$$
$$+ \{\hat{b}_2 X_1/2[1 - K(INC)]^2\}(\partial K/\partial INC)$$

Evaluating $\partial\hat{P}^*/\partial INC$, using Equation (11) at the observational means, reduces the estimated impact of income from Regression (1) by about 12 per cent and its impact from Regression (4) by about 24 per cent. Using the adjusted measures of income's impact, the Table 2 office and hospital visit fee elasticities are similar to Table 1's. However, unlike the Table 1 regressions, the average revenue INC coefficients are positive and significantly different from zero with associated elasticities in excess of unity. One would expect INC to perform somewhat better in the K equations because other reimbursement variables collinear with INC (PRIVH and MMED) are not included. Moreover, the sample differs since estimates of K are not available for all states. But even considering these factors, the implied impact of income on average revenue appears high and should be interpreted cautiously.

Estimates of impact of the physician-population ratio (MDPOP1) are approximately the same as Table 1's. The number of physicians in other fields per 10,000 population (MDPOP2) enters the lab fee and one of the average revenue equations. The sum of the MDPOP1 and MDPOP2 coefficients is significant (negatively) at the 1 per cent level in the average revenue but not in the lab fee equation. As before, parameter estimates of the FMG and LIC10 variables are generally insignificant. The WAGE coefficients in the office and hospital visit regressions are virtually the same as those in corresponding Table 1 regressions. Those in the average revenue equation are somewhat higher. The GRP coefficients are not significant individually but are positive and significant at the 5 per cent level or better in four out of five regressions. Although significant, the associated elasticities are low.[32] Those corresponding to the sum of GRP1 and GRP2 in the office and hospital visit fee regressions are in the 0.1 range. The higher of the two group elasticities from the average revenue regressions is almost 0.3.

Fee-setting Dynamics

Although the data base covers only four years, an attempt was made to study fee-setting dynamics. Fees may move toward P* with a lag because physicians are uncertain about P*'s precise level or they may be motivated by a desire (based on ethical considerations) to spread price changes over a period of years. A simple adjustment mechanism is provided by the partial equilibrium adjustment model.

$$(12) \quad P_t - P_{t-1} = \lambda(P^* - P_{t-1}) \qquad 0 < \lambda \leqslant 1$$

As is well known, λ is estimated by including a lagged dependent variable as an explanatory variable. Ordinary least squares (OLS) results in estimates that are both seriously biased and inconsistent.[33] Eliminating the 1967 observations and using OLS, the implied values of λ for general practitioner office and hospital visit fees are 0.41 and 0.22, respectively, with associated t ratios in excess of 9.0. Employing a method developed by Nerlove for obtaining consistent estimates of λ (described in Nerlove and Schultz, 1970), the implied values of λ exceed 0.9, with associated t ratios below 1.0 in all regressions. The results presented in the above tables are based on the assumption of immediate adjustment. The estimate of λ using the Nerlove technique supports this assumption. But in view of the low t value associated with this estimate, this finding does not merit much confidence. Transformations of the data required by the Nerlove procedure clearly reveal that there is relatively little information of a temporal nature in this sample.

4. DISCUSSION, CONCLUSIONS, AND POLICY IMPLICATIONS

The empirical results indicate that third-party reimbursement has a much more consistently positive and a greater impact on average revenue than on usual physician fees. The Medicare variable is the only consistently reliable reimbursement variable in the usual fee equations, but the elasticities associated with the Medicare parameter estimates in these equations are low. This finding implies that health insurance principally affects the type of care rendered under such standard headings as a follow-up office and/or hospital visit, the extent to which price discrimination is practiced, collection ratios, as well as the number and complexity of procedures performed per visit. Unfortunately, it is not possible to determine which of these is relatively important. As mentioned above, price discrimination is quantitatively unimportant and cannot *per se* be held responsible for the observed patterns.

Two previous studies provide conflicting evidence on the impact of health insurance on physicians' usual fees. Using aggregate time series data, Feldstein (1970) reports a long-run elasticity (based on significant insurance parameter estimates) of a measure of the average price of physicians' services with respect to an insurance variable in the 0.3 to 0.5 range. Feldstein's results are consistent with the results for average price reported above. Steinwald and Sloan (1974) report that insurance has an impact on general practitioner, surgeon, and internist fees but not on those of obstetricians-gynecologists or pediatricians. The significance of major medical insurance receives particular attention in that study. The major medical coefficients are similar to those reported here, but the Steinwald-Sloan coefficients are far more significant. Both studies find small usual fee-major medical elasticities. Although Newhouse (1970) does not present the results of usual fee regressions that contain an insurance variable (in that study, the percentage of population with insurance), he points out that this variable has an insignificant effect on his usual fee measures.

Although previous studies of physicians' fees have reported some significant income parameter estimates, the implied responsiveness of fees to income varies. Parameter estimates reported in Feldstein (1970) and Steinwald and Sloan (1974) imply a lower degree of responsiveness than do those for office and hospital visit charges in this study. Newhouse (1970) reports price elasticities in the 0.7 to 0.9 range, a somewhat greater impact. However, Newhouse's estimates come from regressions that include only one to three independent variables. Since several potential influences on fees are not represented in Newhouse's regressions, such as factor prices, it is almost certain that his income parameter estimates are biased upward. Based on available evidence, it would appear that usual fee-income elasticities in the 0.5 to 0.6 range are more likely. Unfortunately, no conclusion on the impact of per capita income on average revenue is warranted on the basis of this study's empirical evidence.

Medical school enrollments have increased substantially in recent years, as have the number of graduates of foreign medical schools practicing in the United States. One factor responsible for public support of medical education is the presumption that increases in the physician-population ratio will at least temper physician fee inflation.

Some past research tends to contradict this rationale for public support of medical education. The physician-population ratio has a positive impact on the average physician fee in the Feldstein (1970) study, but the t ratios associated with the physician-population ratio parameter estimates are always less than 1. In Huang and Koropecky (1973), the rate of change of the physician-population ratio has a positive impact on the rate of change in physicians' fees, but the associated t ratio is far less than 1. In regressions with the rate of change in Medicare physicians' fees over the period 1967–

1969 as the dependent variable, physician-population ratio has a negative, insignificant impact in one equation, but is positive and significant in another. Huang and Koropecky (1973) emphasize the second results, concluding that "the reasons might be that supply creates its own demand; physicians reduce their working hours; physician density correlates with better information about markets and what they will bear" (p. 35). According to the way the model (on which these conclusions are based) is specified, not only does the physician-population ratio force the physician's price up, but since the ratio is specified to interact with last year's price, the positive effect of the ratio on fees is strengthened with each successive price increase. This pessimistic implication is not plausible since it implies that fees in high-ratio states will continue to diverge from fees in low-ratio states without end.

Newhouse (1970) reports that the physician-population ratio has a positive and significant impact on usual physicians' fees. His results would provide the strongest case for a positive impact, but since his model omits several plausible fee determinants, in particular factor prices, it is not clear that his positive sign on the physician-population ratio coefficient truly represents the partial effect of the physician stock.

The results presented in the preceding section support the view that increases in the physician stock will temper fee increases, at least in the general practitioner and surgeon submarkets. However, the magnitude of the fee response is low. Steinwald and Sloan (1974) show a similar result. Given the policy importance of this finding as well as the contradictory evidence from past studies, it would be useful to conduct additional tests on the influence of the physician-population ratio on fees.

Many policy-makers and experts on health care delivery advocate group medical practice. Tests presented in this study for the impact of group practice on fees are inconclusive. A significantly positive group-practice effect appears in regressions with relatively few explanatory variables. But even the elasticities associated with these estimates are low.

An objective of this study at its outset was to study fee-setting dynamics. Although there is some descriptive evidence to suggest a slow adjustment speed, there are no reliable estimates of the lag structure based on statistical analysis. Unfortunately, analysis of a time series of four cross-sections has not improved the state of knowledge on this subject.

Although variables expressing such physician characteristics as age, board certification status, and location of medical school have been measured with precision in this study, these variables demonstrate no systematic effect on fees. Given a similar pattern in Steinwald and Sloan (1974), it appears that these variables have at best a minor influence on physician fees. Nevertheless, studies that include a more comprehensive list of physician characteristics variables (for example, physician property income and children) should be conducted.

APPENDIX: REIMBURSEMENT AND WAGE VARIABLES

This appendix describes the reimbursement and wage variables more fully.

Methods for Constructing Three Reimbursement Variables

Three reimbursement variables have been constructed: private health insurance benefits per capita population (PRIVH); the fraction of medical expenditures paid by insurance, both private and public (K); and the percentage of the population with major medical insurance (MMED).

An explicit expression for PRIVH is:

$$(13) \quad PRIVH = \frac{BLUSBEN + \gamma_B \cdot Z \cdot BLUBEN}{POP \cdot PI}$$

$$\frac{+ \gamma_C(COMBEN - DISPAY - INDBEN) + \gamma_I INDBEN}{POP \cdot PI}$$

where BLUSBEN = Blue Shield health insurance benefits; BLUBEN = Blue Cross plus Blue Shield health insurance benefits; COMBEN = commercial health *and* disability insurance benefits; DISPAY = disability insurance benefits; INDBEN = insurance benefits of independent health insurance plans (for example, union plans, prepaid group practices); γ_B, γ_C, and γ_I = the fraction of health insurance benefits for expenses *other* than hospitalization (therefore, primarily for physicians' services) with subscripts identifying Blue Cross-Blue Shield, commercial insurers, and independent plans, respectively. State population and the state price index are POP and PI. Although Blue Cross usually reimburses hospital services, Blue Shield's reimbursements are primarily for physicians, except in a few states. In some of these states there is no Blue Shield organization, and Blue Cross makes payments to physicians; in a few others, Blue Shield financial data contain payments to hospitals. In either of these two cases, Blue Cross-Blue Shield benefit payments to physicians are multiplied by γ_B. The variable Z assumes the value of 1 in such cases. When Blue Shield adequately represents reimbursement for physicians' services (as in most states), Z equals zero.[34]

Direct estimates of commercial health insurance benefits are not available and must therefore be constructed from a published series that provides commercial health *and* disability insurance benefit payments by state and year (Health Insurance Institute, 1968–1971). Estimates of disability payments (DISPAY)[35] and benefits of independent plans (INDBEN) are subtracted from COMBEN.[36] All data with the exception of the γ's are for states and the years 1967–1970.[37] The γ's are national averages constructed from Mueller (1971).[38]

$$(14) \quad K = \frac{\text{PRIVH} + \text{MCARE} + \text{MCAID}}{\text{EXP}}$$

where EXP is an estimate of private and public expenditures on physicians' services in the state. Explicitly,

$$(15) \quad \text{EXP} = \frac{\text{PEXP} + \text{OPDEXP}}{\text{POP} \cdot \text{PI}}$$

PEXP and OPDEXP are expenditures on physicians' services in private practice and expenditures on physicians' services in hospital outpatient departments.[39]

$$(16) \quad \text{MMED} = \frac{\text{COMMED} + \mu\text{BLUCOV}}{\text{POP}} \cdot 100$$

Unpublished estimates of persons with commercial major medical coverage by year and state (COMMED) have been provided by the Health Insurance Institute. Comparable data for 1967–1970 for the Blues are not available. Therefore, estimates of Blue Cross-Blue Shield major medical are derived by multiplying Blue Cross-Blue Shield enrollment by state and year (BLUCOV) by the *national* ratio of the Blues' major medical to basic plan enrollment (μ), which is available for the years 1967–1970.

Insurance Regressions

Most of the variation in each of the above three reimbursement variables may be explained by per capita income (INC), the percentage of employees who are members of unions (UNION), the percentage of manufacturing firms with 2,500 employees or more (SIZE), the percentage of persons employed in nonfirm occupations (NONAG), the percentage of nonagricultural employees who work in manufacturing (MANU) or government services (GOV), the number of restricted activity days per capita population (RAD), the percentage of persons in the state aged 65 and over (PAT65), and dummy variables for the years 1968, 1969, and 1970.

Several mechanisms underlie the relationship between income and demand for health insurance. If risk aversion diminishes at higher income levels, so should the demand for health insurance. However, as Feldstein (1973) points out, higher income generates an increased demand for medical care; insurance companies are not likely to take this positive income elasticity on utilization into account when establishing premium schedules. Moreover, tax savings from insurance purchases favor the more affluent. (Feldstein and Allison, 1972; Mitchell and Vogel, 1973.) Group purchases of health insurance are much cheaper than those by individuals, and even among group purchases, there are scale economies. This places unions, large firms, and governmental agencies at an advantage. Persons employed in agriculture are least likely to be able to purchase group insurance. Since the health insurers do not (or cannot at a reasonable cost) fully control adverse selection by adjusting rates and/or by the sale of the policies themselves, persons with lower-health status (measured by RAD) are expected to demand more insurance.

The population age variable (PAT65) performs a different role in each of three health insurance equations. The PAT65 coefficient in the PRIVH (private health insurance benefits) equation may be negative since older persons have less private health insurance coverage. It is likely to have a positive impact on K since Medicare reimbursements are part of K's numerator. The PAT65 variable has been excluded from the MMED equation because it is not clear what effect it would have. Although coverage for persons over age 65 is not included in commercial major medical coverage, it was not possible to completely eliminate enrollment of those over age 65 from the estimated series for the Blues.[40]

Both private and public coverage for physicians' services expanded rapidly during 1967–1970. Growth in private coverage may reflect the very rapid increase in physicians' fees relative to the Consumer Price Index during 1966 and 1967; or, since the increase in major medical insurance was particularly dramatic, an increasing realization by the public that "first dollar" coverage under basic plans offers inadequate protection against serious risks. Dummy time variables account for (but do not explain) structural changes in the demand for insurance during this period.

Table 1 contains the insurance regressions. The K regressions are based on fewer observations since expenditure data are not available for several states and years. Judging by the R^2's, the equations explain most of the variation in all three dependent variables.

Per capita income has a significantly positive impact on both PRIVH and MMED, with respective elasticities (at the means) of 0.66 and 1.07. The most likely reason for INC's negative coefficient in the K regression is that the income elasticity of non-covered medical expenditures is relatively high. Per capita income obviously has a positive impact on PRIVH, and other studies (Feldstein, 1973; Stuart, 1972) indicate that MCARE and MCAID, the other components of K's numerator, respond positively to income.

The variables UNION, SIZE, and NONAG outperform the other two variables related to group insurance purchasing (MANU and GOV). The first three variables exert positive impacts in all but one case (SIZE in the MMED equation). But the elasticity associated with SIZE in that case is virtually zero (-0.04). The health status variable (RAD) is never significant. PAT65 behaves as expected. The year dummy variables reveal a dramatic increase in coverage for physicians' services, particularly in 1969 and 1970.

Predicted values from the PRIVH and MMED equations represent these variables in the empirical analysis of fee determinants. Given the high degree of association between INC and MMED ($r = 0.78$), use of predicted MMED values in the fee regressions would increase multicollinearity unduly. Therefore, actual values were used.[41]

Medicare

Medicare supplemental medical insurance per capita (state) population (MCARE) is best described as the product of three ratios: (1) the fraction of the population age 65 and over; (2) the fraction of the age group over 65 that is enrolled in the supplemental insurance program; and (3) supplemental insurance expenditures per enrollee. The first of the three is a demographic variable. As is well-known, medical needs increase with age.

Appendix

TABLE 1 Insurance Equations[a]

Dependent Variable	INC	UNION	SIZE	NONAG	MANU	GOV	RAD	PAT65	1968	196?	1970	Constant	
1. PRIVH	0.0039c	0.23a	11.2c	0.065	0.042	0.13	0.34	-0.15	-0.15	1.61	3.97c	13.26	$R^2 = 0.66$
	(0.0009)	(0.03)	(2.1)	(0.083)	(0.040)	(0.07)	(0.24)	(0.16)	(0.64)	(0.66)	(0.65)	(8.05)	$F_{(11,180)} = 32.0^c$
2. K	-0.00007	0.0017	0.37c	0.014b	-0.0004	0.0056	0.0005	0.030c	0.058b	0.082c	0.139c	-0.33	$R^2 = 0.59$
	(0.00004)	(0.0012)	(0.09)	(0.006)	(0.0019)	(0.0062)	(0.0096)	(0.006)	(0.025)	(0.025)	(0.026)	(0.37)	$F_{(11,84)} = 10.9^c$
3. MMED	0.0132c	0.092	-6.96b	0.31b	0.082	-0.18	-1.41c	(—)	0.53	2.9c	7.22c	8.95	$R^2 = 0.78$
	(0.0014)	(0.048)	(3.36)	(0.14)	(0.067)	(0.12)	(0.40)	(—)	(1.04)	(1.0?)	(1.07)	(12.9)	$F_{(10,181)} = 64.4^c$

[a] Standard errors in parentheses.
[b] Indicates 5% significance level (two-tail test).
[c] Indicates 1% significance level (two-tail test).

According to Feldstein (1971a), the second component reflects a number of factors—the proportion of individuals over 65 who are white, over age 75, live in cities of over 100,000 population, Medicaid payments of Medicare deductibles and coinsurance, state per capita income, and the proportion of the current population under age 65 with surgical and medical insurance—"a measure of habit persistence in the purchase of insurance" (Feldstein, 1971a, p. 6).

Variations in supplemental expenditures per enrollee, the third component of MCARE, reflect both the quantity of services rendered to enrollees and reimbursement per unit of service under the program. Reimbursement policies are particularly important, because if the program operated according to congressional intent, it would be impossible to argue that MCARE is an exogenous determinant of physicians' fees.

The law establishing Medicare requires that physicians be reimbursed on the basis of "customary, prevailing, and reasonable" criteria. For purposes of this discussion, the essential part of this formula involves the "prevailing" charge. If Medicare carriers, commercial insurance firms, or Blue Cross-Blue Shield organizations followed the congressional intent, they would define "prevailing" charges by applying a standard percentile to the community's cumulative distribution of physicians' fees. All fees below or at the percentile would satisfy the "prevailing" criterion. Also, the carrier would update community fee profiles frequently so that its profile would adequately represent the current distribution. Then as fees rose, so would reimbursement per unit of service.

But there is fairly conclusive evidence that Medicare carriers generally lacked the necessary data for constructing "prevailing" charges for specific procedures at the outset of the program.[42] As a result, fee schedules were often used to determine the reasonable charge.[43] When prevailing charges were based on a community fee distribution, carriers employed varying percentiles in the community fee distribution to define "prevailing," from the 75th to the 95th percentile. Judging from AMA data on the distribution of fees, these differences in percentiles imply substantial differences in "prevailing" charges. In 1967, for example, the 75th percentile of the national distribution of fees for a follow-up office visit and a routine hospital visit corresponded to between $7 and $8 for an office visit and between $9 and $10 for a hospital visit. Fees at the 95th percentile were $14 and $15, respectively. Fee schedules established by Blue Shield for reimbursing hospital visits under their regular plans were generally $5.[44] Huang and Koropecky

(1973) indicate that carriers also differed with respect to updating fee schedules and/or community fee profiles.

Intercarrier variation in reimbursement methods during the early years of the Medicare program justifies considering MCARE exogenous in analyzing fee behavior covering the 1967–1970 period. Actual reimbursements reflect deliberate carrier policies to a far greater extent than physician fee levels existing in the community.

Wages

The U.S. Department of Labor, in Its *Area Wage Surveys*, provides data on wages for selected occupations. Physicians typically employ female personnel with nursing skills and/or with secretarial-clerical skills. Wage data are available for metropolitan areas, not states. To convert the wage series into a usable state series, industrial nurse and secretarial wages (by metropolitan area) have been regressed on the population of the metropolitan area and dummy variables to represent the years 1967–1970 and the nine census divisions.[45] The regressions (not shown) explain most of the variation in both series ($R^2 = 0.72$ for nurses and 0.51 for secretaries). Given parameter estimates of these equations, a wage series by physician field, state, and year has been constructed. Each field-state-year observation reflects the distribution of physicians by community size for that observation, the year, and the appropriate census division. Since secretarial-clerical employees represent the dominant non-physician labor input to physicians' practices (Kehrer and Intriligator, 1974), the secretary wage represents WAGE in the fee equations.

NOTES

1. U.S. Department of Health, Education, and Welfare (1972).
2. Monroe and Roback (1971).
3. U.S. Department of Commerce (1973).
4. Alevizos, Walsh, and Aherne (1973).
5. See Fein (1967), for example, on the alleged advantages of groups. Todd and McNamara (1971) provide data on the formation of groups.
6. That study is an extension of a suggestion in Newhouse (1973); namely, that large medical groups may be relatively inefficient.
7. Number of observations in the 1967–1970 AMA sample: general practitioners, 3,404; surgeons, 2,225; internal medicine, 1,895; obstetrics-gynecology, 774; and pediatrics, 754.

An alternative to aggregating is to conduct the analysis at the level of the individual physician. However, data corresponding to the physicians' market area are needed for several independent variables. If data for an inappropriately defined area are merged with records on individual physicians, the parameter estimates will be biased toward zero. This bias is less likely to occur if the observational unit is the state. An analysis of physicians' fees based on another AMA sample and a somewhat different method has been conducted at the micro level (Steinwald and Sloan, 1974). A useful by-product of the present investigation is a comparison of the results at two different levels of aggregation. There are certain conditions under which aggregation is inappropriate. Theil (1971) states the precise conditions under which aggregation bias will arise.

8. U.S. Department of Health, Education, and Welfare (1972).

9. The quantity of services demanded is specified to depend on the mean fee. There are other dimensions of physician costliness, but in view of the information available, it is not possible to consider these. For example, some physicians are more likely to recommend revisits for a specific diagnosis and/or admit patients to a relatively expensive hospital.

The physician's fee structure may reflect differences in the relative marginal costs of providing specific services. For example, the hospital visit fee may increase relative to a routine office visit fee as the distance between the hospital and the physician's office increases. Unfortunately, the data are not yet available in sufficient detail to capture variation in the marginal costs of providing specific services.

10. Unless otherwise indicated, the data are from the American Medical Association.

11. There are alternative measures of physician experience. Among these are years since graduation from medical school, years practiced in current specialty, and age. The principal advantage of LIC10 is that it reflects experience in the geographic area of current practice as well as years in medicine and current specialty. It represents experience in the area imperfectly since some physicians may secure licenses in several states soon after graduation (particularly in those states known to be restrictive, such as California and Florida). No single measure of physician experience is fully adequate, but fortunately all are positively correlated. So as an empirical matter, it does not make much difference which variables are selected.

12. For statistical evidence, see Health Insurance Association of America (1972). The percentage of population with basic insurance was included in regressions not presented in this paper. The variable tended to enter with a negative sign. A possible explanation of this result is given below.

13. This point is discussed in greater detail in Phelps (1975). He argues there that the direction of causation (positive or negative) from medical care prices to insurance cannot be deduced.

14. The proportions for other major fields are higher: pediatricians, 5 per cent; obstetricians-gynecologists, 19 per cent; internists, 22 per cent; and general surgeons, 55 per cent.

15. Davis and Russell (1972) indicate that hospital admissions are positively related to the price of hospital outpatient services. The same measure was used in this study.

16. The 10 per cent estimate is based on Goldstein (1972). Capital costs, particularly those relating to space, have traditionally been considered relevant only in the long run. However, some economists have correctly questioned the

premise that labor is always variable whereas capital varies only in the long run. (See Oi, 1962, for example.)

17. The dependent variables in both studies are measures of the physician time input. The negative effect of income on the physician's time input implies a positive effect on the physician's imputed wage.

18. The AMA has included questions on both property income and children on its most recent survey of physician's practices (PSP8 conducted in late fall 1973).

19. Some sociological and psychological evidence related to physicians' choice of speciality is available (see Sloan, 1968). This body of literature might be useful for predicting specific types of cases the physician prefers, but is not really relevant for studying output and price decisions.

20. Feldstein (1970, 1972) emphasizes that physicians' price and output decisions are motivated by a desire to select interesting cases. Although it is clear that the physician would on balance prefer to have some variety in the cases he treats, and, like other professionals, probably seeks to avoid disagreeable customers, the *empirical* importance of this factor to an inquiry into physician price and output setting is questionable. The references Feldstein cites (Friedson, 1971; Martin, 1957) do not specifically model the case selection process, nor does one gain from these studies the impression that case selection is a particularly important variable of choice, once the physician is established in a particular setting. The Martin study refers to medical students, not to physicians in private practice. If the physician wanted to make meaningful changes in the mix of patients he sees, he would probably do better to change his specialty and/or practice mode, since there are substantial interspeciality and intermode differences in patient mix. Data presented in Sloan (1973) indicate that "type of patient" has a role in practice mode choice, but is less important than other factors such as "professional independence," "regularity of hours," and "income potential."

21. Fixed costs in this context pertain to those associated with maintaining even the smallest-scale practice. These are probably relatively unimportant in comparison to the marginal costs. As seen below, the model as specified predicts that marginal, not fixed, costs affect the physician's price.

22. Studies of physician fee-setting before Steinwald-Sloan found that several variables in their regressions behaved in a manner inconsistent with a "standard" maximizing model of the type generally used by economists. The Steinwald-Sloan study, using better data than had previously been available, reports signs on such variables as patient income and the physician-population ratio that are consistent with profit maximization.

Equation (4) results in a price equation that may be readily estimated. This would not be the case for a price equation derived from a utility function. Nonlinearities arise with the use of plausible utility functions when price-setting behavior is assumed. The comparative statics solutions, assuming an objective such as Equation (4)'s or a utility function, are essentially the same. To calculate π as defined by (4), the physician subtracts the value he assigns to C_2 from his net practice earnings. Both π and C_2 are measured in dollars.

23. A reasonable objection to the model presented in this section is the assumption that the total cost function is linear. It is easily seen that this simplifying assumption does not alter the essential form of the model. Let $C = d + eQ + fQ^2$. Then $\pi = Q(a_1Q + aX) - d - eQ - fQ^2$, where X stands for the demand shift variables specified above. Differentiating with respect to Q, $Q^* = (-aX + e)/[2(a_1 - f)]$ (I). The general form of the numerator is unchanged; the denominator contains the term $(a_1 - f)$ instead of a_1. $P^* = [a_1e + a(1 -$

$a_1)X]/[2(a_1 - f)]$ (II). The term $(a_1 - f)$ appears in both the numerator and denominator of (II), but not (6). However, the functional form of the price equation is unaffected, and regression analysis cannot be used as a basis for choosing between (6) and (II).

The terms a_1 and f correspond to Professor Huang's β_1 and α_1. (See his comment on this paper.) The essential difference between the model he proposes and the one presented in this paper is that his assumes that the physician is a price-taker in a competitive market whereas mine assumes he has some monopoly power and sets prices. The latter assumption is a more plausible one. My $(a_1 - f)$ may be negative in much the same way that his $(\beta_1 - \alpha_1)$ may be negative.

24. Equations' (8) and (9) specification implies that the average equals the marginal coinsurance rate. The assumption is made necessary because of the lack of data by state and year to develop marginal rates. Sloan and Steinwald (1974) present data on the relationship between average and marginal coinsurance rates. The average is much less than the marginal coinsurance rate for the appendectomy fee. The two rates are much closer in the case of office visits. The fee equation would optimally contain a marginal coinsurance rate and a variable measuring physician firm demand schedule shifts attributable to indemnity coverage. This latter point is discussed in greater length in Sloan and Steinwald (1975) and in a forthcoming physician fee study by these authors (using AMA data specifically collected to measure the effect of third-party reimbursement methods on physicians' fees). Insurance variables defined similar to K have been used in Davis (1974), Feldstein (1970, 1971b), Fuchs and Kramer (1972), and Rosett and Huang (1973). Probably no one is fully satisfied with this type of variable, but it is the best available.

25. According to an AMA survey, almost 39,000 physicians practiced in groups in 1969 compared with about 188,000 in patient care, office-based practice. See Todd and McNamara (1971) and Haug and Roback (1970).

26. Some groups have apparently recognized potential disincentives inherent in group practice and have centralized decision making to some degree. See Sloan (1974a).

27. Price level data come from the U.S. Department of Labor (1971). This source gives cost-of-living data for selected cities and for nonmetropolitan locations by census area. The index is constructed as follows: (1) for states for which only one city is listed, cost-of-living data for the city are taken as representative of all metropolitan areas in the state. Data for the census area in which the state is located are used for nonmetropolitan location. The index is then constructed by multiplying the metropolitan data by the percentage of population living in urban areas of the state and the nonmetropolitan data by 1 minus this percentage. Finally, the index is annualized by dividing the state index by the Consumer Price Index for the year (1967 = 100). The resulting index varies by both state *and* year; (2) for states for which two cities are listed, the larger one is assumed to be representative. All other calculations are the same as #1; (3) for states for which no cities are listed, the closest city is taken to be representative. All other steps are the same.

In a few preliminary regressions, the price index was included as a separate independent variable as an alternative to deflating. The index's coefficient was not significant, and including this variable has little effect on the other estimated coefficients.

28. If fees have a positive impact on major medical coverage, the MMED elasticities reported in the text are biased upward. There are two reasons for

believing that there is little or no upward bias. First, in the Steinwald-Sloan study, individual physician fees are regressed on MMED, which is defined for the physician's state, as in the present study, and the MMED elasticities are virtually the same. It is unlikely that the fee of the individual physician feeds back onto a state average, particularly in view of the intrastate variation in fees. Second, Phelps (1976) includes a medical care price variable in a regression with the maximum payment under major medical insurance as the dependent variable. The t value associated with the medical care price and its square is 0.91. This evidence suggests that major medical coverage is not sensitive to medical care prices.

29. The test is from Kmenta (1971), p. 372.
30. No cost-side (or equivalent supply) variables enter Equation (10).
31. Regression (4), 1.08; Regression (5), 1.11.
32. The fact that there are fewer variables in the Table 2 regressions probably accounts for the increased significant levels.
33. Monte Carlo experiments reported in Nerlove (1971) demonstrate that this bias is severe.
34. The source of the Blue Cross-Blue Shield data is Blue Cross-Blue Shield, *Fact Book*, 1967–1970.
35. These data are available for the years included in the analysis in the January issues of the *Social Security Bulletin*.
36. Independent plan benefit data come from Reed, Anderson, and Hanft (1966) and Reed and Dwyer (1971). The surveys refer to 1965 and 1969. Data for 1967, 1968, and 1970 were obtained by linear interpolation.
37. Plus the exception noted in the preceding note.
38. Table 15. These data correspond to 1969. Judging from similar tables in other years, the γ's change very slowly. $\gamma_B = 0.296$; $\gamma_C = 0.390$, and $\gamma_I = 0.586$.
39. Sources of PEXP and OPDEXP are U. S. Department of the Treasury *Business Income Tax Returns*, 1970–1972; and American Hospital Association, *Hospitals*, "Guide Issue," 1969–1971. When only a single value for a given state was missing, the missing value was filled by linear interpolation. If more than one value is missing, the state has been eliminated from regressions using K.
40. Marmor (1968), U.S. Senate, Committee on Finance (1970), and Huang and Koropecky (1973).
41. See Note 28 for further discussion of this issue.
42. According to Huang and Koropecky, the vast majority of Medicare carriers used fee schedules in 1967.
43. Huang and Koropecky (1973).
44. Reed and Carr (1970). Medicare fee schedules may have been somewhat higher than schedules for regular business. See U.S. Senate, Committee on Finance (1970).
45. The nurse and secretary regressions are based on 255 and 300 observations, respectively.

REFERENCES

1. Alevizos, G., R.J. Walsh, and P. Aherne, *Socioeconomic Issues of Health* (Chicago: American Medical Association, 1973).
2. American Hospital Association, *Hospitals*, Guide Issue, 1969–1971.

3. Bailey, R.M., "Economics of Scale in Medical Practice," in H. Klarman (editor), *Empirical Studies in Health Economics* (Baltimore: Johns Hopkins Press, 1970), pp. 255–273.
4. Blue Cross and Blue Shield, *Fact Book*, 1967–1970.
5. Davis, K., "The Role of Technology, Demand and Labor Markets in the Determination of Hospital Costs," in M. Perlman (editor), *The Economics of Health and Medical Care* (London: Macmillan, 1974), pp. 283–301.
6. _____, and L.B. Russell, "The Substitution of Hospital Outpatient Care for Inpatient Care," *Review of Economics and Statistics*, 54 (May 1972), pp. 109–120.
7. Fein, R., *The Doctor Shortage: An Economic Diagnosis* (Washington, D.C.: The Brookings Institution, 1967).
8. Feldstein, M.S., "An Econometric Model of the Medicare System," *Quarterly Journal of Economics*, 85 (February 1971a), pp. 1–20.
9. _____, "Hospital Cost Inflation: A Study in Nonprofit Price Dynamics," *American Economic Review*, 61 (December 1971b), pp. 853–872.
10. _____, "The Rising Price of Physicians' Services," *Review of Economics and Statistics*, 52 (May 1970), pp. 121–133.
11. _____, "The Rising Price of Physicians' Services: A Reply," *Review of Economics and Statistics*, 54 (February 1972), pp. 105–107.
12. _____, "The Welfare Loss of Excess Health Insurance," *Journal of Political Economy*, 81 (March 1973), pp. 251–280.
13. _____, and E. Allison, "Tax Subsidies of Private Health Insurance: Distribution, Revenue Loss and Effects," mimeo., 1972.
14. Friedson, E., *Profession of Medicine* (New York: Dodd, Mead, and Co., 1971).
15. Fuchs, V.R., and M.J. Kramer, *Determinants of Expenditures for Physicians' Services in the United States, 1948–68* (New York: National Bureau of Economic Research, 1972).
16. Goldstein, M., *Income of Physicians, Osteopaths, and Dentists from Professional Practice* (Washington, D.C.: Social Security Administration, Office of Research and Statistics, Staff Paper No. 12, 1972).
17. Haug, J.N., and G.A. Roback, *Distribution of Physicians, Hospitals and Hospital Beds in the U.S., 1969* (Chicago: American Medical Association, 1970).
18. Health Insurance Association of America, *A Current Profile of Group Medical Expense Insurance in Force in the United States* (New York: The Association, 1972).
19. Health Insurance Institute, *Source Book of Health Insurance Data* (New York: The Institute, 1968–1971).
20. Huang, L., and O. Koropecky, *The Effects of the Medicare Method of Reimbursement on Physicians' Fees and on Beneficiaries' Utilization*, Vol. II, Part I (Washington, D.C.: Robert R. Nathan Associates, 1973).
21. Kehrer, B.H., and M.D. Intriligator, "Allied Health Personnel in Physicians' Offices: An Econometric Approach," in M. Perlman (editor), *The Economics of Health and Medical Care*, pp. 442–458.
22. Kimbell, L.J., and J.H. Lorant, "Physician Productivity and Returns to Scale," mimeo., 1973.
23. Kmenta, J., *Elements of Econometrics* (New York: Macmillan, 1971).
24. Marmor, T.R., "Why Medicare Helped Raise Doctors' Fees," *Transaction*, 5 (September 1968), pp. 14–19.
25. Martin, W., "Preferences for Types of Patients," in R.K. Merton, *et al.*, *The*

Student Physician (Cambridge, Massachusetts: Harvard University Press, 1957), pp. 189–197.

26. Mitchell, B.M., and R.J. Vogel, *Health and Taxes: An Assessment of the Medical Deduction* (Santa Monica: The Rand Corporation, 1973).

27. Monroe, K.E., and G.A. Roback, *Reference Data on Socioeconomic Issues of Health*, revised edition (Chicago: American Medical Association, 1971).

28. Mueller, M.S., "Private Health Insurance in 1969: A Review," *Social Security Bulletin*, 34 (February 1971), pp. 3–18.

29. Nerlove, M., "Further Evidence on the Estimation of Dynamic Economic Relations from a Time Series of Cross-Sections," *Econometrica*, 39 (March 1971), pp. 359–382.

30. _____, and T.P. Schultz, *Love and Life Between the Censuses* (Santa Monica: The Rand Corporation, 1970).

31 Newhouse, J., "The Economics of Group Practice," *Journal of Human Resources*, 8 (Winter 1973), pp. 37–56.

32. _____, "A Model of Physician Pricing," *Southern Economic Journal*, 37 (October 1970), pp. 174–183.

33. Oi, W., "Labor as a Quasi-Fixed Factor," *Journal of Political Economy*, 70 (December 1962), pp. 538–555.

34. Owens, A., "How Much Unpaid Service Doctors Still Provide," *Medical Economics* (April 16, 1973), pp. 88–91.

35. Phelps, C., "Demand for Reimbursement Insurance" (this volume), 1975.

36. Reed, L.S., A.H. Anderson, and R.S. Hanft, *Independent Health Insurance Plans in the United States, 1965 Survey* (Washington, D.C.: Social Security Administration, ORS Research Report No. 17, 1966).

37. _____, and W. Carr, *The Benefit Structure of Private Health Insurance* (Washington, D.C.:Social Security Administration, ORS Research Report No. 32, 1970).

38. _____, and M. Dwyer, *Health Insurance Plans Other Than Blue Cross or Blue Shield Plans or Insurance Companies, 1970 Survey* (Washington, D.C.: Social Security Administration, ORS Research Report No. 35, 1972).

39. Rosett, R., and L. Huang, "The Effect of Health Insurance on the Demand for Medical Care," *Journal of Political Economy*, 81 (March 1973), pp. 281–305.

40. Shortell, S.M., *A Model of Physician Referral Behavior: A Test of Exchange Theory in Medical Practice* (Chicago: Center for Health Administration Studies, University of Chicago, Research Series No. 31, 1971).

41. Sloan, F.A., *Economic Models of Physician Supply*, Ph.D. dissertation, Harvard University, 1968.

42. _____, "Effects of Incentives on Physician Practice Performance," in J. Rafferty (editor), *Health, Manpower and Productivity* (Lexington, Massachusetts: D.C. Heath, 1974a).

43. _____, "A Microanalysis of Physicians' Hours of Work Decisions," in M. Perlman (editor), *The Economics of Health and Medical Care* (1974b), pp. 302–325.

44. _____, "Physician Supply Behavior in the Short Run: An Analysis of 1960 and 1970 Census Data," *Industrial and Labor Relations Review* (July 1975).

45. _____, *Supply Responses of Young Physicians: An Analysis of Physicians in Residency Programs* (Santa Monica: The Rand Corporation, 1973b).

46. _____, and B. Steinwald, "The Role of Health Insurance in the Physicians' Service Market," *Inquiry* (December 1975).

47. Steinwald, B., and F.A. Sloan, "Determinants of Physicians' Fees," *Journal of Business*, 47 (October 1974), pp. 493–511.
48. Stuart, B., "Equity and Medicaid," *Journal of Human Resources*, 7 (Spring 1972), pp. 162–178.
49. Theil, H., *Principles of Econometrics* (New York: John Wiley, 1971).
50. Todd, C., and M.E. McNamara, *Survey of Medical Groups in the United States, 1969* (Chicago: American Medical Association, 1971).
51. United States Department of Commerce, *Statistical Abstract of the United States* (Washington, D.C.: Department of Commerce, 1973).
52. United States Department of Health, Education and Welfare, Social Security Administration, *Medical Care Costs and Prices: Background Book*, (Washington, D.C.: Social Security Administration, 1972).
53. United States Department of Labor, Bureau of Labor Statistics, *Area Wage Surveys* (Washington, D.C.: Bureau of Labor Statistics, bulletins for years 1967–1970).
54. United States Department of Labor, Bureau of Labor Statistics, *Handbook of Labor Statistics* (Washington, D.C.: Department of Labor, 1971).
55. United States Department of the Treasury, Internal Revenue Service, *Business Income Tax Returns* (Washington, D.C.: Internal Revenue Service, 1970–1972).
56. United States Senate, Committee on Finance, *Medicare and Medicaid: Problems, Issues, and Alternatives* (Washington, D.C.: U.S. Senate, 1970).

8‖ COMMENTS

Lien-fu Huang
Howard University

In his paper, Professor Sloan developed a model of physician fee-setting that he tested with a four-year time series of state cross-section data. The physician was treated as a firm that produces health services for consumers. That is, facing the consumers' demand function and his own cost curves, the physician determines the quantity and the price of his services that will maximize his business profit.

The explanatory variables that Professor Sloan employed in his demand function included insurance reimbursement factors such as the reimbursement of private health insurance for physicians' services; the major medical insurance population; Medicare part B reimbursements and Medicaid expenditures for physicians' services, or the overall proportion of the physicians' expenditure that was reimbursed (K); and some selected socioeconomic demand factors of the physicians' potential patients.

In his cost functions, besides the quantity of services produced, Professor Sloan included the physician's age and wages paid to non-physician personnel as independent variables.

The price equation employed can be derived in terms of all the independent variables in the demand and cost functions after the physician's business profit is maximized. In the empirical study, average annual revenue per visit and average usual charge were used as dependent variables representing the price variables. Several regressions were estimated. The results indicated that third-party reimbursement has a relatively greater impact on average revenue than on usual physicians' fees. Among the reimbursement factors, only the Medicare variable was consistently reliable in the usual fee equations, although the impact elasticities associated with the Medicare parameters were generally very low. Among other socioeconomic variables, only the physician-population ratio and the non-physician wage factor were relatively consistent and reliable.

In general, as in his other studies, Professor Sloan's paper has many noteworthy aspects, including a clear statement of the hypotheses to be tested and a careful comparison of the results with those reported by other investigators. However, I am not sure what policy implications can be derived from this research since the empirical results were generally insignificant or inconsistent.

In this paper, I would like to offer the following criticisms with respect to Professor Sloan's paper.

1. THE BASIC MODEL

Sloan's treatment of the physician as a health service firm and his use of the traditional profit maximization theory to explain the physician's behavior pattern are inappropriate. Here, I agree with Professor M. Feldstein's argument (1970) that "the physician is an individual who determines his quantity and price to maximize utility and not profit," and, "a simple profit maximization model does not allow for the physician's preferences for leisure time as well as income." The physician's utility function can be defined as follows:

$U = f$ (business profit, leisure time, professional ethical feeling, number of medically interesting cases, etc.)

His behavior pattern is affected by the several variables in the utility function, and business profit is only one of these. It is generally agreed that the marginal utility of leisure time to a physician is very high because of his income status. The profit maximization model ignores the physician's professional ethical feeling, precluding the refusal of care to certain cases or considering patients' costs when prescribing treatments. Nor can this model explain the fact that some physicians apply price discrimination to select medically interesting cases for the purposes of training and research. Profit incentive could be a strong factor in his utility function, but the physician's behavior is too complicated to be explained by the simple model of profit maximization.

Professor Sloan's demand function included some supply factors as independent variables, such as the physician-population ratio, physician qualification status, and the percentage of various sizes of group practice. This created an identification problem in his real demand function; namely, that it is not possible to distinguish the demand from the supply function.

The traditional model of demand and supply market determination that follows should not be ignored in this study:

$$D = \beta_1 p + \beta_2 X_1 \qquad\qquad \beta_1 < 0$$
$$S = \alpha_1 p + \alpha_2 X_2 \qquad\qquad \alpha_1 > 0$$
$$D = S$$

where D and S represent the quantity of physicians' services demanded and supplied, respectively, and X_1 and X_2 signify the exogenous demand and supply variables. X_2 may include non-physician cost inputs (e.g., wage, rent, and capital), the physicians' relative income factors, the physicians' qualification status, the physicians' average time input, the physician-population ratio, and the medical school enrollment, etc. From this model, the physician fee equation is derived as:

$$P = \frac{1}{\alpha_1 - \beta_1}(\beta_2 X_1 - \alpha_2 X_2)$$

This is a reduced-form equation in which the variation in P is explained in terms of the totality of exogenous demand and supply variables. In this equation $(\alpha_1 - \beta_1)$ is positive. If β_2 is positive, then the increase in the exogenous demand factors will tend to increase the physician fee. If α_2 is positive, then the increase in the exogenous supply factors will tend to lower the physician fee. Sloan's final price regressions are, in fact, the estimation of this type of model, although he started from a profit maximization hypothesis.

This type of model is most commonly employed in market research. Fuchs and Kramer (1972) have successfully applied this type of model to estimate the demand and supply functions for physician services. Their data was composed of a cross-section sample of thirty-three states. M. Feldstein (1970) also used this model, but he failed to obtain the proper signs for price parameters in the demand and supply equations. However, as he stated clearly in his paper, his "estimates are based on the rather small sample of quite imperfect data," and "the conclusion should be treated as preliminary and subject to revision." Feldstein had a time series sample of only nineteen years. Besides, his price and insurance factors could be overly massaged. Fuchs commented that Feldstein's result probably is "the failure to take account of technological change" (1970).

The AMA's data used by Sloan include a much larger sample of time series and cross-section data than were used by Feldstein and Fuchs. Probably, by using the above model, Sloan could have obtained completely different results.

2. THE EMPIRICAL RESULTS

In Sloan's paper, three reimbursement variables have been selected: private health insurance benefits per capita (PRIVH); a fraction of medical expenditures paid by insurance—both private and public (K); and the percentage of population with major medical insurance (MMED). The parameters of these coefficients are hardly significant. The results contradicted almost all the previous studies, including Huang and Koropecky (1973), M. Feldstein (1970), and Fuchs and Kramer (1972), each of which indicated that the insurance reimbursement factors have significant impact on the demand for physicians' services and fees.

Sloan's measurement of the third-party insurance reimbursement variables may contain serious errors, and therefore the true impact relationships were disturbed and biased. For example, he defined:

$$\text{PRIVH} = \{\text{BLUSBEN} + \gamma_B \cdot Z \cdot \text{BLUSBEN} + \gamma_c (\text{COMBEN}$$
$$- \text{DISPAY} - \text{INDBEN}) + \gamma_I \text{ INDBEN}\}$$
$$\div (\text{POP} \cdot \text{PI})$$

where BLUSBEN equals Blue Shield insurance benefits, BLUSBEN represents Blue Cross plus Blue Shield health insurance benefits; COMBEN is commercial health and disability insurance benefits; DISPAY is disability insurance benefits; INDBEN signifies insurance benefits of independent health insurance plans; and γ_B, γ_C, and γ_I represent the fraction of health insurance benefits for expenses other than hospitalization, with subscripts identifying Blue Cross-Blue Shield, commercial insurors, and independent plans, respectively. Since Professor Sloan did not have any information concerning the value of γ_B, γ_C, and γ_I by state and year, the national averages were used for all the samples. If the interstate variations of γ_B, γ_C, and γ_I are significant, then the measurement error of PRIVH is serious. Similar measurement errors and distortions of the true impacts arose for K and the major medical insurance enrollment (MMED).

Also, Sloan's insurance benefit payments were deflated by each individual state's consumer price index. State consumer price indexes vary substantially from one state to another. In the regression analysis of the pooling of time series and state cross-section data, it could be more appropriate to use a time dummy variable in order to hold the time factor constant, rather than to use each individual state's CPI as a deflator.

In his general specification price equation, Sloan also brought in such Medicare and Medicaid factors as the reimbursement variables and found that the Medicare variable was the only reliable and consistent one. This indicated that Medicare reimbursement and other private health insurance reimbursements have different impacts on the inflation of the general physician's fee. The results could be attributable to the Medicare methods of reimbursement or psychological impacts of the governmental system. Huang and Koropecky (1973) obtained similar results. They used the 1952–1969 BLS physician fee index and found that the insurance reimbursement, inflation factor, and Medicare dummy variable could explain the increase in physicians' fees up to 88 per cent. All the coefficients in their model are stable and significant, and the Medicare system contributed roughly 3 per cent of the increase in physicians' fees per annum by increasing the coverage of population and introducing the Medicare methods of reimbursement. In fact, these methods alone may have contributed 1.8 per cent to the increase in overall physicians' fees per annum. More careful investigation of the Medicare impact on physicians' fees and more detailed analysis of its causes are needed in Sloan's paper.

One of the most controversial conclusions in Professor Sloan's paper is that the physician-population ratio has a statistically significant negative impact on physicians' fees. The conclusion implied that the increase in medical education and the supply of physicians can at least temper fee inflation. In empirical studies of this type, this conclusion is unique and important. Previously, Feldstein (1970) found that the increase in the physician-population ratio is inclined to have a positive impact on the increase in physicians' fees. Fuchs and Kramer (1972) found that this ratio has a very significant positive impact on the demand for physicians' services, causing a positive impact on the increase in physicians' fees. Huang and Koropecky (1973) found that the ratio of physicians in private practice to population has a statistically significant positive impact on the increase in Medicare physicians' fees. They applied a nonlinear type of price adjustment model and found that the physicians' population ratio has a positive impact, and last year's price has a negative impact on the increase in Medicare physicians' fees. In a total of eight regressions these results are all statistically significant and consistent (pp. 30–31). These empirical results imply that the physicians' population ratio may push up the price, but the price will rise at a decreasing rate. Given other socioeconomic factors, the physicians' fees in the high-price state will converge to the fees in the low-price state. In his paper, Professor Sloan made two comments on Huang and Koropecky: First, that they obtained some negative and insignificant impacts of physicians' population ratio on the growth in Medicare physicians' fees; second, that their result implies that the fees in high-ratio states will continue to diverge from fees in low-ratio states without end. Both of these comments could be misinterpretations of the model and the results in Huang and Koropecky's study.

The positive impact argument of the physicians on the increase in physicians' fees was expressed mainly in three hypotheses: permanent excess demand for physicians' services (Feldstein, 1970), self-generation of demand by physicians (Fuchs and Kramer, 1972; Huang and Koropecky, 1973), and the physicians' maintenance of target income levels (Newhouse, 1970).

In Huang and Koropecky's study, the factors influencing the increase in Medicare physician fees were investigated. The data base consisted of a 5 per cent sample of Medicare physicians' actual charges grouped by state for the period of 1966–1969. They found that different methods of Medicare reimbursements, the standard deviation of the physicians' fees, the previous year's fees, and census region to be very important determinants. The standard deviation of physicians' fees had a consistently significant positive impact on the increase in Medicare physicians' fees in all the regressions they estimated. This implies that a large dispersion of price distribution will generate a significant incentive for physicians who charge lower fees to catch up to physicians charging higher fees. This would cause prices to rise faster where the dispersion was greater. If this argument is verified, the policy implication is profound. Fee inflation can be reduced if a method of regulation or reimbursement can be designed so as to narrow the dispersion of physicians' fees.

Huang and Koropecky used a dummy variable to indicate geographic region in their estimation of Medicare price equations. They found that during the three-year period surveyed, given all other social, economic, and insurance factors, western states had an 8 per cent higher rate of change than nonwestern states in Medicare physicians' fees.

With the exception of the methods of reimbursement, Sloan's AMA data were comparable to those used by Huang and Koropecky. I believe that he could have obtained results similar to Huang and Koropecky's given the use of the variables that they employed.

REFERENCES

1. Feldstein, M.S., "The Rising Price of Physicians' Services," *Review of Economics and Statistics*, 52 (May 1970), pp. 121–133.
2. Fuchs, V.R., and M.J. Kramer, *Determinants of Expenditures for Physicians' Services in the United States, 1948–68* (New York: National Bureau of Economic Research, Occasional Paper No. 117, December 1972).
3. Huang, L.F., and O. Koropecky, "The Effects of the Medicare Method of Reimbursement on Physicians' Fees and on Beneficiaries' Utilization," Vol. II, Part I (Washington, D.C.: Department of Health, Education, Welfare, Social Security Administration, SS Pub. No. 92-73 (10-73) 1973).
4. Newhouse, J. "A Model of Physician Pricing," *Southern Economic Journal*, (October 1970), pp. 174–183.

Gail Wilensky

Institute for Public Policy Studies and
Department of Economics, University of Michigan

Frank Sloan's paper is an interesting attempt to estimate empirically physician fee-setting behavior. But because of a variety of problems, most of which can be attributed to less than ideal data, it is not clear whether many of the results from this paper can be accepted *per se* with much confidence. The study does, however, provide some interesting comparisons with a previous study carried out by Steinwald and Sloan on a less aggregated basis.

I have two general reservations about the approach taken in the paper plus a few difficulties either with the way a variable is constructed or with the way a result is interpreted.

The first reservation involves the use of data that are aggregated at the state level. The rationale for the aggregative data base is clear. It permits the pooling of data from a variety of sources. In addition, reimbursement data are available only on an aggregate basis. Finally, it eliminates the need for explaining all unexpected signs in terms of errors in attributing aggregative data to the micro level. On the other hand, the use of aggregate data makes it more difficult to interpret the results. The most serious problem involves the construction of a third-party reimbursement variable. One specification contains three variables: private health insurance expenditures on health care other than hospital in the state (PRIVH), Medicare SMI expenditures, and Medicaid expenditures on physicians. Another involves the sum of the above three divided by per capita health expenditures in the state. Obviously neither specification is a true price for a given case and it is not clear what effects you are observing when you aggregate.

There are essentially three distinct problems with the private health expenditure variable, although not all of these are aggregation problems *per se*. The first problem is that the approximation is at best an average price rather than a marginal price, even though we generally postulate that behavior is influenced by what occurs at the margin. The existence of a variety of limits, floors, and exclusions could cause the marginal price to deviate substantially from the average price. The second and perhaps most important problem is that it is unlikely that the level and/or type of insurance is invariant across individuals. This means that the only "price" variable we can observe is the percentage of private health expenditures in a particular state covered by insurance, even though there is reason to believe that the distribution of net prices across individuals may be important. Third, even if everyone had the same insurance package, the use of the average percentage of the nonhospital health bill in the state covered by insurance would produce measurement errors, since the physician's fees against which this percentage would apply would differ. Thus, I believe that there are substantial problems with the third-party reimbursement variable as it now stands. Nonetheless, I would agree with the author that his variable is an improvement over using the percentage of the population with some form of insurance coverage, the latter being a variable that has been used in several earlier studies.

The second reservation involves the lack of a very well-specified model of physician fee-setting. Although not all that much being done here is different from what is being done elsewhere, in part by the author, the lack of a well-specified model makes some of the estimation appear to be more ad hoc than I think was the case and increases the difficulty of interpreting some of the results. In addition, I am very uneasy about the treatment of major medical insurance (MMI). First, we are told that major medical insurance is endogenous to the system and then that actual rather than predicted values of major medical insurance are used in the Table 1 regressions because of collinearity between MMI and income. Irrespective of the sign and significance of the variable, the primary conclusion one is left with is that a serious identification problem remains.

In addition to the above two points, I have difficulty with a few other variables or their interpretation. The most important one involves the private health expenditure variable. In some initial estimations, Sloan found that the PRIVH variable was consistently negative in the office and hospital visit fee regressions although it was always positive in the average revenue equation. Since the negative coefficient was regarded as being highly implausible, the decision was made to exclude it from the final regressions for office and hospital visit fees. First, it is unclear whether or not the variable was significant. Second, the seriousness of this finding, given the purpose of the study, is not made sufficiently explicit. A major purpose of the study is to estimate the impact of third-party reimbursement on the physician's fee-setting. In the first specification of third-party reimbursement, there are problems with all three components. The Medicaid variable performs poorly. The Medicare variable is generally significant but it is a proxy for several distinct factors and is therefore difficult to interpret. Finally, PRIVH, which represents three fourths of third-party reimbursements, has an implausible sign and is excluded from the fee regressions. Thus I find it difficult to accept the suggestion that the impact of private third-party reimbursement on usual charges is relatively unimportant and the major effect is reflected in average revenue. Aside from the fact that the variable was not a good reflection of the net price or average cost that a physician's patients faced, it seems to me that we just do not understand the effect of PRIVH on usual charges. I was also disturbed that no attempt was made to explain the negative coefficient, given the importance of this variable. Was it just inadequate data or a reflection of something else that was going on? For example, one possibility is that there is a relatively long lag between the time Blue Shield or other private carriers increase their rates and inflationary pressures in the medical sector, particularly during this period. If physicians feel obligated to stick to the established fee schedule but bill separately for component services that previously had been included in their "office visit" fee or which they previously had not done, we could justify the positive coefficient for average revenue and a negative or insignificant relationship to fees.

At a considerably lesser order of importance, I find the experience variable and the age variable a little strange. Approximating experience in terms of whether or not a physician has been licensed less than ten years in his current state of practice does not seem very promising. In the first place, it makes little sense unless you assume that the physician's current state of practice was also his first state of practice. In addition, it is unclear why a binary variable of this nature should be particularly helpful. Similarly, it is not obvious why we would want to use the percentage of physicians over age 55 as a variable. Although it is essentially a human capital equation, it could be that there are a lot of physicians over 55 because the area is a geographically declining one, in which case it is not a human capital equation at all. The use of at least the percentage over 55 and the percentage under 40 would seem to be an improvement. Any information about the age distribution in an earlier year would also be helpful.

As indicated at the outset, I think that this is an interesting attempt to explain variations in fee-setting, but in the end, I do not think very much can be said about either the impact of reimbursement or about fee-setting dynamics, two of the major interests of the study. The major difficulty in both cases I think is data inadequacies. Perhaps the most interesting finding both here and in Sloan's earlier disaggregative study is a small but negative relationship between physician-population ratio and physician fees. The implication is that the physicians' services market, at least for general practitioners, may work a little more like an ordinary economic market than others have found.

Finally, I believe that the only way we will be able to estimate the relationship between third-party reimbursement and physician fees is when the private health insurance expenditure data are available on a disaggregative basis. In particular, what is needed is a weighted average of the average price, or better yet the net price prevailing in a physician's market area. Such information is difficult to collect, would require a well-designed survey, and could probably only be derived accurately from physicians' billing records.

PART THREE

National Health Insurance

9

BERNARD
FRIEDMAN
Northwestern University

Mortality, Disability, and the Normative Economics of Medicare

ABSTRACT

Medicare subsidizes the purchase of health services by elderly persons. This paper supposes that several insurance alternatives may be compared, or experience monitored, using a social welfare function that recognizes gains from risk spreading, cash transfers, and improved health status. A particular measure of welfare gain, an "equivalent transfer," is derived and applied to the Medicare experience.

Econometric analysis suggests that, owing to Medicare, some improvement in mortality and disability is evident in 1969. Whether these health improvements are "large" is a question for statistical hypothesis testing, but also it is a tractable question of parameter values in the equivalent transfer formula.

1. INTRODUCTION

Medicare is one of several conceivable programs for improving the opportunity for elderly persons to spread individual monetary risk.

365

Each elderly person, under Medicare, is partially reimbursed for certain expenses in what may be called a system of matching grants conditional on validation by physicians and other health professionals. A matching grant, instead of a more neutral cash transfer, is a natural instrument of policy by a central authority wishing to partly overrule individually perceived values.[1]

This paper formulates the assessment of Medicare and some limited alternatives by a central authority. Individual risk preference and individual valuation of cash transfers are to be honored, but the improvement of health status is taken to be a matter for outside valuation.[2] The relevance of such a formulation for applied welfare analysis will be briefly discussed in this section. Then in Section 2 a particular measure of welfare gain, an "equivalent transfer," is derived. The application of this measure to monitoring the early results of Medicare is sketched. The next two sections of the paper apply econometric models for estimating improvements associated with Medicare in mortality and disability.

The problem for statistical inference is the adequate specification and testing of stochastic disturbance properties of age-specific rates. Each age-specific mortality rate should not be treated as an independent time series, since over time different individuals are observed, with different histories appearing elsewhere in the data. A related shortcoming is inherent in the cohort approach of epidemiology—technology is dated in time, affecting different cohorts at different ages. These two observations motivate the statistical tests in Section 3. Mortality rates for ages in five-year intervals, and for years at five-year intervals ending in 1969, suggest a significant improvement for elderly white males associated with Medicare. The result for older white women is less clear. Disability rates for both elderly men and elderly women over the period 1959-1971 show meaningful improvements relative to younger persons.[3] Whether health gains are substantial is a question for statistical hypothesis testing and also a tractable question of parameter values in the equivalent transfer formula.

The volumes of expert testimony and position papers during the early 1960s indicate that the purchase of additional medical care for the elderly was regarded as a key social goal.[4] Such a goal is furthered more by Medicare than by either of the two following insurance alternatives: (1) A floor on disposable income for nonhealth consumption, implemented by a subsidy with a means test; (2) A system of cash indemnities that "compensates" for health impairment without encouraging the purchase of particular services.

It is possible to criticize either of the insurance alternatives on the grounds of practicality or human dignity. In addition, neither of these alternatives offer the potential leverage of a reimbursement program for promoting efficient supplier behavior. Finally, the case for reimbursement contracts can be advanced directly, without prejudging whether experience indicates such contracts to be cost effective. The premise is that the high cost to a consumer of keeping well informed about health leads to overly long delays in seeking medical attention.

2. A NORMATIVE MODEL FOR QUANTITATIVE ASSESSMENT OF MEDICARE

The central features of Medicare to be treated here are (1) a transfer of resources to the elderly; (2) a presumably better spreading of monetary risk among the elderly; (3) presumably better average levels of health for the elderly. The purpose of this section is to derive a measure of welfare change that combines information on the above three phenomena. The measure may be called an "equivalent transfer" and may be used to compare hypothetical programs or to monitor the welfare change of a given program. The equivalent transfer is derived with a particular social welfare function.

Economists use a social welfare function (SWF) to specify exactly the information and ethical prescriptions that seem to be relevant for a decision by some absolute authority. The SWF may be completely irrelevant for understanding or participating in the political process of voting. The economic content of voting is limited to the self-interest of each and every person who votes. A program like Medicare has an effect on persons who do not vote.[5] More important, Medicare seems appropriate for the SWF approach if costs of information about the efficacy of medical care are drastically lower for a central planning authority.[6] The use of a SWF does not prejudge whether, as a result, a reimbursement program would be found inferior to cash indemnity insurance.

If we ignore program features that involve redistributing or comparing the preferences of different individuals, the SWF applies to a representative individual. Analyses containing this limitation have become conventional in the context of intertemporal and life-cycle phenomena.

The representative individual is here assumed to be required to save out of his current income while young, building up a sum of money, G. At a critical age, the saving ends and the individual receives an annuity together with a reimbursement contract for the purchase of medical services. At this critical age, the future consumption of other goods and services per period is determined by the following variables:

y = annuity income, plus actuarial value of the government reimbursement per year

z = out-of-pocket ("direct") expense on covered medical services, a random variable

π = premium charges per year for health insurance plus the actuarial value of government reimbursement

c = consumption of goods and services other than medical care.

From the above, assuming no borrowing or lending,

(1) $\quad c = y - \pi - z$

and c is a random variable.[7] The number of future periods that the individual will enjoy, and his health status while alive, are obvious concerns to him. In this analysis, however, a planning authority will be assumed to partially overrule individual valuation of medical services and health.

Define T to be an average health status variable perceived by the planning authority and assume that $u(c)$ is a function that displays the individual's degree of risk aversion.

The function $T \cdot E\left[u(c)\right]$, which is a product of expectations, will be taken as the social perception of individual welfare at the critical age. This objective function is assumed to be unique except for origin and scale. It preserves the degree of risk aversion displayed by u. The variable T may be interpreted as the effective number of periods in which $E\left[u(c)\right]$ is enjoyed.[8] This objective function is somewhat analogous to the human capital criterion of benefits from health programs.[9]

Suppose that two programs, labeled 1 and 2, or two situations (say, before and after Medicare), are to be compared. Required changes in the quantity of saving before retirement will be ignored in the welfare comparison. A measure of the welfare gain to the elderly for situation 2 is the "equivalent transfer" τ defined by

(2) $\quad T_2 \cdot E\left[u(c_2 - \tau)\right] = T_1 \cdot E\left[u(c_1)\right]$

The measure τ is the amount of nonmedical consumption whose loss in situation 2 leaves the objective function at the same value as in situation 1. The introduction of an arbitrary constant or scale factor in the objective function would not change τ.[10]

Further analysis of τ depends on a parametric specification of risk aversion. The following function with constant absolute risk aversion will be assumed:

(3) $\qquad u(c_i) = 1 - \exp\left[-R(y_i - \pi_i - z_i)\right]$

where R is the parameter measuring the degree of risk aversion.[11] It is now possible to solve (2), letting $\omega = T_2/T_1$ and $K = e^{-R(y_1 - \pi_1)} E(e^{Rz_1})$, to obtain

(4) $\qquad \tau - (y_2 - y_1) - (\pi_2 - \pi_1) + \dfrac{1}{R}\log\left[\dfrac{E(e^{Rz_1})}{E(e^{Rz_2})}\right] + \dfrac{1}{R}\log\left(\dfrac{\omega + K - 1}{\omega K}\right)$

This specific measure provides a means for comparing dollars of cash transfer with relative improvement in average health status.[12] For constant τ, the rate of substitution between ω and y_2 is

$$\left.\frac{dy_2}{d\omega}\right|_{\tau\text{constant}} = -\frac{1}{R}\left[\frac{(1-K)}{\omega(\omega+K-1)}\right] < 0 \text{ when } \omega > 1$$

There is some evidence that plausible values for R currently lie in the range 10^{-4} to 10^{-3}. Consider $R = 5 \cdot (10)^{-4}$. Then a hypothetical 1 per cent improvement in health status raises τ by $172 at $K = 0.1$. Notice that relatively small values of K are appropriate given typical values of R and y_1.

For comparisons with and without Medicare, information on the z_1 distribution may be obtained from a 1962 survey by social security (see Epstein and Murray, 1967). Complete information on the z_2 distribution is not readily available, although it is presumed that direct cost risk has been greatly reduced.[13] The increased premium cost $\pi_2 - \pi_1$ has been rather high. There are two components of π_1, previous public reimbursement π_1^g, and the cost of previous private insurance. According to Cooper et al. (1973), average per capita reimbursement under all public programs to the elderly was $131 in fiscal 1966, and it rose to $498 in fiscal 1969. Medicare is a program for which $y_2 - y_1 = \pi_2 - \pi_1^g$; there is no lump cash transfer. There is an indirect cash transfer, that portion of premiums $\pi_1 - \pi_1^g$ representing previous private insurance that is discontinued. This transfer may be guessed for 1966 by using the benefit ratio for all private insurance, which implies an average reimbursement to the elderly of $109.[14]

Conceivable alternative programs could use a lower π_2, say π_2^*, by reimbursing only "catastrophes" and in addition raise cash benefits to y_2^* with the same total cost if $y_2^* - y_2 = \pi_2 - \pi_2^*$. Whether such a strategy would promote much less average health improvement is a key question. The rest of this paper will concentrate on econometric attempts to assess health status change.

3. MEDICARE AND AGGREGATE MORTALITY EXPERIENCE

This section deals with a test of whether there was a biased improvement in U.S. mortality after 1966—biased in favor of persons over age 65. A specification of the statistical properties of aggregate mortality is applied to the data classified by year, 1934–1969, and by age, 35 and over in five-year age intervals. The statistical specification is an application of econometric methods that does not seem common in mortality studies. The deterministic core of the model is the Gompertz view of the aging process after maturity, known in demography since 1825.

Causality cannot be established at the level of aggregation used here. The more modest objective of a model is to monitor some potentially stable relationship suggested by firmer knowledge at a lower level. For a particular disease process, a reimbursement program like Medicare would promote earlier treatment and more intensive consumption of medical services.[15] When health results are compared for different dates in time, technological or environmental change may swamp the price effects. The inference of technical change from the stochastic properties of an otherwise stationary relationship is nothing new in econometrics.[16]

Per capita expenses on personal health care for the elderly rose from $440 in fiscal 1966 to $720 in fiscal 1969, a gain of 64 per cent. For younger persons, the increase was only 32 per cent.[17] Expenses for hospital care accounted for $160 of the increase for the elderly, a rise of nearly 100 per cent. In the first year of the program, it seems that as much as half of the increased hospital expense of $46 represented previous "charity" care.[18] After the first year, total expense continued to rise rapidly.

The Health Interview Surveys provide additional information on the changes in use of health services by different age groups. The relative increase in hospital care for the elderly represented higher admission rates and longer stays, as shown below.[19]

	1963–1965		1968–1969	
	Discharge Rate per 1,000	Mean Stay	Discharge Rate per 1,000	Mean Stay
All ages	128.3	8.3	125.6	9.1
Age 45–64	147.9	11.0	143.1	11.3
Age 65+	186.3	12.7	232.6	15.3

The increased discharge rate and mean stay for the elderly were not uniform across disease categories. Certain diseases of the heart, the largest single category of discharges, rose from 11.2 per cent of discharges to 12.8 per cent. Other categories showing an increased share of discharges were diseases of the eye, respiratory conditions, arthritis, and diseases of bones and joints. Marked increases in mean stay occurred for infective and parasitic diseases, mental and personality disorders, and diseases of the nervous system. These categories of increased hospital care suggest that declines in mortality may be only a small part of health improvement.

Recently, econometric studies of mortality have dealt with regional variation in age-specific or age-adjusted mortality rates. Differences in environment, medical care, income, education, and racial composition are taken to be causal determinants of differences in regional death rates. Auster, Leveson, and Sarachek (1969) estimate an elasticity of mortality for whites with respect to health expenditure of about −0.1, with a standard deviation almost as large in absolute value. The independent effect of higher average income seems to be an increase in average mortality. Silver (1972) found no significant association between state and local government spending for health and mortality in SMSA's.

The quantitative information generated by these studies would not seem applicable to the problem at hand—predictions by age of mortality over time. A relationship with an age-adjusted dependent variable cannot be an aggregate of the same relationship for each age group.[20] Moreover, an age-specific death rate changes over time partly because it refers to different people with different histories.

The series in Figure 1 seems to display a change in trend after 1966, which can be compared with other age-specific series. Yet the various age-specific series are not independent because of the aging process. Biometricians often present mortality data organized by cohort—i.e., the mortality rate for the same group of people compared over time as the group ages. After age 35, cohorts seem to follow Gompertz' Law—the logarithm of mortality is linear in age.[21] Five recent cohort curves are plotted in Figure 2.

FIGURE 1 Mortality for Age 65–69; All Races and Sex (per 100,000)

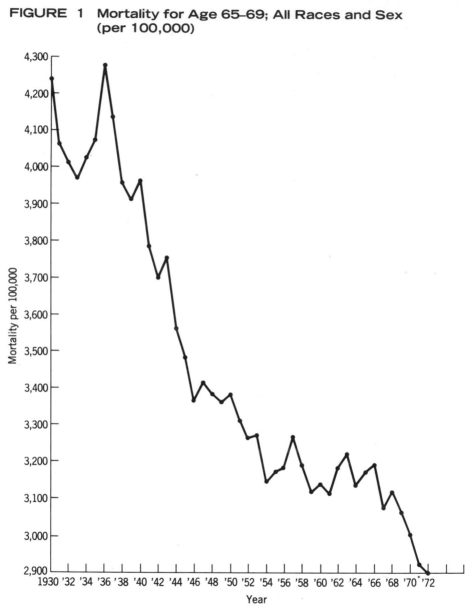

SOURCE: U.S. National Center for Health Statistics.

*Calculated from preliminary 10% sample for 1970–1972.

FIGURE 2 The Logarithm of Mortality as a Function of Age: Cohort Curves, All Races and Self, Combined

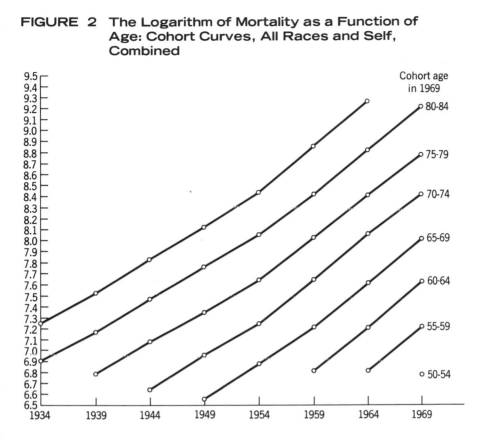

Define the following variables:

m_{it} = mortality rate for cohort i in year t
a_{it} = the age of cohort i in year t
c_i = a cohort-specific constant
B = a constant common to all cohorts

Then Figure 2 might be described with a cohort model that is a complete reconstruction of independent time series,

(5) $\qquad m_{it} = c_i B^{a_{it}}$

Further refinement in the cohort model is suggested by data such as in Figure 3, reprinted from Moriyama and Gustavus (1972). It seems that more recent cohorts after age 35 have a lower c_i and a higher B; that is, they begin at a lower rate but rise faster. A more careful inspection of this phenomenon reveals a flaw in the pure cohort model. Two cohort curves in Figure 3 cross the previous

FIGURE 3 Cohort Mortality, White Female

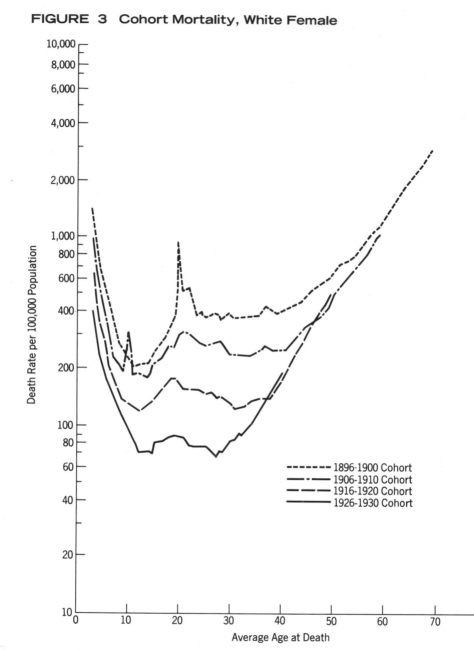

SOURCE: Moriyama and Gustavus (1972).

cohorts at the same calendar date. In Figure 2, the older cohorts seem to abruptly change slope after 1954.

A modification of the cohort model with a proportional shift in all mortality rates at each date will now be discussed. Let m_{at} be the mortality rate for the group age a in year t, and let m_{-1} stand for $m_{a-1,t-1}$. Then suppose that

$$(6) \qquad m_{at} = (1 + \lambda_t) \cdot B \cdot m_{-1} + u_{at}$$

where u_{at} is a random disturbance with mean zero. Because each m_{at} is an observed relative frequency between 0 and 1, and because each observation is for a group of different size, the disturbance u_{at} will be heteroskedastic, but with easily estimated variance.[22] A further stochastic property of u_{at} is suggested in discussions of epidemics—that u_{at} may be negatively correlated with $u_{a-1,t-1}$.

The model (6) was estimated by the established two-step, generalized least squares procedure. Since 1969 is the latest year for which mortality by five-year age interval is tabulated, the years used are 1969, back by five-year intervals through 1934.[23] In each year ten age groups are used, the youngest being age 35–39.[24] Separate analyses were made for white males and for white females.

A test of the effect of Medicare is whether the shift parameter, λ, for 1969 is significantly lower for the elderly than a separately estimated value for the young.[25] Since λB is an unrestricted linear parameter in (6), significance tests may be easily obtained with the t statistic. In Table 1 are the relevant parameter estimates. The overall fit of the model is extremely close, and a maximum likelihood search for a first-order negative correlation between u_{at} and $u_{a-1,t-1}$ produced too small a value to be meaningfully different from zero.

The relative improvement for older white males in 1969 is statistically significant at the 5 per cent level, while the hypothesis of equal parameters in the female case cannot be rejected. Tables 2

TABLE 1 Estimates of Shift Coefficients λB for 1969 (standard errors in parentheses)

	$(\lambda \hat{B})$ Under Age 65	$(\lambda \hat{B})$ Age 65–84	$\hat{B}$
White male	.14 (.04)	.03 (.03)	1.436 (.018)
White female	.06 (.09)	.15 (.06)	1.437 (.033)

TABLE 2 Actual and Predicted Mortality Rates for White Males (per 100,000)

Age[a]	Actual 1964	Actual 1969	Predicted 1969	95% Interval
42	414	425	390	± 10
47	688	685	628	16
52	1,133	1,108	1,044	28
57	1,801	1,774	1,720	46
62	2,694	2,758	2,734	73
67	4,104	4,010	4,089	198
72	5,876	6,107	6,230	165
77	8,402	8,557	8,919	237
82	12,698	12,191	12,754	339

[a]Midpoint of five-year interval.

and 3 compare actual mortality rates in 1969 with predicted values derived by fitting through 1964 and assuming that λ for 1969 will be the same as for 1964. These comparisons have the same obvious indications as the parameter tests.

It is puzzling that a gain for older men is apparent but not for older women. Table 3 indicates that mortality was meaningfully lower for older women in 1969 than in 1964, but there was also a strong decrease predicted by cohort experience. The test for nega-

TABLE 3 Actual and Predicted Mortality for White Females (per 100,000)

Age	Actual 1964	Actual 1969	Predicted 1969	95% Interval
42	234	241	238	13
47	367	365	367	19
52	562	551	576	31
57	831	819	882	47
62	1,260	1,231	1,304	70
67	2,087	1,966	1,978	106
72	3,364	3,278	3,276	176
77	5,600	5,301	5,281	284
82	9,794	8,998	8,792	473
89				

tively autocorrelated residuals did not indicate misspecification of Constant B in (6). The difference in result by sex will not be seen in the disability data of the next section.

The extent of improvement in mortality for white males is not immediately suitable for the welfare assessment in (4). If we take T to be the sum of annual survival rates, then T will rise somewhat less than in proportion to the fall in mortality. In particular, for a mortality reduction of about 5 per cent at every age, suggested by Table 1, ω would be about 1.03. This ignores improvement in health status of the living, to be discussed below.

4. DISABILITY AND THE CONSUMPTION OF HEALTH SERVICES

This section reports a study of disability using interview data collected by the National Center for Health Statistics. Reductions in disability augment social welfare gains stemming from mortality reduction, and the extent of one type of improvement might not be easily inferred from the extent of the other.[26]

The first data to be examined are age-specific disability rates over time, 1959–1971. The data suggest relative gains for older men and women since 1965. The disability measure used here is the number of restricted activity days, R, defined as days in which usual activities are substantially reduced because of illness or injury.

In Figure 4, average R is plotted over time for four age-sex classes. In the preceding section I stated that a set of age-specific time series should not be treated as if each were independent. Here, however, the age categories are too broad and the time series too short to adequately treat the autoregressive properties of disability. Instead, it seems more plausible to test for a stable contemporaneous relationship between R and the utilization of health services.

Annual expenditures on personal health care per capita have been calculated by Cooper et al. (1973). These may be converted to constant dollar units with the BLS price index for medical care. Values of per capita real expense, PRE, for different age groups are available after 1966. For this period, per capita real expense for persons over age 65, PREA, has been regularly about 2.5 times PRE for the entire population. Survey evidence for 1962 showed PREA $\approx$ 1.5 PRE. This factor was assumed to hold throughout 1959–1965.

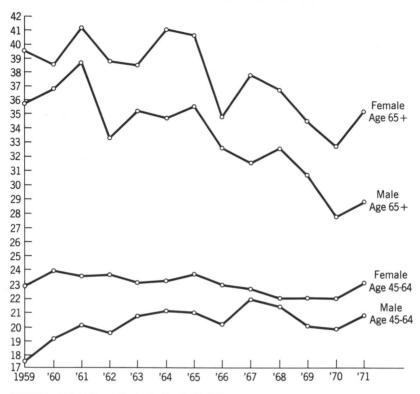

FIGURE 4   Restricted Activity Days per Person

SOURCE: U.S. National Center for Health Statistics.

During the brief time period covered in Figure 4, there is not a significant relationship between R and PRE for persons aged 45–64. For females, however, the trend lowers beginning in 1966, which is almost significant.

For the elderly, the data support a significant relationship between R and PREA. The regression of R on PREA yields a coefficient estimate for men of -0.018 (t statistic -5.2), and for women -0.013 (t statistic -3.4). If the effect of Medicare is taken to be the rise in PREA from 1.5 PRE to 2.5 PRE, then in 1969 the program is associated with a decline of 5.7 disability days for men and 4.1 days for women. These declines would have been 18 per cent and 11 per cent, respectively. These estimates are crude and upwardly biased by the omission of variables such as income or social security cash benefits, since other goods and services may be purchased that reduce disability. Over a longer time series, the problem of exogenous technical progress might be treated by distinguishing cause-specific disability rates.

One possible means of combining information on disability reduction with information on mortality reduction will now be discussed. The aim is to construct a useful scalar measure of relative improvement, ω, to use in (4).

Recall that $\omega = T_2/T_i$, where each T_i is a factor multiplying the annual expected utility of consumption of goods other than health services. Let S_{ti} be the probability of survival to year t under program i. Let a_{ti} be a factor that reduces utility of those alive depending on the level of average disability; specifically, let

$$u_{ti} - 1 = \frac{\text{disability days in year } t}{365}$$

One particular way of formulating the planning agency's tradeoff between survival and disability is

(7) $$T_i = a_{ti} + \sum_{t=1}^{L} S_{ti} a_{ti}$$

where $S_{ti} = 0$ for all $t > L$. Perhaps the major reservation in advocating such a measure is a suspicion that it would not be appropriate for situations wherein mortality increases despite improvements in the health of the living. In the practical application here, changes in mortality will be seen to govern the scalar index ω.

In the following table (7) is used to compute values of ω for men and women aged 65–69 in 1969, r being the relative decline in mortality rates and d the relative decline in disability days.

Men				Women			
r	d	T	ω	r	d	T	ω
0	0	11.32		0	0	16.44	
.03	.10	11.64	1.028	.03	.10	16.87	1.026
.06	.10	11.85	1.047	.06	.10	17.13	1.042
.03	.20	11.75	1.038	.03	.20	17.04	1.036
.06	.20	11.97	1.057	.06	.20	17.31	1.052

The importance of disability and health status measures seems destined to grow. Further use of the Health Interview Surveys will treat disability as an outcome of environmental events, the use of medical services, and the lagged effects of past behavior. A preliminary approach to production function analysis in survey data is reported below. The results were not encouraging; they suggest refinements in research methods and the need for longitudinal samples.

Previously, Grossman (1972, pp. 55–66) has reported estimates of the determinants of cross-sectional variation in disability. After application of two models with disability as a dependent variable, he suggests that the more convincing interpretation of the data is given by a model of the demand for "flows" of good health.[27]

Grossman's attempt to estimate with consistent methods the effect of medical care in reducing disability did not yield reliable results.[28] My preliminary study led to a similar conclusion.

The Health Interview Survey for 1969 provides the number of restricted activity days for an individual during the two weeks prior to interview. Each quarter of the year, however, is a separate random sample of the U.S. population. Therefore, average disability for subpopulation i in a two-week period, $\bar{R}_i$, is seasonally unbiased. The method of choosing subpopulations will be considered below. The probability of a disabling condition does not depend on contemporaneous use of medical care, and by analogy to Gompertz' Law is assumed to rise exponentially with age. The length of disability, given its occurrence, is assumed to depend negatively on the intensity of medical care.

Define the following averages for subpopulation i:

MDV = number of physician visits (12 mos.)
HOS = number of hospital days (12 mos.)
HI = proportion with hospital insurance
HG = proportion with education at least through high school graduation
INS = 0.25 (HI) + (1-HI) a crude estimate of average net price of medical care.

Let the prefix L for any variable name denote a logarithmic transformation.

In the absence of data on past use of medical care, I attempted to specify the static production function over groups

$$(8) \qquad L\bar{R}_i = \alpha_0 + \alpha_1 AGE_i + \alpha_2 LMDV_i + \alpha_3 LHOS_i + \alpha_4 LHG_i + u_i$$

Problems of identification and simultaneity bias must now be discussed, and methods for grouping and consistent estimation described. In reality, there are a variety of illnesses, each with a different established method and intensity of medical treatment. Some conditions that are treated with more than average intensity may nevertheless have worse than average disability results, which, of course, carries no implication that the choice of treatment was inefficient. One suspects, therefore, correlation between amount of care and the residual in (8). Identifying information may not be present in the sample—e.g., variables that affect MDV and HOS but are not correlated with the residual in (8). I assumed that income and price of care are variables that may be used as instruments in estimating (8). Only a crude measure of price was available.

The population over 45 was classified into 9 age categories and 7 income groups, yielding 63 subpopulations. The grouping strategy, in addition to removing seasonality, sought to use an instrumental technique to purge LMDV and LHOS of correlations with u. Classification by age may not advance the above strategy, so (8) was estimated by two-stage least squares with LINS, LHGP, AGE, and income dummy variables used as the exogenous variables. The computed estimates of α_2 and α_3 were positive, which seems primarily to reflect a failure to identify the true parameters of a production relation.

Fruitful research on cross-sectional variation in disability may be aided by cause-specific analysis, or supplementary information on regional quality variation and standards of medical care. The longer-term effects of differences in intensity or quality of medical care may require repeated interviews with the same individuals.

CONCLUDING REMARKS

It was not the purpose of this paper to conclude whether Medicare is or was better than some other program. The purpose was to demonstrate the feasibility of deriving and usefully combining information on health status, cash transfers, and risk bearing. The social welfare function suggested in this paper is one of an infinity of formulations. The need to use some such precise formulation for planning government intervention in personal health decisions seems obvious.

NOTES

1. The dominant private insurance plans also cover health loss with a matching grant. The welfare formulation in this paper is not meant to explain how the private insurance system or Medicare arose, but may be relevant to the question of why they survive.
2. The effect of higher taxes and higher prices for health services on younger persons will not be considered.

3. Despite the short time span, the data suggest a break in trend after 1965 that is consistent with a stable relationship between real per capita health expense and days of restricted activity. A cross-section multivariate analysis in 1969, however, did not permit the identification of such a "production" relationship.

4. See H. Somers and A. Somers, *Medicare and the Hospitals: Issues and Prospects* (Washington, D.C.: The Brookings Institution, 1967), Ch. I.

5. Each person who votes may weigh his own potential gain or loss against the gain or loss of others. Pauly (1971) suggests that the existence of such consumption externalities is the key impetus behind public reimbursement programs for medical care. In the general analysis of government there will be many SWF's. Rothenberg (1961) argues that the community can come to a prior agreement on a single SWF to be implemented by neutral technocrats.

6. The problem of adverse selection and other high private transaction costs argue for public administration of insurance, but this is not synonymous with the application of a SWF.

7. The exposition may be carried through with an addition to y of the annuity value of other assets as long as these are unaffected by program change. Also, c is assumed to be non-negative.

8. The same objective function may be offered with the following justification: Assume that each period has independent and identically distributed outcomes of current expense and that individual utility is the sum of utility in all periods lived. Then, average summed utility will be

$$E\left[u(c)\right] \cdot (1 + S_1 + S_2 + \ldots)$$

where S_j is the probability of survival to period j, averaging over all initial conditions.

9. Both criteria are weighted sums of future planner-perceived gains to the representative individual. Use of the human capital criterion does not typically recognize risk preference. See, e.g., Weisbrod (1961) and Rice (1966). Both criteria override individual preferences with regard to discounting the future, and individual subjective probabilities. Discounting could be incorporated in the SWF used here.

10. The concept is analogous to "certainty equivalence." Therefore, extrapolation to situations with no risk would suffer from a recognized drawback—consumer preferences may be somewhat incomparable between the case of no risk and some risk.

11. The specification of Constant R has been applied in discussions of health insurance by Zeckhauser (1970), Friedman (1971), Feldstein (1972), and Arrow (1974).

12. Suppose that T is the sum of survival rates given in an earlier note. If the entire survival curve is shifted up by proportion $r > 1$, then ω is slightly less than r; specifically,

$$\omega = r - (r - 1)/T_1$$

13. This conclusion may depend on the precise manner of treating free care in the pre-Medicare period. The appropriate z_1 distribution is what would have been observed in the year for which all comparisons are made, in this paper 1969.

14. Elderly persons were likely to have insurance with less extensive reimbursement, but were likely to be paying higher premiums for individual coverage. In 1969 they might have been paying more than this amount in the absence of Medicare.

15. This distinction may have practical relevance for a minority of diseases such as

cancer. The distinction attempts to recognize that consumer response to lower prices may be more directly relevant to early treatment than to the mode of treatment. The behavior of physicians as decision-making agents with some leeway to exercise their own preferences may show a more complicated response to public programs. See Fuchs (1972, Ch. 4) and Friedman (1974).

16. An early example in the literature on economic growth is R. Solow, "Technical Change and the Aggregate Production Function," *Review of Economics and Statistics*, 39 (1957), pp. 312–320.

17. During this period the CPI medical care component rose by about 15 per cent. The expenditure data are from Cooper *et al.* (1973).

18. See R. Lowenstein, "Early Effects of Medicare on the Health Care of the Aged," *Social Security Bulletin* (April 1971).

19. The utilization data in this section are from "Age Patterns in Medical Care, Illness, and Disability," *Vital and Health Statistics*, Series 10, Nos. 32 and 70.

20. This particular problem could be corrected in the linear case by age-adjusting all the independent variables. The question of proper pooling is more serious. Silver computes a coefficient of concordance between separate rankings of regions for age-specific mortality. The values for this statistic are quite low in 1960, and are more troubling for men than for women.

21. Since Gompertz' initial suggestion, more complicated models and speculations have been offered. For most of these formulations, the rate of increase in mortality is approximately constant from "maturity," falling off gradually at older ages. See Spiegelman (1968), pp. 163–170.

22. If the true value of m_{at} is μ, then the variance at u_{at} is $\mu(1 - \mu)/n_{at}$, where n_{at} is number alive at beginning of year t.

23. I must thank Joan Klebba, National Center for Health Statistics, for helpful assistance with these data.

24. The open-ended group, age 85+, was ignored.

25. A three-year period may be too soon to capture the effect of earlier treatment of serious illness, as the trend in Figure 1 suggests. When later data become available, the possibility must be considered that technical or environment change has been slanted in favor of the elderly. For example, a decline in the proportion of cigarette smokers may have occurred more rapidly and with greater effect among the elderly.

26. Fuchs has discussed the extent of correlation between mortality and disability measures across regions. See "Some Economic Aspects of Mortality in the United States," National Bureau of Economic Research, 1965, mimeo. The possibility should not be overlooked that over time, reduced mortality at older ages might raise the average observed disability of the living.

27. Of primary interest to Grossman is the stock of health that represents both the capitalization of future flows and the lagged effects of past investment choices.

28. The regression used a NORC sample of 550 members of the labor force in 1963 with some disability days.

REFERENCES

1. Auster, R., I. Leveson, and D. Sarachek, "The Production of Health, an Exploratory Study," *Journal of Human Resources*, 4 (Fall 1969), pp. 411–436.

2. Cooper, B., N. Worthington, and M. McGee, *Compendium of National Health Expenditure Data*, Department of Health, Education and Welfare, Publication No. (SSA) 73-11903, Washington, D.C.

3. Epstein, Lenore A., and Janet H. Murray, *The Aged Population of the United Sates—The 1963 Social Security Survey of the Aged*, Resarch Report No. 19, Social Security Administration, Washington, D.C., 1967.

4. Feldstein, M., "The Welfare Loss of Excess Health Insurance," *Journal of Political Economy*, 81 (March–April 1973), pp. 251–280.

5. Friedman, B., *A Study of Uncertainty and Health Insurance*, Ph.D. dissertation, Massachusetts Institute of Technology, 1971.

6. ———, "A Test of Alternative Demand-Shift Responses to the Medicare Program," in M. Perlman (editor), *The Economics of Health and Medical Care* (London: Macmillan, 1974).

7. Fuchs, V. (editor), *Essays in the Economics of Health and Medical Care* (New York: National Bureau of Economic Research, 1972).

8. ———, "Some Economic Aspects of Mortality in Developed Countries," in M. Perlman (editor), *The Economics of Health and Medical Care* (London: Macmillan, 1974).

9. Grossman, M., *The Demand for Health: A Theoretical and Empirical Investigation* (New York: National Bureau of Economic Research, Occasional, Paper 119, 1972).

10. Moriyama, I., and S. Gustavus, *Cohort Mortality and Survivorship: U.S. Death Registration States, 1900–1968*, Vital and Health Statistics, Series 3, Number 16, U.S. Public Health Service, Washington, D.C., 1972.

11. Palmore, E. (editor), *Normal Aging* (Durham, North Carolina: Duke University Press, 1970).

12. Pauly, M.V., *Medical Care at Public Expense* (New York: Praeger, 1961).

13. Rice, D., *Estimating the Cost of Illness*, U.S. Public Health Service, Health Economics Series No. 6, Washington, D.C., 1966.

14. Rothenberg, J., *The Measurement of Social Welfare* (Englewood Cliffs, New Jersey: Prentice-Hall, 1961).

15. Silver, M., "An Econometric Analysis of Spatial Variations in Mortality Rates by Race and Sex," in V. Fuchs (editor), *Essays in the Economics of Health and Medical Care* (New York: National Bureau of Economic Research, 1972), Ch. 9.

16. Spiegelman, M., *Introduction to Demography*, Revised Edition (Cambridge, Massachusetts: Harvard University Press, 1968).

17. Sullivan, D., "Disability Components for an Index of Health," *Vital and Health Statistics*, Series 2, Number 42, U.S. Public Health Service, Washington, D.C., 1971.

18. Weisbrod, B., *The Economics of Public Health* (Philadelphia: University of Pennsylvania Press, 1961).

19. Zeckhauser, R., "Medical Insurance: A Case Study of the Trade-off Between Risk Spreading and Appropriate Incentives," *Journal of Economic Theory*, 2 (March 1970).

9 ‖ COMMENTS

Stuart H. Altman and Ira Burney
Department of Health, Education, and Welfare

Bernard Friedman's paper is really two very interesting papers. Unfortunately, the bridge between them is not as strong as it could be. The first is an application of welfare theory to provide a framework for analyzing Medicare. The second is an empirical investigation of the effects of Medicare on the health status of the aged. In these brief comments the model and its assumptions are reviewed, other important issues to consider are identified, and the empirical results are examined.

Friedman proposes an intriguing model to compare the welfare of the aged before and after Medicare. The novel aspect of the model is the attempt to incorporate three health-related features into the welfare function. They are (1) consumption of medical services, (2) risk spreading, and (3) health status. The concept of "equivalent transfer," τ, which purports to measure the monetary value of welfare gains in these three features, is developed. One of the basic ramifications of the model is that all welfare gains are attributed to Medicare.

The model is a two-period life-cycle formulation. It assumes that a representative individual (in period 1) saves out of current income. At the critical age (period 2), all saving ends and the individual receives an annuity and a reimbursement contract for the purchase of medical services.[1] Future consumption of goods and services is governed by two other variables: (1) Z, a random variable reflecting out-of-pocket expenses for noncovered medical services, and (2) π, average spending on health insurance premiums, both public and private. Assuming no borrowing, lending, or saving, consumption of goods and services other than medical care, C, is defined by the identity[2] $C = y - \pi - Z$.

With this consumption identity, Friedman specifies an objective function. It is $T \cdot E\left[u(c)\right]$, the product of average health status T as perceived by the central planning authority and the expected value of a utility function $u(c)$. Friedman comments that this objective function is "the social perception of individual welfare at the critical age." To compare welfare of the aged before and after Medicare, Friedman incorporates the equivalent transfer τ into the objective function. The definition of τ is embodied in the following equation

$$T_2 \cdot E\left[u(c_2 - \tau)\right] = T_1 \cdot E\left[u(c_1)\right]$$

The authors are Deputy Assistant Secretary for Health Planning and Evaluation, and Staff Economist, Department of Health, Education, and Welfare. The views expressed here are those of the authors and do not necessarily represent the views of the Department. The authors would like to especially acknowledge the helpful comments of George Schieber.

where subscripts 1 and 2 refer to pre- and post-Medicare, respectively. Friedman describes τ as "the amount of nonmedical consumption whose loss in situation 2 leaves the objective function at the same value as in situation 1." Positing a negative exponential utility function with the property of constant absolute risk aversion, Friedman solves the above equation for τ.

The model is an intriguing conceptual approach that incorporates the consumption of medical services, risk spreading, and health status in comparing the welfare of the aged before and after Medicare. However, in examining Medicare (or other public programs) there are some other important issues to consider. For example, under what circumstances should the government intervene in the private market? If government intervenes, what policy instruments should be employed? What are the total (i.e., general equilibrium) effects of intervention on the rest of society? Friedman's formulation does not address itself to these fundamental issues.

In the case of Medicare, one key reason for public intervention was the failure of the private market to provide health insurance for the elderly. Largely out of the labor force, the elderly lacked the opportunity to purchase health insurance at group rates. In addition, experience rating, the competitive tool of the commercial companies, forced the Blues to abandon community rating, which to a certain extent had allowed some aged persons to purchase protection at reasonable rates. Finally, an institutional feature of the market is that unlike life insurance, one cannot purchase health insurance on an annuity basis. For these reasons an adequate market for health insurance for the aged failed to develop. Distributional considerations provide yet another, albeit interrelated, rationale for the creation of Medicare, since many elements of society had empathy with the elderly, a majority of whom are poor. If these distributional considerations are viewed in a more global framework, one should consider the welfare of the givers as well as the receivers.[3]

Inasmuch as public intervention can lead to greater efficiency under these circumstances, the question becomes, "What policies should be used?" When Medicare was being debated, several approaches—subsidies for the purchase of private insurance, creation of insurance pools, and having the government act as underwriter—were considered. It would be useful to develop a model to compare the implications of these alternative mechanisms. Such a model could also be useful in addressing some of the important questions in the current national health insurance debate.

The second part of Friedman's paper is an empirical investigation of whether the health status of the elderly improved after Medicare. Indeed, these results are encouraging, although they are far from definitive. First, he attempts to measure improvements in mortality. Because this measure ignores improvements in the health status of the living, changes in disability are also measured. Finally, mortality and disability are integrated to obtain a comprehensive indicator of the change in health status.

Friedman acknowledges the problem of attempting to discern causality with aggregate mortality data but aspires to a less grand objective of finding an associative relationship. The critical assumption of this approach is that *all* the change in health status is attributed exclusively to one program—

Medicare. Changes in health status arising from other programs such as housing subsidies, food stamps, cleaner environments, and increases in real income (Social Security benefits) are not properly accounted for.

Two tests of improvement in mortality of the aged are performed with cohort mortality data. In the first test a modified cohort mortality model is estimated for white males and females. Although the model indicates improvements in mortality for white males, the hypothesis of no improvement or indeed retrogression in mortality for white females cannot be rejected.

The second test applies the model to mortality data for each of eight cohorts up to 1964. The estimated equation is then used to predict what 1969 mortality would have been if the underlying pre-Medicare trends continued. A test of the effect of Medicare is whether the actual 1969 mortality rate is significantly different from the predicted 1969 mortality. Friedman finds that for white males there is a significant difference for six cohorts (four cohorts under age 65 in 1969 and the oldest two over 65). For white females, the actual is significantly different from the predicted for only one of the nine cohorts (age 62).

Although these results are encouraging, they are hardly unambiguous. In view of the insignificant result for white females, it may be premature to attribute improvements in mortality for males to Medicare, especially since so many other social programs were changing at the same time. In any case, it may also be that a three-year period is too short to detect improvements in health status, especially for the aged, who have many chronic conditions that might be affected only slightly by medical care.

Since improvements in mortality do not take into account improvements in the health of the living, changes in disability are also considered. In a crude model, Friedman regresses days of restricted activity for the aged on real per capita expenditures for the aged and reports highly significant results. Friedman suggests that in 1969 Medicare is "associated with a decline of 5.7 disability days for men and 4.1 disability days for women." These results should be interpreted cautiously since other important variables may be omitted from the model. Moreover, there is a problem of causality, and "free care" in the pre-Medicare period may not be adequately accounted for.

Friedman then attempts to combine mortality and disability to determine the likely range of the relative improvement in health status. He uses one of many possible sets of assumptions, and in view of the value judgments this specification presumes, several alternative combinations might have been more helpful. Friedman computes the relative improvement in health after Medicare for several possible values of the improvement in mortality and disability. Unfortunately, he does not use the relative improvement in health to calculate τ, the dollar value of welfare gains.

In summary, Friedman has presented an interesting model to analyze the welfare effects of Medicare on beneficiaries. To the extent that his empirical results can be attributed to Medicare, they reflect favorably on the program. Nevertheless, the model is limited in applicability and leaves untested many other important aspects of a national health financing system.

NOTES

1. That is, the Medicare reimbursement contract reimburses eligible persons for specified medical services if these services are rendered by recognized providers.
2. It is unclear how this model relates to the institutional features of Medicare. For example, Part A of Medicare (primarily for institutional services) is mandatory and is financed by a payroll tax on employers and currently employed workers. Benefits are paid out of current income and indeed this feature may be viewed as an intergenerational transfer of wealth. Part B (primarily for noninstitutional services) is a voluntary program financed by premiums set annually and paid by both the beneficiary and government general revenues. Indeed, one can make an analogy between the government and private employers if we consider Part B as a large group policy with premiums paid by both enrollees and by government contributions.
3. See especially Irwin Garfinkel, "Is In-Kind Redistribution Efficient?," *Quarterly Journal of Economics,* 87 (May 1973), pp. 320–330.

Victor R. Fuchs

National Bureau of Economic Research
and Stanford University

I shall limit my comments to Friedman's attempt to determine the effect of Medicare on mortality. This is, as he points out, a hazardous undertaking. The available data cover only three full post-Medicare years, 1967–1969, possibly too short a period for any significant changes in mortality to emerge. In the short run death rates are subject to many random influences such as influenza epidemics or variations in the severity of winter weather.

Even if a longer period were available, however, the problem of establishing a causal connection between Medicare and mortality change would be formidable. For the population as a whole, long-run trends in mortality are determined primarily by environmental and behavioral changes and by advances in medical technology, not by changes in quantity of medical care. From 1900 to the mid-1930s, age-adjusted mortality of U.S. whites decreased at an average rate of about 1.3 per cent per year. The decline, which was only slightly more rapid for females than for males, was mostly the result of rising real income and of basic public health measures. Very little was attributable to advances in medical science or increased quantity of medical care.

From the mid-1930s to the mid-1950s, age-adjusted death rates fell at a much faster rate: 1.7 per cent per year for white males and 2.9 per cent per year for white females. The acceleration was the result of rapid advances in medical technology, particularly the development of anti-infectious drugs.

Around 1954–1955 there was an abrupt change in trend (pointed out by Friedman in his cohort charts). Since then, the age-adjusted male death rate has been approximately constant. The female rate has continued to decline but at a much slower pace: 0.7 per cent annually.

To test for the effects of Medicare, Friedman employs a cohort model with observations at five-year intervals back to 1934. Regressions through 1964 yield predicted age-specific mortality for 1969 that he compares with actual mortality. He finds a significant result for males but not for females.

A close examination of Friedman's Table 2 reveals a curious pattern of deviation between actual and predicted mortality rates in 1969, with the relative deviation decreasing systematically with age, as shown in my Table 1 below.

By splitting the population at age 65, Friedman finds a significant "Medicare effect," but if the population were split at 55 or 75, a significant difference between the older and younger ages would also emerge. There may be some real phenomena at work that are systematically reducing mortality more with increasing age, or the pattern may result from some bias in the cohort model. But the conclusion of a Medicare effect seems premature.

Friedman's cohort model is only one of several imperfect approaches that can be followed to test for Medicare effects. The mortality of any population in a given year is a function of its age, the state of medical science, the quantity of care available, the current environment, plus a host of past medical and environmental variables and previous mortality experience. Because cohort, age, and year are linked in an identity relationship, it is not possible to completely identify their separate effects.

I have attempted to test for a Medicare effect on mortality by fitting regressions of the form In $M = a + bT$ to annual data for the periods 1955–1965 and 1967–1969.[1] In no case can we reject the null hypothesis of no difference between the periods. The F values are typically very small.

I have also used the 1955–1965 regressions to derive predicted values for the Medicare years. The percentage difference between the actual and the predicted values for these years is shown in Table 2. Again, there is no evidence that Medicare has had a significant effect on the mortality of the aged.

I do not find this result very surprising. Current changes in mortality, in my view, are determined primarily by nonmedical factors. During the decade of the 1960s, for instance, the death rate for emphysema for white males ages

TABLE 1 Relative Deviation between Actual Mortality and Friedman's Predicted Mortality, White Males, 1969

Age	$(A - P)/P$
42	+9.0%
47	+9.1
52	+6.1
57	+3.1
62	+0.9
67	−1.9
72	−2.0
77	−4.1
82	−4.4

SOURCE: Table 2 in Friedman's paper.

TABLE 2 Percentage Deviation between Actual and Predicted Death Rates, 1967–1969[a]

Sex	Age	1967	1968	1969	Average 1967–1969
Males	45–54	−1.4	+0.1	−2.3	−1.2
	55–64	+0.4	+2.5	+0.2	+1.1
	65–74	−1.5	+0.8	−2.4	−1.0
	75–84	−1.4	+1.4	+0.5	+0.2
Females	45–54	−0.3	+2.2	−0.6	+0.5
	55–64	+1.2	+5.1	+3.3	+3.2
	65–74	+0.3	+2.4	+0.7	+1.1
	75–84	−2.8	+0.2	−1.5	−1.4

[a] Predicted values based on regressions fitted to annual data, 1955–1965.

65–74 more than doubled, the rate for lung cancer increased by 25 per cent, and the rate for arteriosclerotic heart disease went up by 15 per cent. These increases were not the result of a deterioration in the quantity or quality of medical care. During the same decade there were substantial (more than 25 per cent) decreases in the death rates for cancer of the large intestine, rectum, and prostate. The medical profession has no firm explanation for these declines and they are not believed to be the result of more medical care.

To pursue seriously the question of the effect of Medicare on mortality, several different approaches should be tried. For instance, it would be desirable to disaggregate by cause of death. Particular attention could then be paid to those categories wherein there is some reason to believe that increased access to medical care should make a difference (e.g., infectious diseases). It might also be useful to disaggregate by state and region. There was probably some geographic variation in the impact of Medicare on utilization of care by the aged, and one could test for a relation between such utilization and changes in mortality. Along the same lines, it might be useful to look at recent mortality experience in countries that did not experience any shift in care for the elderly.

These comments, which have been limited to mortality, do not do justice to the ambitious scope of Friedman's paper. They reflect my own belief in the need for more intensive investigation of sharply defined questions.

NOTES

1. The year 1966 is omitted because Medicare was partially in effect.

   M = age-sex-specific death rates
   T = time

10

KAREN DAVIS and ROGER REYNOLDS
The Brookings Institution

The Impact of Medicare and Medicaid on Access to Medical Care

Medicare and Medicaid, initiated in 1966 under the Johnson Administration, were in the forefront of the Great Society programs designed to help the poor and disadvantaged enjoy the fruits of a growing and prosperous economy. They received the largest and most rapidly growing share of budgetary resources of all social programs enacted during that period. In fiscal 1975, governmental expenditures under the federal-state Medicaid program are expected to be $13 billion, providing medical care services for 25 million low-income people; Medicare is expected to spend $15 billion on medical care services for 24 million elderly and disabled people.

Concern with the high cost of these programs has almost eclipsed the substantial achievements of the programs in increasing access to medical care services by many persons who formerly had to seek charity care or do without much-needed care. To gain better

The views expressed here are those of the authors and not necessarily those of the officers, trustees, or other staff members of The Brookings Institution. Financial support for this study has been provided by the Robert Wood Johnson Foundation.

perspective on the benefits of these programs, this paper will address three major questions:

1. What impact have Medicare and Medicaid had on use of medical services by the poor and elderly, particularly in relation to other persons with similar health problems?
2. What factors account for uneven utilization of medical services by persons eligible for Medicaid?
3. To what extent do socioeconomic and demographic characteristics continue to affect the utilization of health services by the elderly?

1. IMPACT OF MEDICARE AND MEDICAID ON USE OF MEDICAL SERVICES

Recent evidence indicates that Medicare and Medicaid have led to marked improvements in contact with the medical system by poor persons and greatly increased the access of the elderly of all income classes to institutional services such as hospital and nursing home care. Andersen *et al.* (1972) report that in 1970, 65 per cent of low-income persons saw a physician during the year, compared with 56 per cent in 1963.[1] They also point out that poor pregnant women began increasingly to visit physicians earlier—71 percent of low-income women received medical attention in the first trimester of pregnancy in 1970 as against 58 per cent in 1963. Results from National Health Surveys show that, while 11 out of every 100 elderly persons were hospitalized in 1962, 16 were hospitalized in 1968.[2]

Furthermore, these changes in use of services were not part of an overall pattern. Utilization by higher-income persons remained stable over the period or declined slightly. Therefore, the poor made striking gains in use of services relative to higher-income groups. As shown in Table 1, in fiscal 1964 high-income persons paid 19 per cent more visits to a physician than low-income persons; by 1971, more low-income persons than high-income persons were using such services.

There also were significant redistributions in institutional care. Pettingill (1972) reports that although days of hospital care for the aged increased at an annual rate of between 6 and 13 per cent in the first three years following the inception of Medicare, days of care by persons under age 65 declined steadily.[3] The share of hospital days spent by the elderly increased by six percentage points over

TABLE 1 Physician Visits per Capita, by Age and Family-Income Group, Fiscal Year 1964, Calendar Year 1971

Age and Income Group[a]	1964	1971
All ages	4.5	5.0
Low income	4.3	5.6
Middle income	4.5	4.7
High income	5.1	4.9
Ratio, high income to low income	1.19	.88
Under 15 years		
Low income	2.7	4.0
Middle income	2.8	4.1
High income	4.5	4.8
Ratio, high income to low income	1.67	1.20
15–64 years		
Low income	4.4	5.8
Middle income	4.7	4.9
High income	4.9	4.8
Ratio, high income to low income	1.11	.83
65 years and older		
Low income	6.3	6.7
Middle income	7.0	6.4
High income	7.3	7.5
Ratio, high income to low income	1.16	1.12

SOURCES: U.S. Department of Health, Education and Welfare, National Center for Health Statistics, *Volume of Physician Visits by Place of Visit and Type of Service*, United States, July 1963–June 1964, Series 10, No. 18, (1965) and unpublished tabulations for 1971.

[a] Low income is defined as under $4,000 in 1964 and under $5,000 in 1971. Middle income is defined as $4,000–$6,999 in 1964 and $5,000–$10,000 in 1971. High income is defined as $7,000 and above in 1964 and $10,000 and above in 1971.

this period. In later years, hospital care of younger age groups began to increase relatively faster, as might be expected as the adjustment to Medicare ended and private insurance coverage of the under age 65 group continued to expand.[4] In addition, Loewenstein has found that Medicare induced a marked increase in the use of extended care facilities by the elderly.[5] Administrative cutbacks in this benefit in 1969 later moderated these gains.

Although these data and studies give solid support to the contention that Medicare and Medicaid have been largely successful in achieving their goal of ensuring access to medical care services for covered persons, they are subject to several qualifications.

First, Medicaid does not provide medical care services for all poor persons, but only those falling within certain welfare categories, such as single-parent families, and the blind, disabled, and aged. In 1974, an estimated 9 million persons with incomes below the poverty level, or about 35 per cent of the poor, were ineligible for Medicaid. Therefore, gains in use of medical services may not be widely shared by all poor persons.

Second, greater equality in utilization of medical services among income classes may be misleading because poor persons generally have more severe health problems than higher-income persons, and persons receiving welfare are less healthy as a whole than other poor persons. Comparisons among persons of similar health status can therefore be expected to indicate much wider differences in use of services among income classes.

Third, even if utilization of services is adjusted for health needs of the population, the poor may still not participate in "mainstream" medicine, receiving care of comparable quality, convenience, and style to that received by more fortunate persons. Poor persons may continue to be treated in crowded and dreary clinics, enduring long waits and receiving few amenities. Care may be discontinuous, episodic, fragmented, and impersonal if patients see different physicians or health personnel at each visit. Any given level of care, as measured by physician visits or days of care in a hospital, may be less effective in terms of meeting the patient's health needs than the same level of care received by higher-income patients in more amenable settings.

Finally, even if Medicare and Medicaid have assisted poor and elderly persons as a whole in receiving care comparable to that received by others, racial discrimination or variations in the availability of medical resources may lead to a very uneven distribution of benefits among eligible persons.

To sort out the simultaneous influence of health status, income, coverage under public programs, sociodemographic factors, and availability of medical resources requires sophisticated techniques of analysis. Before turning to such an analysis, however, it is instructive to review briefly evidence on utilization rates and types of care received by persons of various income classes, once some adjustment is made for welfare eligibility and health status.

Welfare Status and Use of Medical Services

Although the poor as a whole have made marked gains in the use of medical services relative to higher-income groups, not all poor persons have received benefits from the Medicaid program. For those excluded from coverage, utilization of physician services lags well behind other poor persons and higher-income persons.

Data from the 1969 Health Interview Survey (HIS) of the National Center for Health Statistics permit some comparison of medical care utilization of poor persons receiving welfare and other poor persons. This categorization provides a rough indication of coverage under Medicaid, but several problems should be kept in mind. At the beginning of 1969, eleven states did not have Medicaid programs (although all but two states had programs in effect at the beginning of 1970), so that some persons, although eligible for public assistance, were not receiving medical assistance at that time. Furthermore, some states covered medically needy persons under Medicaid as well as public assistance recipients, so that some of the utilization of services by poor persons not on welfare may be influenced by the Medicaid program. Nevertheless, examining these two groups of poor persons provides some rough evidence of utilization of medical services by persons eligible for Medicaid relative to other poor persons.

As shown in Table 2, data from the 1969 HIS indicate that persons with incomes below $5,000 who were not on public assistance averaged 4.7 physician visits compared with 6.6 visits for those poor on welfare. The physician visit rate for poor persons not on welfare was actually less than that of persons with incomes above $15,000—even before adjusting for the greater health problems of the poor. Thus, the conclusion that the poor now use services more than do higher-income persons is at least partially misleading because it does not distinguish among those eligible for Medicaid and other poor persons.

Health Status and Use of Services by Income Classes

More important, however, is the fact that comparing use of medical services among income classes is misleading in any attempt to determine whether the poor now have equal access to medical care with higher-income persons inasmuch as such a comparison does not adjust for the more serious health problems of the poor.

TABLE 2 Physician Visits by Family Income, Public Assistance Status, and Age Group, 1969[a]

	All Persons		Under 17 Years		Age 17–44		Age 45–64		Age 65 and over	
	Unadjusted	Adjusted for Health Status	Unadjusted	Adjusted for Health Status	Unadjusted	Adjusted for Health Status	Unadjusted	Adjusted for Health Status	Unadjusted	Adjusted for Health Status
All family incomes	4.6	4.6	3.8	3.8	4.4	4.4	4.9	4.9	6.6	6.6
Under $5,000	4.9	3.7	3.0	3.0	4.8	4.2	5.8	4.0	6.5	6.1
Aid	6.6	4.5	3.7	3.5	8.9	5.9	11.2	5.2	9.0	6.4
No aid	4.7	3.6	2.8	3.0	4.5	4.1	5.4	3.9	6.3	6.1
$5,000–9,999	4.2	4.6	3.6	3.9	4.3	4.5	4.8	5.2	6.1	6.8
$10,000–14,999	4.4	4.9	4.2	4.2	4.4	4.6	4.5	5.1	6.8	7.5
$15,000 and over	4.8	5.2	4.6	4.5	4.4	4.8	4.7	5.5	9.6	10.4
Ratio, aid to no aid, income under $5,000	1.40	1.25	1.34	1.19	2.00	1.42	2.08	1.32	1.43	1.05
Ratio, income over $15,000 to no aid, income under $5,000	1.02	1.44	1.67	1.53	1.00	1.17	.87	1.40	1.52	1.72

SOURCE: Estimated from the 1969 Health Interview Survey, National Center for Health Statistics. See Appendix 2 for regressions.

[a] Excluding individuals reporting family income unknown, those under 17 for whom head of household education was unknown, and those 17 and older for whom individual education was unknown.

There are many dimensions of ill health and the "medical need" for care, ranging from discomfort, pain, and debilitating conditions to potentially fatal medical problems. Holding constant for health status in an examination of utilization patterns among income classes is difficult, both because data on these dimensions of health are limited and because the range and intensity of these conditions differ markedly so there is little consensus on which measures are most analytically appropriate.

A crude adjustment, however, can be made using data supplied in the 1969 HIS. The survey includes data on several dimensions of health status, including chronic conditions and limitation of activity that may be considered indicators of a "health stock" and number of days during the year in which activity is restricted, which reflects the incidence of more episodic illness. Obviously, even these measures of health status can vary markedly since two illnesses of the same duration may reflect quite different needs for medical care. Furthermore, some needs for medical care, such as maternity care, may be accompanied by very little restriction of activity. In spite of the limitations of these measures, however, they do permit us to gain some insight into the effect of substantial differences in need for services among income classes.

Table 2 indicates physician visit rates for persons of different income classes if they were to experience the average level of chronic conditions and restricted activity days of persons in their broad age group. These results were derived from ordinary least squares regressions reported in Appendix 2, Table 1.[6]

Adjustment for health status leads to a striking change in utilization patterns. Instead of following a U-shaped pattern with low-income persons using services more than middle-income persons, utilization increases uniformly with income. Poor persons eligible for welfare use physician services about the same as middle-income persons with comparable health problems, whereas those low-income persons not on public assistance lag substantially behind other poor and middle-income persons in use of services. Children in families with incomes above $15,000 visit physicians 53 per cent more frequently than poor children not on welfare, whereas high-income elderly persons see physicians more than 72 per cent more often than poor elderly persons not on welfare.

Quality and Convenience of Medical Care

Although the poor, particularly those on welfare, have made marked gains in use of medical services relative to other income groups, there is evidence that the poor do not obtain care in the same setting, from the same kind of physicians, and with the same ease and convenience as higher-income persons. Instead, the poor—whether on welfare or not—are much more likely to receive care from general practitioners than from specialists, in a hospital outpatient department rather than in a physician's office, and after traveling long distances and waiting substantially longer for care.

As shown in Table 3, the poor receive 70 per cent of their care from general practitioners, compared with 41 per cent for persons with family incomes over $15,000. Few poor children receive care from pediatricians. Higher-income women of child-bearing age are also twice as likely as are poor women to be cared for by specialists. The proportion of care received from specialists does not vary appreciably among the poor on welfare and other poor.

Some differences among income classes also exist in the place in which care is obtained. Persons with family incomes above $15,000 receive 87 per cent of their physician care in private settings (office, home, or telephone call to private physician) compared with only 80 per cent for those with family incomes below $5,000. The poor on welfare are even less likely to receive care in private settings— only 75 per cent.

It is hazardous to draw inferences about the quality and adequacy of care from these differences in the extent of specialist care and differences in the setting of treatment. It may well be, contrary to common belief, that specialist care for children and pregnant women is no more efficacious than care from a general practitioner;

TABLE 3 Percentage of Physician Visits to Selected Kinds of Physicians, by Income, 1969

	General Practitioner (all ages)	Pediatrician (under 17 years)	Obstetrician/ Gynecologist (women 17–44 years)
All persons	59	32	21
Under $5,000	70	18	13
Aid	73	21	6
No aid	70	17	14
$5,000–9,999	61	30	23
$10,000–14,999	51	40	24
$15,000 and over	41	39	23

SOURCE: Calculated from the 1969 Health Interview Survey, National Center for Health Statistics.

and care in a hospital outpatient department, incorporating the best of recent medical research, may be better than care from a private physician long since departed from medical school.

Nevertheless, it is fair to conclude that the poor do not receive the same kind of medical care received by most middle-income citizens. One manifestation of the pursuit of a desirable level of care and differences in the place in which care is obtained is the less convenient care received by low-income persons. The poor spend 50 per cent more time traveling and waiting to see a physician than do higher-income persons. Combined waiting and traveling time is also higher for the poor on welfare, a total of 81 minutes per visit compared with 66 minutes for other poor persons (and 43 minutes for those with family incomes above $15,000). In addition to the higher prices for medical care, the poor also face substantial burdens on the nonmonetary resources of their households in seeking medical care. Furthermore, although welfare recipients for the most part pay no monetary price under Medicaid for health services, they have assumed higher nonmonetary costs.

2. DISTRIBUTION OF MEDICAID BENEFITS

Although it is clear that the poor have made striking gains relative to higher-income groups in using medical services, it is also true that not all the poor have shared equally in these gains. Persons not receiving public assistance lag substantially behind Medicaid recipients in use of services. But even for those covered by Medicaid, program data suggest that benefits are very unevenly distributed. In this section we explore in greater detail the sources of variations in use of services among public assistance recipients and their experience relative to other low-income persons.

Medicaid is a federal-state program in which states have considerable leeway to determine eligibility for benefits, range of medical services covered, and limits on benefits for any given type of service. About half the states provide coverage for medically needy persons who, although not sufficiently poor to qualify for public assistance, are unable to meet the costs of medical bills.[7] Although all states are required to provide certain basic services such as hospital and physician care, some states also provide a wide range of supplementary services such as drugs, dental, and clinic services.

These optional features of the Medicaid program give rise to substantial interstate variation in benefits. In 1970 payments per child recipient, for example, ranged from $43 in Mississippi to $240 in Wisconsin.[8] Furthermore, most states in the Deep South cover only about one-tenth of poor children, whereas in the Northeast nearly all poor, and many near-poor, children receive services. Similar variations in benefits characterize the adult Medicaid categories.

Medicaid benefits not only are unevenly distributed by state, but whites and urban residents receive a disproportionately large share of them. Payments per white recipient are 75 per cent higher than payments per black recipient.[9] Rural residents get few benefits from the program. For example, poor children in rural areas have only 11 per cent of their medical expenditures met by Medicaid, compared with 75 per cent for poor children in central cities.[10]

These sources of variation in benefits may interact and reinforce one another. For example, benefits in the South may be low because of the high incidence of black or rural poor persons who receive little or no benefits because of family composition or discriminatory administration of the program. Similarly, the low proportion of benefits going to these groups may, in part, be a reflection of their greater concentration in states choosing to maintain only limited Medicaid programs.

Furthermore, some of the variation in benefits may be attributable to factors associated with location or race such as education, health status, or availability of medical resources. To better understand the independent influence of each of these factors, econometric techniques are used below to estimate the utilization of hospital and physician services by public assistance recipients.

Factors Determining Utilization of Medicaid Services

Recipients of Medicaid benefits make no direct payment for services, and physicians are required to accept state-established reimbursement levels as payment in full for services. Therefore, there is no price mechanism by which quantity of services demanded is necessarily equated with quantity of services that providers are willing to supply.

Actual utilization of services, therefore, is the outcome of a rationing process that may be affected by desires of physicians regarding the patients they prefer to treat, willingness of patients to provide the time and effort required to obtain services, and procedures established by states administering the program that may affect both the total quantity of services available and the distribution of those services among recipients. In addition, use of services may be related to alternatives available to recipients and providers. For example, poor persons in areas with charity hospital facilities, but with few physicians willing to participate in the program, may substitute hospital care for care from private physicians. Willingness of physicians to participate, on the other hand, may be influenced by numbers of physicians in the area, demand for their services by non-poor patients, and level of Medicaid reimbursement (which varies from state to state).

A complete model of utilization under Medicaid, therefore, would include (1) patient characteristics, including health status, age, sex, race, education, family size, and working status; (2) measures of physician preferences among patients, which might include many of the same patient characteristics as above; (3) availability of medical resources both to the entire population and to the poor covered by Medicaid; and (4) features of the program controlled by the states.

This model of the utilization of medical services under Medicaid was estimated with data on 3,163 public assistance recipients in the 1969 HIS.[11] The survey provides much of the detail on individual characteristics that is required for this analysis. The health status variables used were chronic conditions and restricted activity days. Rather than single variables indicating age and head of household education, dummy variables were used for several age and education groups to capture nonlinearities in these effects. In addition, another dummy variable was entered for females age 17 to 44 to reflect the greater utilization of prenatal and maternal care by this group. Cross-product terms of race and region were specified to more accurately indicate where racial inequalities may occur.[12]

Geographical identification of individuals interviewed in the survey is limited. Using what information was provided on the location of individuals, measures of the availability of physicians and short-term general hospital beds per 1,000 population were included as follows: for persons living in the twenty-two largest SMSA's, figures for these particular areas were used; for other persons, figures for the census region broken down by SMSA and non-SMSA residence were inserted.[13]

Variation attributable to state program features is reduced by restricting the sample to public assistance recipients, excluding medically needy persons covered by Medicaid in some states. In addition, the analysis focuses on hospital and physician services, two basic services required by law and for which states may be expected to less frequently impose stringent restrictions on benefits.

A possible source of bias that may continue to exist in the results relates to the absence of Medicaid programs in eleven states at the beginning of the year of the survey. Since seven of these states were in the South, an attempt was made to alleviate this problem by introducing a dummy variable for residence in the South. This effort, however, proved to have no significant impact on the results and is not included in the results reported.

For comparison purposes, similar estimates of utilization are presented for low-income persons (family income below $5,000) not receiving public assistance.[14] This is a heterogeneous group, including some medically needy Medicaid recipients, some working poor with private health insurance, and some poor without either public or private coverage. Although the incidence of Medicare and private insurance coverage in this group might be expected to have a substantial impact on the utilization of services by this group, such information was not available in the survey. Part of the role played by insurance coverage may, however, be reflected in the variable that reflects working status.

For each dependent variable—physician visits in the two weeks prior to the interview and hospital episodes and days for the preceding year—a large number of values are concentrated at zero. Since the classical least squares regression model is inappropriate in such cases, the Tobit estimation technique was used for this analysis.[15]

Econometric Results for the Poor

The results of the Tobit estimation of physician and hospital utilization for public assistance recipients and other low-income persons are presented in Table 4. Chi-squares show that the characteristics included in the estimates contribute significantly to the explanation of the utilization of health services in all cases.

As shown in Table 4, both health status variables—restricted activity days and chronic conditions—are highly significant in explaining utilization by public assistance recipients and other low-income persons. The impact of health status is illustrated more clearly in Table 5, which gives the expected values for physician visits, hospital episodes, and hospital days for varying hypothetical levels of health status, with other independent variables held

TABLE 4 Tobit Results—Public Assistance Recipients and Other Low-Income Persons, 1969[a]

	Public Assistance Recipients			Other Low-Income Persons		
	Physician Visits	Hospital Episodes	Hospital Days	Physician Visits	Hospital Episodes	Hospital Days
Constant	−1.898	−2.842	−65.37	−3.362	−3.288	−54.52
	(7.04)	(4.44)	(5.14)	(28.36)	(15.91)	(17.49)
Restricted activity	0.135	0.137	2.63	0.198	0.130	1.99
days	(9.99)	(8.87)	(8.71)	(32.31)	(22.53)	(23.32)
Chronic conditions	0.316	0.196	3.21	0.341	0.252	3.93
	(7.82)	(4.23)	(3.53)	(19.21)	(15.28)	(15.97)
Age 17–44	−0.363	−0.157	1.81	−0.164	0.242	4.67
	(1.32)	(0.51)	(0.30)	(1.62)	(2.57)	(3.28)
Age 45–64	−0.172	0.065	3.71	−0.181	0.391	6.47
	(0.87)	(0.28)	(0.81)	(2.19)	(5.09)	(5.59)
Age 65 and over	−0.424	0.121	5.92	−0.144	0.578	9.36
	(2.15)	(0.53)	(1.31)	(1.75)	(7.57)	(8.14)
Female	−0.003	−0.380	−7.81	0.149	−0.199	−3.47
	(0.02)	(2.52)	(2.62)	(2.60)	(3.73)	(4.34)
Female, age 17–44	0.952	1.960	29.33	0.519	1.241	15.30
	(3.19)	(5.83)	(4.49)	(4.88)	(12.83)	(10.49)
Head of household	−0.091	0.205	4.91	0.129	0.181	2.35
education, 9–12 yrs.	(0.76)	(1.51)	(1.83)	(2.45)	(3.77)	(3.25)
Head of household	0.565	0.001	−1.88	0.097	−0.053	−0.93
education, > 12 yrs.	(1.94)	(<0.01)	(0.26)	(1.17)	(0.69)	(0.79)
Family size	−0.136	−0.105	−2.37	−0.078	0.006	0.01
	(4.28)	(2.88)	(3.26)	(5.06)	(0.42)	(0.05)
Working	0.060	−0.099	−0.57	−0.019	−0.323	−5.32
	(0.26)	(0.38)	(0.11)	(0.32)	(5.77)	(6.29)
Black–South	−0.242	−0.740	−10.50	−0.449	−0.510	−6.44
	(1.61)	(3.77)	(2.71)	(5.60)	(6.71)	(5.60)
Black–outside South	−0.336	−0.173	−1.33	−0.050	−0.086	−1.37
	(2.30)	(1.04)	(0.41)	(0.54)	(0.96)	(1.02)
Physicians	0.108	−0.187	−2.04	0.261	−0.066	0.24
	(1.01)	(1.47)	(0.82)	(5.39)	(1.44)	(0.36)
Hospital beds	—	0.164	4.42	—	0.023	1.12
		(1.11)	(1.52)		(0.52)	(1.64)
Chi-square	391	331	294	2274	1730	1734

NOTE: t statistics in parentheses.
[a] Persons with family income under $5,000.

TABLE 5 Annual Predicted Utilization for Low-Income Persons by Health Status and Welfare Eligibility, Adjusted for Other Characteristics, 1969

| | Health Status[a] | | | | | |
| | Public Assistance Recipients | | | Other Low-Income Persons | | |
	Good	Average	Poor	Good	Average	Poor
Physician visits	4.09	4.95	7.10	2.69	3.36	5.12
Hospital admissions	.141	.162	.210	.090	.108	.151
Hospital days	2.40	2.72	3.47	1.18	1.42	2.04

[a] Average health status is defined as at the mean level of restricted activity days and chronic conditions for all low-income persons. Good health status is that at half the means. Poor health status is that at twice the means.

constant at their mean values for the whole low-income population. In every case public assistance recipients make more use of services than other low-income persons. For example, a poor person who is average with respect to health status would receive 52 per cent more physician visits and undergo nearly twice as many days of hospital care as a similar poor person not on welfare. Thus, by reducing the price of care to zero, Medicaid has had a substantial impact on utilization of those poor who are eligible for Medicaid benefits.

Although poor persons with more severe health problems make much wider use of medical services, public assistance recipients are somewhat less sensitive to health status as a determinant of utilization than other poor persons. This occurs largely because of the high levels of utilization among Medicaid recipients in relatively good health. For example, as health status deteriorates from "good" to "poor," physician visits by public assistance recipients increase by 74 per cent compared with 90 per cent for other low-income persons.

Similarly, public assistance recipients show little sensitivity to age as a determinant of either inpatient or outpatient care, after adjustment for health status. Only among the elderly, who receive significantly less ambulatory care than other public assistance recipients, does age have a significant impact. On the other hand, substantial differences occur by age for other poor persons. Children receive more ambulatory care than adults age 45 to 64 and hospitalization increases uniformly with age, even with adjustment for health status.

The dummy for women of ages 17 to 44 proves a good proxy for the special health care needs of females of child-bearing age for both groups. In this area the contrast in the amount of care received by Medicaid recipients and other poor women is especially sharp. The expected number of physician visits by females from 17 to 44 years old, for instance, is 8.8 and 4.7 per year for members of each group, respectively, when other variables are held constant at their mean values. As shown earlier, although women in this age group eligible for Medicaid have made substantial gains in the amount of care received, these gains are not equally reflected in the proportion of care received from specialists. Nonetheless, it can be assessed that maternity care has been one area in which Medicaid has been especially successful in meeting an important deficiency in the health care of the poor.

Females in other age groups have not shared equally under Medicaid. This suggests that the time constraints of women on public assistance may be more binding because their services are more needed in the home. The effect of the constraint of nonmonetary resources in welfare households is also evident in the results for the family-size variable. Family size proves a significantly stronger constraint on the use of health services for Medicaid recipients than for other low-income persons. The interpretation of the last two variables is supported by evidence earlier cited on the higher traveling and waiting time spent by public assistance recipients.

The effect of constraints on household resources is also evident in the results for the variable indicating normal working status. Individuals not on public assistance who are regularly employed received significantly less care in hospitals than other poor persons. Among public assistance recipients, the working-status variable has no discernible effect largely because such a small proportion of the welfare population is in the labor force.

Interpretation of the results for head of household education must be tentative, although they do tend to show that persons in households in which the head has more education recognize the benefits of more health care, but also organize to receive care on a more efficient basis. For public assistance recipients, differences based on head of household education are apparent for those with education between nine and twelve years for hospitalization and those with better than a high school training for ambulatory care. Although prices do not serve as an incentive for such persons to be more efficient in obtaining care, as was also reflected in the relatively strong influence of family size, nonmonetary constraints play a significant role in determining utilization in such households. In other low-income households, education of the head seems to contribute to utilization if it is limited to some high school level training. That the level of utilization should not differ between those in households where the head has more than and less than a high school education may reflect distortion created by the households in which the head is highly educated but is deferring medical attention with the expectation that the household's income will improve.

None of the availability variables substantially affect the utilization of health services, with the exception of ambulatory care received by non-welfare poor persons. In part, this may reflect the inappropriate measure of these variables, since the poor may be restricted to a subset of all providers such as county hospitals or those physicians practicing in low-income neighborhoods. There are also two economic forces that may contribute to this result. First, since Medicaid patients do not pay for the care, providers, especially with regard to ambulatory care, lack the ability to affect the utilization patterns of these persons by ordinary economic means. Second, hospitals may be quite arbitrary in their hospitalization of poor persons in seeking to fulfill their occupancy goals and charity obligations. Such behavior is plausible since low-income persons receive a large amount of ambulatory care at hospital outpatient departments, thus affording hospitals wide leverage over whether to admit these patients for inpatient treatment if there is a slack in occupancy levels.

Separate estimates of utilization were obtained omitting the availability measures and including dummy variables for nonmetropolitan residence in the South and outside the South. Ambulatory care was lower in the rural South, but rural poor outside the South did not use ambulatory services significantly differently from urban poor (see Appendix 3, Table 1). However, the rural South variable was not significant when the availability measures were also included (see Appendix 3, Table 2), perhaps because of the collinearity inherent in the construction of the availability measures.

The race variables reveal that the benefits of Medicaid have not been shared equally by blacks and whites even after individual and family characteristics have been taken into account. Black Medicaid recipients in all areas receive less ambulatory care, and black hospitalization rates are also lower in the South.[16] As shown in Table 6, blacks do receive more care with Medicaid than they would without it; the improvement in ambulatory care is greatest in the South and in hospital care outside the South. Medicaid also

TABLE 6 Annual Predicted Utilization for Low-Income Persons, by Welfare Eligibility, Region, and Race, Adjusted for Other Characteristics

	Public Assistance Recipients			Other Low-Income Persons		
	Physician Visits	Hospital Episodes	Hospital Days	Physician Visits	Hospital Episodes	Hospital Days
White	5.28	0.176	2.87	3.51	0.114	1.50
Black— South	4.23	0.089	1.73	2.33	0.067	0.95
Black— outside South	3.88	0.151	2.70	3.36	0.105	1.37

markedly increases utilization by whites. Outside the South, differences between the races are in fact greater for Medicaid recipients than for other low-income persons. Outside the South there is no significant difference in the number of physician visits between blacks and whites not on public assistance, whereas among welfare recipients physician visits among whites are 24 per cent higher than among blacks, holding other variables constant at the mean values for all low-income persons. White welfare recipients are admitted to hospitals nearly twice as often as black welfare recipients of similar characteristics in the South, while among non-welfare recipients admissions for whites are 70 per cent greater than for blacks.

Although it is not possible on the basis of this analysis to determine definitely what accounts for the racial differences, some explanations can be ruled out. For example, since education, family size, working status, and availability of medical resources are held constant, racial differences cannot be traced to these factors. The most plausible explanation for the difference is discrimination. Discrimination can be either overt or institutional.[17] Overt discriminatory practices are apparently still prevalent in some communities. For example, in one Alabama town, the four white physicians all maintain segregated waiting rooms, keep black patients waiting until all white patients have been seen, and then allocate the remainder of the working day to the care of black patients. Those patients for whom time does not permit treatment are requested to return the following day. Waiting times for black patients average between four and six hours.[18] Such discriminatory practices obviously limit utilization by blacks.

Frequently, however, discrimination is institutionalized, arising from segregated housing patterns, or past overt discriminatory practices that affect current patterns of physician location, hospital staffing patterns, referral patterns, and patient preferences. Hearings on Civil Rights Act enforcement in Medicare and Medicaid recently held by the House Judiciary Committee indicate that institutional discrimination is widespread. Among the causes cited are convenience of some institutions to black communities, familiarity with some institutions from past associations, absence of a private physician causing patients to turn to charity hospitals, short supply of physicians in minority neighborhoods, and patients not informed or aware that Medicaid benefits are available in private hospitals. Some practices, such as ambulance drivers taking black accident victims to charity hospitals and expansion of hospital staffs restricted to specialists (whereas black physicians tend to be general practitioners), may be either overt or "statistical" discrimination depending on whether the rules governing these decisions are devised for the purpose of excluding blacks from some facilities or simply work out on average to exclude blacks.[19]

In summary, substantial differences exist in the manner in which health services are allocated among persons eligible for Medicaid and other low-income persons. Health status, however, is the major determinant of utilization for both groups, although public assistance recipients' use of services is somewhat less sensitive to health status than that of other low-income persons. The poor not receiving public assistance receive substantially fewer services than those on welfare, even after adjustment for health status is made. Differences by age in utilization that are evident for the poor not on welfare are not apparent for those receiving public assistance. There is evidence that nonmonetary effects have substituted for monetary allocation of services among Medicaid recipients. As a result blacks, females other than those of child-bearing age, and those in large families have not equally shared the gains made under Medicaid.

3. DISTRIBUTION OF MEDICARE BENEFITS

Unlike Medicaid, Medicare is a uniform, federal program providing medical care benefits to all elderly persons covered by the social security retirement program. Although the same set of benefits is available to all covered persons regardless of income, race, or geographical location, wide differences also exist in the Medicare program in the use of services and receipt of payments on the basis of each of these factors. It was originally hoped that the removal of financial barriers to medical care would enable all elderly persons to receive medical care services largely on the basis of medical need. Yet, those elderly population groups in the poorest health are the lowest utilizers of medical care services under the program— the poor, blacks, rural residents, and residents of the South.

Data from the Medicare program indicate that in 1968 estimated potential reimbursement for supplemental medical insurance services per person enrolled was twice as high for elderly persons with incomes above $15,000 as for persons with incomes below $5,000. About half of this difference reflects differences in quantity of services, whereas the other half represents a higher payment level for services (which in turn may be accounted for by a more expensive mix of services, better care, or pure price differences). Whites receive 60 per cent more payments for physician services than elderly blacks, and more than double the payments per elderly black person enrolled in the South, with nearly all the difference representing differences in percentage of eligible persons receiving reimbursable services.[20] Elderly persons in nonmetropolitan counties average $250 from Medicare annually compared with $360 for the elderly in metropolitan counties with a central city.[21] Regional differences are also substantial. Physician benefits in the West were 40 per cent higher than in the South in 1968. About three-quarters of the variation in these benefits on the basis of location reflects differences in quantity of services received.[22]

Part of these large differences may be attributable to factors associated with income, race, and location—factors such as education, health status, and availability of medical resources. Again, to investigate the role played by each of these several factors, an econometric analysis of utilization of medical services by the elderly was made using the 1969 HIS.

Unlike the Medicaid program, Medicare beneficiaries pay a substantial portion of the cost of physician services. The elderly are required to pay the first $60 of physician expenses during the year ($50 in 1969), 20 per cent of all allowed charges in excess of the deductible, and any excess of the actual charge for a service over that determined by Medicare as reasonable. In 1972, on about 56 per cent of Medicare claims, physicians agreed to charge no more than Medicare allows; on the rest, they were not so restrained.[23] The price mechanism, therefore, may play a stronger role in allocating services to Medicare beneficiaries.

Two groups of elderly, however, are not subject to the deductible and coinsurance amounts: those elderly Medicaid recipients whose states "buy" them Medicare coverage and those elderly purchasing supplementary private health insurance. Unfortunately, the 1969 Health Interview Survey, although noting eligibility for public assistance, does not indicate which elderly persons have private insurance as well as Medicare. Since higher-income elderly persons are more likely to purchase supplementary private insurance, including income in an examination of utilization of medical services by the elderly will capture both the direct effect of income and possible lower net prices faced by higher-income persons who purchase insurance. The dummy variable for public assistance recipients should capture the effect of zero price for those elderly covered by Medicaid and Medicare.

Health status is measured, as in the Medicaid model, by restricted activity days and chronic conditions, as well as a dummy variable indicating some limitation of activity attributable to chronic conditions. Several additional proxies for health status are age, sex, and working status. The dummy variable for elderly persons who consider working as their usual activity may also reflect a greater time constraint for working persons. Since Medicare program data indicate that blacks in the South receive fewer benefits than blacks in other areas, and still less than whites, separate race dummies for the South and areas outside the South were included in the analysis. Because of the limited education of the elderly, education was captured by a dummy variable for all persons with nine or more years of education rather than more refined educational classes.

Availability of medical resources, measured by physicians per 1,000 persons and short-term general care hospital beds per 1,000 population, was also introduced into the model. The appropriateness of including both supply and demand variables in a market in which price plays a major role has been addressed in other studies. With respect to physician services, Feldstein (1970) theorizes that the physician sets both price and supply such that excess demand exists for his services, whereas the consumer is simply a price-taker.[24] Fuchs and Kramer (1972) suggest alternatively that demand is supply-induced. An increase in physicians per capita is likely to reduce travel and time costs to the patients. In addition, they argue, physicians may inflate demand when supply has some slack by using their discretionary power to recommend to a patient his need for more care.[25] Again, with respect to hospital utilization, several possible arguments are the existence of excess demand, the physician-agent relationship, and the incompleteness of that relationship because of peer group pressure on the physician.[26]

Data used in the analysis are also from the 1969 Health Interview Survey of the National Center for Health Statistics. In 1969, the survey included 11,970 persons age 65 and over. Observations were excluded from this analysis for persons for whom either family income or education was unknown or not reported, reducing the sample size to 10,573. Like in the Medicaid estimates, Tobit regression analysis is employed.

Econometric Results for the Elderly

Tobit regression results are given in Table 7 for physician visits, hospital days, and hospital episodes. Chi-square tests indicate the equations to be statistically significant.

All indicators of morbidity contribute positively to utilization and are highly significant. Age, however, has a negative coefficient in the physician visit equation and positive coefficients in the hospital equations. Measures of morbidity apparently control for health status sufficiently to permit the age variable to act predominantly as a measure of the physical accessibility of services to the elderly. Thus, the very old are less likely to seek ambulatory care but compensate somewhat by utilizing more institutional care.

Computed annualized values of physician visits are shown in Table 8 for different incomes and health status levels, holding other independent variables constant at their mean values. The striking observation is that health status does play the predominant role in determining the number of physician visits a person will make. Morbidity measures of twice the mean levels typically cause slightly less than twice as many visits as average morbidity characteristics. This relationship is stable for all income classes. Physician visits vary more among income classes for persons in better health, but no one in good health, for example, will ordinarily receive more physician services than an elderly person whose health is only average.

When adjustment is made for health status, physician visits increase uniformly with income. As shown in Table 8, persons in average health and with incomes above $15,000 made 70 per cent more physician visits than low-income persons in similar health and not receiving public assistance. The increase in utilization for higher-income persons may occur either because the cost-sharing provisions of Medicare are less of a deterrent to use as income rises

TABLE 7 Tobit Results, Persons Age 65 and Over, 1969

	Physician Visits	Hospital Episodes	Hospital Days
Constant	−1.954	−3.282	−67.34
	(4.85)	(7.42)	(8.53)
Chronic conditions	0.314	0.151	2.23
	(13.91)	(6.90)	(5.71)
Limited in activity	0.302	0.602	11.98
	(3.93)	(8.15)	(9.10)
Age	−0.018	0.008	0.15
	(3.40)	(1.55)	(1.76)
Restricted activity days	0.120	0.115	2.02
	(16.83)	(17.24)	(17.11)
Income $5,000–10,000	0.148	0.253	3.71
	(1.77)	(3.20)	(2.63)
Income $10,000–15,000	0.301	0.398	4.14
	(2.25)	(3.13)	(1.81)
Income $15,000 +	0.720	0.493	7.98
	(5.01)	(3.46)	(3.15)
Public assistance recipient	0.356	−0.056	−1.10
	(2.60)	(0.41)	(0.45)
Family size	−0.066	0.015	0.43
	(2.14)	(0.54)	(0.86)
Female	0.143	−0.062	−1.25
	(2.16)	(0.99)	(1.12)
Individual education, 9 years and over	0.179	−0.021	−0.05
	(2.66)	(0.33)	(0.04)
Working	−0.066	−0.306	−6.08
	(0.68)	(3.13)	(3.45)
Black—South	−0.559	−0.664	−9.85
	(3.40)	(4.16)	(3.47)
Black—outside South	−0.115	−0.050	1.78
	(0.62)	(0.28)	(0.58)
Physicians	0.187	−0.297	−3.35
	(2.80)	(4.49)	(2.86)
Hospital beds	—	0.072	2.29
		(1.20)	(2.12)
Chi-square	899	811	786

NOTE: *t* statistics in parentheses.

TABLE 8 Average Physician Visits for the Elderly, by Health Status and Family Income, Adjusted for Other Determinants

Family Income	Health Status[a]		
	Good	Average	Poor
Under $5,000			
No aid	2.78	5.64	10.47
Aid	3.86	7.52	13.42
$ 5,000–9,999	3.14	6.60	11.70
$10,000 14,999	3.75	7.27	12.98
$15,000 and over	5.35	9.53	16.98

SOURCE: Calculated from Table 7 and tabulations from the 1969 HIS.
[a] Good health is defined as no chronic conditions, limitation of activity, or restricted activity days. Average and poor health are defined at the mean and twice the mean level of the three morbidity indicators used.

or because higher-income persons are more likely to purchase supplementary private insurance and hence face a lower net price.

The significance of the public assistance recipients variable suggests that reduction in net price has a positive impact on use of services. Persons on public assistance, and hence likely to have cost-sharing amounts paid by state Medicaid plans, receive 30 to 40 per cent more services than other low-income persons not receiving public assistance, holding constant for other determinants of utilization such as health status, age, sex, race, and education.

Utilization of hospital services also increases with income; however, the difference in average hospital days between the highest- and lowest-income groups is only 40 per cent as compared with a 70 per cent spread for outpatient visits (see Table 9). The lower income elasticity for hospital care may reflect the greater medical urgency of institutional care so that even lower-income persons will, for the most part, pay the hospital deductible (of $44 in 1969).

Public assistance recipients do not differ significantly in hospitalization from other elderly persons with incomes under $5,000, which is plausible for two reasons. There are no extra benefits for public assistance recipients under the hospital plan similar to the elimination of deductible and coinsurance amounts under the physician plan. In addition, the elderly on welfare are more likely to substitute physician visits for hospitalization, and thus they have less need to enter the hospital than poor persons not on welfare.

Racial differences in the South are substantial. Although their average health status is worse than for the population as a whole,[27]

TABLE 9 Average Hospital Utilization for the Elderly, by Health Status and Family Income, Adjusted for Other Determinants

Family Income	Health Status[a]		
	Good	Average	Poor
	Hospital Episodes		
Under $5,000	.114	.210	.362
$ 5,000–9,999	.140	.250	.427
$10,000–14,999	.159	.285	.472
$15,000 and over	.177	.312	.512
	Hospital Days		
Under $5,000	2.31	4.21	7.21
$ 5,000–9,999	2.78	4.93	8.16
$10,000–14,999	2.85	5.02	8.29
$15,000 and over	3.52	6.06	9.77

[a] See Table 8 for definitions of health status levels.

elderly Southern blacks receive fewer ambulatory services than any income group. Elderly blacks in average health in the South make half as many physician visits (2.91 visits per person) as other persons age 65 and over if their income is under $5,000, and they receive no public assistance and make two-thirds as many visits (6.67 visits per person) as others if they are in the highest-income class. By contrast, differences in use of physicians by race are not evident outside the South. Medicare has made no attempt to insist that physicians not discriminate among patients on the basis of race, arguing that Medicare merely reimburses patients for services received and does not enter into contractual agreements with physicians.

Racial differences in hospital care also exist in the South, although Medicare has attempted to enforce nondiscriminatory practices in hospitals.[28] Elderly blacks in the South in average health spend 2.84 days in the hospital whereas other elderly persons average 4.60 days. This suggests that discrimination in hospitals may be as extensive as that shown by individual physicians in the South, although physicians are not required to assert compliance with provisions of the Civil Rights Act. In regions outside the South, blacks are not hospitalized significantly less than whites.

The availability of more physicians causes elderly persons to visit physicians more often for reasons cited earlier. Table 10 shows, however, that the elasticity of supply is generally lower in those areas where the number of physicians per capita is the lowest (for average characteristics in those areas). An implication of this result is that there is perhaps a surfeit of physicians in the Northeast and urban parts of the West, since a large proportion of small changes in physician manpower in those areas may be absorbed by those covered by Medicare.

The elasticity of hospital episodes with respect to the availability of hospital beds is 0.47, whereas the elasticity estimated from the hospital day equation is 0.94. The hospital day elasticity does not vary much by region, ranging from a low of 0.88 in the West to a high of 1.01 in North Central states and is similar to the elasticity of 0.92 found by Feldstein for the whole population.[29]

The local supply of physicians contributes negatively to admissions, indicating that physicians are inclined to hospitalize only more severe cases among the elderly. Overall, the elasticity of hospital days with respect to physicians is −0.20, confirming Feldstein's suggestion that "better organization of physicians' services for Medicare patients could generally reduce costly hospital admission."[30]

Separate estimates of utilization omitting the availability measures reveals that elderly persons in nonmetropolitan areas of the South make significantly fewer physician visits than the urban elderly, but rural elderly both in the South and outside the South experience somewhat more hospital episodes than the urban elderly (see Appendix 3, Table 3). Including both the availability measures and the geographical variables, however, eliminates the significance of the geographical variables (see Appendix 3, Table 4).

TABLE 10 Elasticities of Physician Utilization with Respect to Physicians per Capita for the Elderly, by Region and Residence for Characteristics in those Areas

	All Regions	Northeast	North Central	South	West
All residences	.80	1.00	.74	.61	.93
Urban	.81	1.02	.77	.62	.94
Rural	.54	.88	.57	.47	.57

SOURCE: Calculated with data from Table 7, tabulations from the 1969 HIS, Haug, Robark, and Martin, and *Distribution of Physicians in the United States, 1970* (Chicago American Medical Association, 1971).

Persons with more than eight years of education received significantly more ambulatory physician services, as did females. Education, although important in explaining physician visits, does not eliminate the significance of income as a major determinant of physician utilization. Neither education nor sex were significant in the hospital equations.

Elderly persons who still regularly work to earn an income are hospitalized less often and for shorter periods. The net effect of the financial constraint posed by losing time from being on the job is 38 per cent fewer hospital days than nonworking persons, holding other factors at their expected values. Working did not have an important effect on ambulatory care.

In summary, once adjustment is made for health status and other determinants, use of medical services increases uniformly with income. Elimination of cost-sharing requirements under the physician plan for Medicaid recipients, however, brings their utilization up to that of the middle-income elderly. The results suggest that discrimination against blacks in the South by physicians and hospitals may be substantial—racial differences cannot be attributed solely to differences in income or education. Use of both physician and hospital services by the elderly is sensitive to the availability of medical services.

4. IMPLICATIONS FOR NATIONAL HEALTH INSURANCE

An analysis of experience with utilization of medical services under Medicare and Medicaid yields three major implications in the current consideration of national health insurance. First, financing medical care can have, and has had, a major impact on helping covered persons receive needed medical care services. The major failure—at least of Medicaid—is not in what it tried to do, but in what was not attempted—namely, widespread coverage of all poor persons regardless of welfare status. As a consequence, those poor persons excluded from Medicaid—estimated at 9 million persons in 1974—have failed to achieve adequate and equitable access to medical services. Extension of medical care financing to these persons, either through reform of Medicaid or national health insurance, should be a top priority.

Second, experience with Medicare reveals that imposition of uniform cost-sharing provisions (deductible and coinsurance amounts) results in wide disparities in use of medical services on the basis of income. However, eliminating these payments for Medicaid recipients enabled them to receive similar amounts of services as middle-income elderly persons. This suggests that eliminating or reducing cost-sharing provisions for all lower-income persons while retaining some cost-sharing for higher-income persons could help to achieve greater equality in access to care.

Third, both Medicare and Medicaid confirm that certain groups of persons, even if covered by medical care financing plans, lag behind in access to care. This is a serious problem for minorities, who appear to continue to face substantial discrimination in the medical care market. Rural residents and persons in the South also face barriers to utilization of services, largely as a result of a limited supply of medical manpower. Supplementary health care delivery programs designed to meet the special needs of these population groups must be an essential part of health care policy. Further research to determine the most effective approaches to improving the access to care of these groups is urgently needed.

APPENDIX 1

Definitions of Independent Variables

Chronic conditions: number of conditions (any departures from state of physical or mental well-being) occurring more than three months prior to interview or classified as chronic regardless of onset.[a]

Limited in activity: 1 if chronic conditions limit the amount or kind of major or minor activity normally performed; 0 otherwise.

Age: age in years at last birthday.

Restricted activity days: number of days in two weeks prior to the interview a person reduces amount or kind of normal activity because of a specific illness or injury.

Income $5,000–9,999: 1 if family income is greater than or equal to $5,000 and less than $9,999; 0 otherwise.

Income $10,000–14,999: 1 if family income is greater than or equal to $10,000 and less than $14,999; 0 otherwise.

Income $15,000 +: 1 if family income is greater than or equal to $15,000; 0 otherwise.

---

[a]See DHEW, "Current Estimates—1969," p. 41.

Family size:　number of related household members; coded 8 if family has more than 8 members.

Public assistance:　1 if person is recipient of public assistance other than social security or pensions at time of interview and family income is less than $5,000; 0 otherwise.

Black—South:　1 if black living in the South; 0 otherwise.

Black—outside South:　1 if black living outside the South; 0 otherwise.

MDPC:　nonfederal patient care physicians per 1,000 population (see Section 1 for source and description of construction of this variable).

BedPC:　number of nonfederal short-term general and other special hospital beds per 1,000 population (see Section 1 for source and description of construction of this variable).

Education 9+ years:　1 if education of individual is greater than 8 years; 0 otherwise.

Work:　1 if major activity in twelve months prior to interview was working to earn a living or working as paid for a family business or farm; 0 otherwise.

Female:　1 if female; 0 if male.

Source (unless otherwise noted above): U.S. Department of Health, Education and Welfare, National Center for Health Statistics, "Current Estimates from the Health Interview Survey–1969," *Vital and Health Statistics* Series 10, Number 63 (Washington, D.C.: U.S. Government Printing Office, 1971).

APPENDIX 2

TABLE 1　Ordinary Least Squares Estimates of Physician Visits, by Age Group, 1969[a]

Physician Visits	All Persons	Under 17	17–44	45–64	65 and over
Constant	1.50	1.02	1.92	0.88	2.27
	(16.52)	(7.07)	(11.91)	(4.00)	(8.13)
Income $5,000–9,999	1.01	0.93	0.32	1.22	0.73
	(9.64)	(5.60)	(1.76)	(4.97)	(1.82)
Income $10,000–14,999	1.28	1.26	0.48	1.21	1.46
	(10.90)	(6.97)	(2.37)	(4.43)	(2.20)
Income $15,000+	1.60	1.58	0.72	1.56	4.36
	(11.78)	(7.44)	(3.08)	(5.34)	(5.94)

TABLE 1   (concluded)

Physician Visits	All Persons	Under 17	17–44	45–64	65 and over
Aid	0.92	0.57	1.76	1.24	0.31
	(3.60)	(1.78)	(3.18)	(1.60)	(0.40)
Restricted activity days	0.08	0.14	0.10	0.06	0.04
	(110.56)	(93.39)	(72.26)	(46.88)	(21.72)
Chronic conditions	1.62	2.86	2.02	1.84	1.56
	(41.46)	(23.47)	(26.36)	(24.49)	(14.17)
$\bar{R}^2$	.12	.19	.14	.13	.08

NOTE: t statistics in parentheses.
[a] Excluding individuals reporting family income unknown, those under 17 for whom head of household education was unknown, and those 17 and older for whom individual education was unknown.

APPENDIX 3

TABLE 1   Tobit Results—Public Assistance Recipients and Other Low-Income Persons, 1969[a]

	Public Assistance Recipients			Other Low-Income Persons		
	Physician Visits	Hospital Episodes	Hospital Days	Physician Visits	Hospital Episodes	Hospital Days
Constant	−1.718	−2.507	−51.29	−2.950	−3.264	−49.05
	(8.03)	(10.25)	(10.57)	(27.89)	(33.31)	(33.20)
Restricted activity days	0.134	0.136	2.60	0.198	0.129	1.99
	(9.95)	(8.81)	(8.63)	(32.32)	(22.50)	(23.29)
Chronic conditions	0.318	0.205	3.32	0.342	0.252	3.93
	(7.88)	(4.44)	(3.66)	(19.20)	(15.29)	(15.96)
Age 17–44	−0.357	−0.162	1.63	−0.160	0.242	4.66
	(1.30)	(0.53)	(0.27)	(1.58)	(2.56)	(3.28)
Age 45–64	−0.172	−0.073	3.65	−0.183	0.395	6.51
	(0.87)	(0.32)	(0.80)	(2.21)	(5.13)	(5.62)
Age 65 and over	−0.410	−0.200	6.85	−0.147	0.580	9.44
	(2.08)	(0.87)	(1.52)	(1.77)	(7.59)	(8.21)
Female	−0.007	−0.393	−8.06	0.150	−0.200	−3.48
	(0.06)	(2.62)	(2.69)	(2.63)	(3.74)	(4.34)
Female, 17–44	0.956	1.961	29.55	0.514	1.241	15.27
	(3.20)	(5.86)	(4.53)	(4.83)	(12.83)	(10.48)

TABLE 1 (concluded)

	Public Assistance Recipients			Other Low-Income Persons		
	Physician Visits	Hospital Episodes	Hospital Days	Physician Visits	Hospital Episodes	Hospital Days
Head of household	−0.126	0.140	3.88	0.123	0.175	2.23
education, 9–12	(1.04)	(1.02)	(1.42)	(2.33)	(3.63)	(3.06)
yrs.						
Head of household	0.522	−0.081	−3.26	0.088	−0.063	−1.16
education > 12	(1.79)	(0.33)	(0.45)	(1.05)	(0.81)	(0.99)
yrs.						
Family size	−0.137	−0.097	−2.33	−0.079	0.008	0.04
	(4.33)	(2.69)	(3.23)	(5.12)	(0.57)	(0.17)
Working	0.055	−0.091	−0.50	−0.020	−0.323	−5.31
	(0.23)	(0.35)	(0.10)	(0.32)	(5.77)	(6.27)
Black—South	−0.168	−0.558	−8.27	−0.454	−0.518	−6.90
	(1.08)	(2.89)	(2.16)	(5.52)	(6.84)	(6.03)
Black—outside	−0.315	−0.129	0.22	−0.025	−0.111	−1.44
South	(2.16)	(0.80)	(0.07)	(0.27)	(1.27)	(1.08)
Non SMSA—South	−0.245	−0.265	−5.13	−0.269	−0.003	−1.47
	(1.61)	(1.45)	(1.42)	(4.41)	(0.05)	(1.77)
Non SMSA—	0.094	0.552	9.34	−0.186	−0.029	−1.49
outside South	(0.60)	(3.18)	(2.70)	(3.06)	(0.52)	(1.78)
Chi-square	394	345	303	2268	1736	1728

NOTE: t statistics in parentheses.
[a] Persons with family income under $5,000.

TABLE 2 Tobit Results—Public Assistance Recipients and Other Low-Income Persons, 1969[a]

	Public Assistance Recipients			Other Low-Income Persons		
	Physician Visits	Hospital Episodes	Hospital Days	Physician Visits	Hospital Episodes	Hospital Days
Constant	−1.887	−1.874	−51.40	−3.302	−3.010	−50.10
	(4.88)	(2.67)	(3.69)	(18.77)	(11.71)	(13.00)
Restricted activity	0.134	0.135	2.60	0.198	0.130	1.99
days	(9.96)	(8.76)	(8.62)	(32.31)	(22.53)	(23.33)

TABLE 2 (concluded)

	Public Assistance Recipients			Other Low-Income Persons		
	Physician Visits	Hospital Episodes	Hospital Days	Physician Visits	Hospital Episodes	Hospital Days
Chronic conditions	0.319	0.203	3.32	0.342	0.252	3.93
	(7.89)	(4.39)	(3.66)	(19.22)	(15.27)	(15.95)
Age 17–44	−0.359	−0.160	1.67	−0.163	0.244	4.70
	(1.31)	(0.52)	(0.28)	(1.61)	(2.59)	(3.31)
Age 45–64	−0.170	0.068	3.64	−0.181	0.391	6.46
	(0.86)	(0.29)	(0.80)	(2.18)	(5.08)	(5.58)
Age 65+	−0.404	0.182	6.81	0.147	0.578	9.36
	(2.04)	(0.80)	(1.50)	(1.78)	(7.56)	(8.13)
Female	−0.073	−0.396	−8.06	0.149	−0.199	−3.48
	(0.06)	(2.64)	(2.70)	(2.60)	(3.74)	(4.35)
Female, age 17–44	0.954	1.967	29.54	0.518	1.238	15.22
	(3.20)	(5.88)	(4.53)	(4.88)	(12.79)	(10.45)
Head of household education, 9–12 yrs.	−0.123	0.131	3.87	0.125	0.175	2.25
	(1.01)	(0.96)	(1.42)	(2.37)	(3.62)	(3.10)
Head of household education, >12 yrs.	0.530	−0.096	−3.28	0.093	−0.066	−1.15
	(1.81)	(0.26)	(0.45)	(1.12)	(0.85)	(0.98)
Family size	−0.134	−0.103	−2.34	−0.078	0.007	0.03
	(4.23)	(2.83)	(3.22)	(5.03)	(0.48)	(0.12)
Working	0.060	−0.103	−0.53	−0.020	−0.324	−5.33
	(0.26)	(0.39)	(0.10)	(0.32)	(5.78)	(6.30)
Black—South	−0.156	−0.605	−8.25	−0.439	−0.522	−6.71
	(0.99)	(3.03)	(2.09)	(5.32)	(6.81)	(5.78)
Black—outside South	−0.321	−0.096	0.18	−0.052	−0.091	−1.47
	(2.19)	(0.57)	(0.05)	(0.55)	(1.01)	(1.09)
Physicians	0.095	−0.198	−0.66	0.226	−0.273	−3.34
	(0.53)	(0.91)	(0.16)	(2.52)	(3.16)	(2.60)
Hospital beds	—	−0.067	0.32	—	0.042	1.56
		(0.41)	(0.10)		(0.83)	(2.04)
Non SMSA—South	−0.151	−0.480	−5.70	−0.062	−0.233	−3.91
	(0.65)	(1.77)	(1.06)	(0.61)	(2.43)	(2.72)
Non SMSA— outside South	0.176	0.403	8.68	−0.015	−0.244	−4.45
	(0.79)	(1.51)	(1.63)	(0.17)	(2.82)	(3.44)
Chi-square	374	337	303	2274	1740	1746

NOTE: t statistics in parentheses.
[a] Persons with family income under $5,000.

TABLE 3 Tobit Results—Persons Age 65 and Over, 1969

	Physician Visits	Hospital Episodes	Hospital Days
Constant	−1.691	−3.403	−62.43
	(4.27)	(9.15)	(9.44)
Chronic conditions	0.315	0.153	2.25
	(13.94)	(7.00)	(5.78)
Limited in activity	0.306	0.603	12.00
	(3.98)	(8.16)	(9.11)
Age	−0.018	0.007	0.15
	(3.42)	(1.51)	(1.75)
Restricted activity days	0.120	0.115	2.02
	(16.82)	(17.23)	(17.11)
Income $5,000–9,999	0.160	0.233	3.41
	(1.91)	(2.95)	(2.42)
Income $10,000–14,999	0.324	0.370	3.65
	(2.42)	(2.91)	(1.59)
Income $15,000+	0.743	0.457	7.42
	(5.18)	(3.21)	(2.93)
Public assistance recipient	0.383	−0.063	−1.14
	(2.79)	(0.46)	(0.47)
Family size	−0.067	0.020	0.48
	(2.17)	(0.70)	(0.96)
Female	0.143	−0.061	−1.24
	(2.16)	(0.97)	(1.11)
Individual education, 9 years and over	0.178	−0.027	−0.29
	(2.63)	(0.42)	(0.25)
Working	−0.065	−0.303	−5.96
	(0.66)	(3.09)	(3.38)
Black—South	−0.521	−0.643	−9.98
	(3.21)	(4.03)	(3.53)
Black—outside South	−0.095	−0.082	1.41
	(0.52)	(0.47)	(0.46)
Non SMSA—South	−0.242	0.169	0.56
	(2.66)	(2.01)	(0.37)
Non SMSA—outside South	−0.005	0.179	1.69
	(0.06)	(2.43)	(1.28)
Chi-square	898	800	799

NOTE: t statistics in parentheses.

TABLE 4 Tobit Results—Persons Age 65 and Over, 1969

	Physician Visits	Hospital Episodes	Hospital Days
Constant	−2.072	−3.107	−63.22
	(4.81)	(6.55)	(7.48)
Chronic conditions	0.317	0.151	2.23
	(14.02)	(6.90)	(5.71)
Limited in activity	0.304	0.603	12.00
	(3.95)	(8.17)	(9.11)
Age	−0.018	0.008	0.16
	(3.45)	(1.57)	(1.79)
Restricted activity days	0.120	0.115	2.02
	(16.82)	(17.24)	(17.11)
Income $5,000–9,999	0.145	0.253	3.72
	(1.73)	(3.20)	(2.64)
Income $10,000–14,999	0.309	0.392	3.99
	(2.30)	(3.08)	(1.74)
Income $15,000+	0.721	0.492	7.94
	(5.02)	(3.45)	(3.13)
Public assistance recipient	0.370	−0.044	−0.82
	(2.69)	(0.32)	(0.34)
Family size	−0.063	0.015	0.43
	(2.05)	(0.55)	(0.86)
Female	0.144	−0.064	−1.30
	(2.17)	(1.02)	(1.17)
Individual education, 9 years and over	0.181	−0.025	−0.14
	(2.67)	(0.39)	(0.12)
Working	−0.066	−0.304	−6.02
	(0.67)	(3.10)	(3.42)
Black—South	−0.491	−0.670	−10.03
	(2.93)	(4.17)	(3.52)
Black—outside South	−0.122	−0.055	1.64
	(0.67)	(0.32)	(0.54)
Physicians	0.257	−0.422	−6.41
	(2.26)	(3.76)	(3.23)
Hospital beds	—	0.079	2.50
		(1.18)	(2.10)
Non SMSA—South	−0.015	−0.159	−3.82
	(0.11)	(1.24)	(1.67)
Non SMSA—outside South	0.180	−0.137	−3.44
	(1.59)	(1.24)	(1.75)
Chi-square	904	813	790

NOTE: *t* statistics in parentheses.

NOTES

1. Ronald Andersen *et al.*, *Health Service Use: National Trends and Variations, 1953–1971*, U S. Department of Health, Education and Welfare, October 1972, tables 5 and 15.
2. Charles L. Schultze *et al.*, *Setting National Priorities: The 1973 Budget* (Washington, D.C.: The Brookings Institution, 1972), p. 225.
3. Julian H. Pettingill, "Trends in Hospital Use by the Aged," *Social Security Bulletin* (July 1972), pp. 3–14.
4. Insurance payments per person under age 65 increased from $62 in 1969 to $100 in 1973, increasing the share of the total health bill paid by insurance from 29.9 per cent to 33.4 per cent. Barbara S. Cooper and Paula A. Piro, "Age Differences in Medical Care Spending," *Social Security Bulletin* (May 1974), pp. 3–14.
5. Regina Loewenstein, "Early Effects of Medicare on Health Care of the Aged," *Social Security Bulletin*, 34 (April 1971).
6. For example, to derive the adjusted figures for the under age 17 group, the coefficient on restricted activity days (0.14) was multiplied by the average number of restricted activity days for all children, and the coefficient on chronic conditions (2.86) was multiplied by the average number of chronic conditions in children. These terms were added to the constant term to derive the under $5,000, no aid, adjusted visit rate. Adjusted visit rates for other income groups are greater than this rate by an amount equal to the corresponding coefficients in Appendix 2.
7. Medically needy persons eligible for Medicaid are those aged, blind, disabled, or families with dependent children whose income net of medical expenses is within 133 per cent of the public assistance support level.
8. Karen Davis, "National Health Insurance," in Barry Blechman *et al.*, *Setting National Priorities: The 1975 Budget* (Washington, D.C.: The Brookings Institution, 1974), Ch. 8.
9. See Karen Davis, "Financing Medical Care: Implications for Access to Primary Care," in Spyros Andreopoulos (editor), *Primary Medical Care* (New York: John Wiley, 1974).
10. Ronald Andersen *et al.*, *Expenditures for Personal Health Services: National Trends and Variations*, 1953–1970, U.S. Department of Health, Education and Welfare, Health Resources Administration, October 1973, Table A-11.
11. The sample excludes fifty-four individuals for whom head of household education was not reported.
12. Detailed specifications of the independent variables used are contained in Appendix 1.
13. Source: Haug, Robark, and Martin, *Distribution of Physicians in the United States, 1970* (Chicago: American Medical Association, 1971).
14. This sample comprised 25,673 individuals. An additional 497 individuals with head of household education unreported were omitted from the sample.
15. James Tobin, "Estimation of Relationships for Limited Dependent Variables," *Econometrica*, 26 (1958), pp. 24–36.

    The tobit model specifies that an index I be generated such that:

    $$Y_j = 0 \qquad \text{for } I_j \leq e_j$$
    $$Y_j = I_j - e_j \qquad \text{for } I_j > e_j$$

    where Y is the value of the dependent variable, I is a linear continuation of the independent variables to which Y is hypothetically related, and e is a $N(0,S^2)$ variable. The predicted expected value of the dependent variable given the index $\hat{I}$ is given by

$$\hat{Y}_j = \hat{I}_j\, F\!\left(\frac{\hat{I}_j}{\hat{S}}\right) + \hat{s}\, f\!\left(\frac{\hat{I}_j}{\hat{S}}\right)$$

where F and f are the standard normal cumulative distribution and standard normal density functions, respectively.

16. White utilization patterns did not show significant regional differences, and hence were constrained to be equal in the South and outside the South.

17. See Ray Marshall, "The Economics of Racial Discrimination," *Journal of Economic Literature* (September 1974), for a discussion of different types of discrimination.

18. Melbah McAfee, "Black Belt Community Health Center," paper presented at Conference on Hunger in the South, University of North Carolina, June 23, 1974.

19. U.S. House of Representatives, Committee on the Judiciary, *Hearings on Title VI Enforcement in Medicare and Medicaid Programs,* September 12, 17, 24, and October 1, 1973 (Washington, D.C.: U.S. Government Printing Office, 1974).

20. See Karen Davis, "Financing Medical Care: Implications for Access to Primary Care," in Spyros Andreopoulos (editor), *Primary Medical Care* (New York: John Wiley, 1974).

21. Eugene C. Carter, "Health Insurance for the Aged: Amounts Reimbursed by State," U. S. Department of Health, Education, and Welfare, Social Security Administration, Office of Research and Statistics, H1-32, October 19, 1971.

22. U.S. Department of Health, Education, and Welfare, Social Security Administration, Office of Research and Statistics, Medicare, 1968: Section 1, Summary, 1973.

23. Charles B. Waldhausen, "Assignment Rates for Supplementary Medical Insurance Claims, Calendar Years 1970–72," Social Security Administration, Office of Research and Statistics, H1-46, June 30, 1973.

24. Martin S. Feldstein, "The Rising Price of Physician Services," *Review of Economics and Statistics,* 52 (1970), pp. 121–133.

25. Victor R. Fuchs and Marcia J. Kramer, *Determinants of Expenditures for Physicians' Services in the United States, 1948–68* (New York: National Bureau of Economic Research, Occasional Paper No. 117, 1972).

26. Martin S. Feldstein, "Econometric Studies of Health Economics," Harvard Institute of Economic Research, Discussion Paper No. 291, 1973.

27. The only exception is for those few blacks in the South in the highest-income class. However, only 1 per cent of the black population in the South has family incomes of $15,000 and above.

28. However, only 3 per cent of participating institutional providers are actually site visited to check for compliance. See House Judiciary Committee Hearings, *op cit.*

29. Martin S. Feldstein, "Hospital Cost Inflation: A Study of Nonprofit Price Dynamics," *American Economic Review,* 61 (1971), pp. 853–872.

30. Feldstein, "An Econometric Model of the Medicare System," p. 9.

10 ‖ COMMENTS

John Rafferty
Department of Health, Education, and Welfare

SUMMARY

The authors' purpose is to address three broad questions pertaining to the Medicare and Medicaid programs in the United States: What impact have these programs had on use of medical services by the poor and the elderly? What factors account for differences in the level of use of Medicaid by those who are eligible? To what extent do social and demographic characteristics affect the use of medical services by the elderly? The first three sections of the paper deal with each of these questions in turn, and a fourth section then discusses the implications of the empirical findings for a national health insurance program.

Section 1, which deals with the general impact of Medicare and Medicaid on use, draws from a variety of sources. The authors indicate that, since enactment of these programs, use of medical services by low-income individuals has increased, and that low-income persons have gained on those with higher incomes. However, as the authors stress in this section of the paper, this general observation may be quite misleading. First, Medicaid provides services only for certain categories of the poor, leaving approximately 9 million poor uncovered. Second, there is evidence that the poor receive lower-quality care and receive it in settings that are less convenient and less pleasant than is the case for the population at large. Third, the authors stress the fact that generalizations about levels of use by the poor and the elderly may be misleading because of differences in health status between these groups and the population at large; they show that, although the relationship between use levels and income levels tends to be U-shaped (with the poor and the wealthy receiving larger amounts of care than those in the middle-income groups), when health status is adjusted for, the relationship is positively sloped throughout.

In sections 2 and 3, which deal individually with Medicaid and Medicare, respectively, an econometric model is estimated. This is presented as an approximation to a more complete model, which is very briefly described, but which is not considered feasible. The model that is estimated for the Medicaid study consists of three independent regression equations, of which the independent variables are physician visits, hospital episodes, and hospital days; twenty independent variables, including measures of health status, measures of resource availability, and sociodemographic variables appear in each equation. The three equations are estimated first for public assistance recipients and then for other low-income persons, using Tobit analysis, and the resulting coefficients are then discussed. Among other things, they show that large variations in use occur among Medicaid eligibles, that blacks lag substantially behind whites, that education increases the use of physician services but not hospital services, that larger families have lower hospitalization rates and ambulatory visits, and that health status is the major determinant of utilization among the poor. However, use of services by public assistance recipients is less sensitive to health status than is use by other low-income individuals, and the poor who are not on public assistance receive far fewer services than those on welfare, even after adjustment for health status and other characteristics.

Similar equations are estimated for the analysis of Medicare benefits in Section 3, although here the equations also include income variables, in an effort to capture not only the direct effect of income but also the possibly lower net prices that are faced by higher-income persons who are more likely to have supplementary insurance. In brief, with respect to Medicare, the authors find that, other things the same, the use of medical services by the elderly increases uniformly with income, but, for those individuals who are also covered by Medicaid as well as Medicare, the elimination of cost-sharing requirements appears to raise their utilization rate to that of the middle-income elderly. The authors find much lower levels of use by blacks in the South, both for physicians and hospital services, which they interpret as evidence of racial discrimination. They find that use of both physician and hospital services by the elderly is sensitive to the availability of medical services, but they also conclude that available hospital beds are rationed equitably between the elderly and other age groups.

In the final section the authors then discuss three general implications of their findings for national health insurance. First, although Medicare and Medicaid have helped covered individuals receive needed medical care, they indicate that Medicaid has failed by not covering all of the poor; coverage for these individuals, therefore, is indicated as a top priority for a national health insurance program. Second, they indicate that the cost-sharing provision of Medicare leads to a wide disparity in use on the basis of differences in income; therefore, a graduated cost-sharing arrangement would increase the equitability of access under a national health insurance plan. Third, experience with Medicare and Medicaid shows that some population groups will lag in utilization even if they are covered, as is the case for minority groups and residents of rural areas at the present time; therefore, supplementary programs for such groups would seem to be required under any national health insurance scheme.

CRITIQUE

In this paper Karen Davis and Roger Reynolds have presented a very substantial amount of useful information on the Medicare and Medicaid programs, information that is not only of considerable policy importance, but also carries significant implications for future research. Since a discussant finds it necessary to focus on the weaknesses in, or the necessary qualifications to, the research under review, such negative comments tend to occupy the major portion of the discussant's time; this, however, should not be allowed to detract from the usefulness of much of the work reported in this paper. Medicare and Medicaid represent the closest approximations to national health insurance in the experience of the United States, and since analyses of these programs have been very few and far between, this broad study is very welcome indeed.

One distinguishing feature of the paper, as alluded to in the summary above, is that it presents and discusses a considerable number of individual findings, far more than can be covered in this brief discussion. As a result, this review will be confined primarily to just a few of the broader, more general, considerations even though this may fail to do full justice to the amount of information the paper presents.

My major concern really has to do with the interpretation of the statistical results. First, I feel that this paper treads dangerously close to what another economist has called the "Regression Humbug Syndrome"; the equations that are estimated here do have the appearance of the reduced forms of supply-demand models, but we are given no explicit theoretical understructure for these regressions, nor a discussion of expected signs. The independent variables that appear in the equations appear to have been determined less on the basis of theoretical reasoning than on the basis of what data were available. In the absence of any explicit hypotheses to be tested, whatever significant relationships do drop out of the regressions are then discussed, and are explained on a more or less *ad hoc* basis. One danger is the tendency to conclude, implicitly, that if no significant relationship appeared, no such relationship exists, which may be quite untrue. This general approach may be more appropriate when the primary objective is prediction; here, however, where our interest is less in prediction than in explanation and understanding of structure, more explicit theoretical underpinnings would be desirable.

One example of the difficulties which may appear in connection with this kind of research approach is the interpretation of the finding of relatively low levels of utilization, of both physicians and hospitals, on the part of blacks in the South. The findings are very striking, and are of considerable interest and policy importance, but the interpretation of the cause of this disparity as clear, out-and-out racial *discrimination* is scientifically premature; at least, that the disparity in use is caused by discrimination cannot really be deduced from the present analysis, for we really don't know the degree to which the disparity is attributable to demand as opposed to supply factors. Indeed, the authors' interpretation does not seem like an entirely unreasonable one, but certainly at least one plausible alternative is that, because of *past* discrimination, blacks do not presently seek out care, so that the actual cause *today* is on the demand side rather than the supply side. This is not trivial, because the appropriate policy for correcting such disparities would be very different in each instance—requiring some kind of civil rights enforcement in the former, and perhaps outreach and educational efforts in the latter case.

The second critical point I'll make also pertains to interpretation of results, and I should hasten to add that although I feel that the point is important, it is a much less pervasive problem in this paper than is the former one. This is simply a reminder that this study employs cross-sectional data, and that it is necessary to be particularly cautious when the results of such an analysis are used in discussions in which our real interest is in variations that actually occurred across time; the appropriateness of cross-sectional data depends on the degree to which those factors that determine the cross-sectional variation can reasonably be assumed to be the same factors that caused the changes over time. I will again give just one illustration of this particular problem, using a case in which I do have empirical reason for believing that the authors' interpretation of their findings is incorrect. This concerns the use of hospital services by the elderly, under Medicare. The authors conclude from the cross-sectional analysis that the elderly "do not receive care at the expense of younger persons needing medical care where supply is most deficient," and that ". . . available beds are rationed equitably among all age groups." Because of the weakness of the supply variables used for these estimates, this conclusion should be somewhat tentative, but nevertheless, it may well be that, cross-sectionally, use by the elderly responds to variations in supply in essentially the same way as use by the population as a whole. However, that is not really the question at issue; rather, we are concerned here with those changes over time that are directly attributable to the provision of health insurance for the elderly, which is not quite the same thing. In fact, I have looked into this specific question using time series data and obtained just the opposite result—that the introduction of Medicare coincided with very dramatic changes in hospital use by the non-elderly. Specifically, for patients under 65, diagnosis-specific lengths of stay were dramatically reduced immediately after introduction of Medicare, and, for this younger group, there was a substantial decline in admissions of the more discretionary types of cases. Whether or not this shift was "appropriate" in some sense is a separate question, but I believe there is no doubt that the increased use of hospitals by the elderly did come at the expense of younger patients, which is the opposite of what is suggested by the cross-sectional results. Thus, I would argue that the Davis-Reynolds finding may itself be quite valid, but its interpretation is not: The factors that determine the response of utilization to availability across regions are not the same as the factors that determined these responses over time when Medicare was introduced; and, the introduction of NHI, which will increase effective demand by some groups more than by others, should therefore also be expected to cause the increase in use by the more favored groups to come at the expense of others. Again, my point is simply that caution is necessary in generalizing these cross-sectional results to changes that occurred over time.

I will limit my critical comments to these two points, but I would like to address one other issue that I feel is very relevant here, an issue that is perhaps regarded by economists as the most pervasive and critical constraint on health economics research. This is the matter of limitations in the availability of statistical data. I believe that the authors of this present paper have effectively mined the data that were available to them, and many of the limitations of their study are a simple function of the limitations in those data.

However, I also think that in health economics we are at a point when we could benefit by observing the research approaches of people in other fields, such as sociology and psychology. Unlike economists, who have been prone to design their research around the data in hand, in these areas the research is often designed first, and then, perhaps as one step in that design process, the survey instrument or the particular mechanism whereby the necessary data will be generated is developed. Although our usual approach—that of massaging the secondary data we are able to acquire from others—has a pleasing ring of efficiency, there is a question involving how often that approach is really cost effective. Therefore, perhaps economists should become more willing to generate the data required to answer the questions they want to raise. This does raise the monetary costs of doing research, but it is pertinent to note that, at the Bureau of Health Services Research, the problem we have faced has been more often a problem of finding research proposals of high technical quality rather than finding the dollars to support well-designed projects based on high-quality data. I feel this point is quite relevant in this specific context; among the many contributions the authors make in their paper is to narrow old questions and identify new ones, but I really doubt if very much can be done about answering those questions without some fairly heroic efforts on the part of researchers themselves to generate the data that will be required.

Dorothy P. Rice
Social Security Administration

As is usual with Dr. Karen Davis' work, this paper is a fine piece of empiricism. The findings are significant in an important sense: two large government programs—Medicare and Medicaid—are shown to have achieved what they set out to do. This may be surprising to some economists because when one searches the literature, one finds time and again that government programs too often fail in their objectives. The paper is important because it compares medical care use for the low-income population receiving welfare and other poor persons, leading to the conclusion that extension of medical care financing to those poor persons excluded from Medicaid should be a top priority reform.

After a few specific comments, I will compare some of the Davis-Reynolds findings with data from the Social Security Administration's Current Medicare Survey for the population aged 65 and over.

With respect to Medicaid, the authors adjust the 1969 Health Interview Survey for health status and show that physician visits increase with income if the low-income persons not on public assistance are separated and their physician use is compared with that of persons with middle and higher family income. Although there is a verbal description of how the "adjusted for health status" physician visits were estimated for Table 2, it is still not clear what the equations in Appendix 2 mean. Therefore, the reader has to trust that the authors did the estimations correctly.

In explaining the factors determining the use of Medicaid services, the authors state ". . . there is no price mechanism by which quantity of services demanded is necessarily equated with quantity of services which providers are willing to supply." Although quantity demanded may not be a function of price, since the Medicaid recipient does not pay for services, the fact that fee schedules vary from state to state means that the quantity supplied may vary from state to state as a function of the fee schedule. The authors appear to recognize that physicians may prefer to treat some patients rather than others but do not explicitly include fees paid as a measure of physician preferences among patients. A variable for this might be included in the regression analysis in Table 4.

With respect to the Medicare program, the authors fail to point out that utilization trends observed for 1967–1969 do not hold for 1969–1971. Pettingill (quoted on page 392) also shows that Medicare admissions per 1,000 population rose at an average annual percentage change of 0.3 from 1969 to 1971 compared with 7.4 between 1967 and 1969. Covered days of care per 1,000 population increased 12.6 per cent per year from 1967 to 1969 but declined 3.4 per cent per year between 1969 and 1971. Average length of covered stay increased 4.8 per cent per year during the earlier period and declined 3.8 per cent per year in the later period. ECF admissions per 1,000 enrollees hit a peak in 1969, increasing by 15.7 per cent over 1968 but declined 10.2 per cent during 1969–1970 and 13.4 per cent during 1970–1971.[1] There was an initial impact of Medicare coverage during the first three years that has reversed direction or tapered off in subsequent years. The implications of these more recent changes are not discussed by the authors.

In the section on "Distribution of Medicare Benefits," Davis and Reynolds discuss data from the Medicare program but could do a great deal to make the actual meaning of their statements clear to the reader. For example, they state that ". . . whites receive 60 per cent more payments for physician services than elderly blacks." It is true that reimbursement for physician and other medical services per person enrolled under SMI in 1968 was 62 per cent higher for whites than for all other races, but there was only a 15 per cent difference in terms of reimbursement per person served.[2] The authors claim "nearly all of the difference" in reimbursement per person enrolled between whites and all other races represents "differences in percentage of eligible persons receiving reimbursable services." The authors should indicate how they determine this point. In 1968, reimbursement per person enrolled was $78.76 among whites and $48.44 among all other races. By definition,

$$\text{reimbursement per person enrolled} = \left(\frac{\text{number served}}{\text{number enrolled}} \right) \times \left(\frac{\text{reimbursement per person served}}{} \right)$$

If we let P = reimbursement per person served

$$Q = \frac{\text{number served}}{\text{number enrolled}}$$

then the difference in reimbursement per person enrolled between whites and all other races can be expressed as

$$\Delta(PQ) = \Delta PQ_0 + \Delta QP_0 + \Delta P \Delta Q$$

where, for example, $\Delta(PQ)$ represents the difference in reimbursement per person enrolled between whites and all other races, P_0 represents reimbursement per person served among all other races, and Q_0 represents the ratio of number served to number enrolled among all other races. With this equation, and assuming that the interaction term is distributed proportionately between the P and Q terms, we can determine the proportion of the difference in reimbursement per person enrolled between the races that is attributable to differences in reimbursement per person served and percentage of enrolled persons receiving reimbursable services. Taking the necessary data from the 1968 summary, we do not find that nearly all the difference stems from the proportion of enrollees served. Twenty-seven per cent is attributable to a difference in reimbursement per person served of $199 among whites and $173 among all other races.

Additional questionable statements are made by the authors with respect to the factors affecting geographical and income differences in Medicare reimbursements. Reimbursement depends on meeting the deductible and determining reasonable charges. Charges for some services may be disallowed more often than for other services and utilization of services may vary by geographic area, income class, etc. The extent to which charges are disallowed for a particular covered service may also vary by characteristics such as geographic area and income class.

Davis and Reynolds argue that economic forces may contribute to lack of significant coefficients among the availability variables in their regression equations for public assistance recipients and other low-income persons. More specifically, "since Medicaid patients do not pay for the care, providers, especially with regard to ambulatory care, lack the ability to affect the utilization patterns of these persons by ordinary economic means." What do the authors mean by "ordinary economic means?" We suspect they do not assume a typical competitive economic market with equilibrium prices and quantities responding to shifts in supply and demand. As the authors indicate, there is no one theory of market behavior that is generally accepted as describing the market for physicians' services. The market for hospital services is also complex, and interpretation of the coefficients of the availability variables requires a detailed examination of the markets for these services.

In their concluding remarks, the authors state that "imposition of uniform cost-sharing provisions (deductible and coinsurance amounts) results in wide disparities in use of medical services on the basis of income." They find utilization among the elderly related to income, but it does not follow that cost-sharing provisions cause these disparities. Furthermore, after accounting for family size in determining whether a given annual family income was low or high, Peel and Scharff (1973) found no difference in the number of SMI services per user with charges between enrollees with high family incomes and those with low to moderate family incomes and no public medical assistance.[3] To the extent that medical care prices vary geographically, equality in access would also require coinsurance rates to vary with prices if an enrollee is not to pay more coinsurance for the same quantity of services where prices are higher.

It may be interesting to compare the Davis-Reynolds findings with unpublished data from SSA's Current Medicare Survey (CMS) of a sample of Medicare beneficiaries interviewed monthly for a period of fifteen months.

Davis and Reynolds find health status in terms of chronic conditions and restricted activity days positively related to utilization, with public assistance recipients using more services than other low-income persons and being less sensitive to health status in their utilization (tables 4, 5). Similar results are observed for Supplementary Medical Insurance enrollees in the accompanying table based on data from our Current Medicare Survey. Utilization of covered services increases as comparative health status deteriorates, with welfare recipients using many more services at each level of health. The gradients are quite steep for both groups, but less so for welfare recipients because of high utilization by welfare recipients with comparatively better health. These conclusions apply both to the percentage of enrollees served and the average number of services per person served. Utilization increases as health status deteriorates both because relatively more persons receive services and each recipient uses more.

Davis-Reynolds and CMS findings (not shown here) are consistent for health status and public assistance, and partly for race. Both surveys show direct relationships between utilization of physicians' care and covered services, respectively, and health status and public assistance. Davis and Reynolds report that blacks in the South make fewer physician visits, but no significant relation for blacks outside the South. But their black-outside South variable compares utilization by blacks outside the South with that of all other persons, including blacks in the South. It is difficult, therefore, to know just what relation exists between utilization by blacks compared with whites. The CMS table shows more covered services per person served for whites in each region, with the differences between whites and all other races greater in the Northeast and West than in the South. (Number of enrollees of all other races in the West is too small, however, to provide a reliable estimate.) Furthermore, the proportion of whites served exceeds the proportion of all other races by more in the Northeast and North Central than in the South.

One final point is worth mentioning. Davis and Reynolds find a negative relation between physician visits and age, whereas CMS shows a positive, although not highly significant, association. As they point out, however, age may capture the effect of health status if the latter is not controlled.

Davis and Reynolds conclude that "supplementary health care delivery programs" designed to meet the special needs of minorities, rural residents,

Covered Medical Services under the Supplementary Medical Insurance Program, by Health Condition and Welfare Status, and by Region and Race, 1969

Health Condition and Region	Total			No Welfare / White			Some Welfare / All Other Races		
	Number Served (000's)	Percentage of Enrollees	Average Number of Services Per Person Served[a]	Number Served (000's)	Percentage of Enrollees	Average Number of Services per Person Served[a]	Number Served (000's)	Percentage of Enrollees	Average Number of Services per Person Served[a]
	Total			_No Welfare_			_Some Welfare_		
All health conditions[b]	13,963	77.7	16.7	11,633	75.6	14.2	2,330	90.3	28.9
Better than others	5,706	71.2	10.7	5,153	69.8	9.7	553	87.6	19.6
Same as others	6,082	80.0	14.7	4,980	78.4	13.2	1,096	88.2	21.6
Worse than others	2,175	92.4	37.7	1,494	90.7	32.8	681	96.6	48.2
	Total			_White_			_All Other Races_		
All regions	15,595	78.7	17.2	14,440	79.1	17.5	1,112	73.9	12.6
Northeast	4,252	80.1	20.3	4,077	80.8	20.5	157	67.1	13.2
North Central	4,406	76.2	16.6	4,191	76.5	16.7	205	70.9	16.2
South	4,536	78.4	14.5	3,841	78.8	14.9	684	75.8	12.0
West	2,402	81.6	17.8	2,332	81.6	18.1	67	82.7	6.9

a Includes in-hospital visits.
b Excludes unknown conditions. Comparative health status is reported by the sample persons at the beginning of the survey.

and persons in the South must be an essential part of health care policy. This statement surely serves to whet the appetite. What are these supplementary programs? Are they medical service, manpower, or health insurance programs? Would they supplement or replace existing programs? How would they be financed?

Medicare and Medicaid have clearly accomplished a great deal toward increasing access to medical care. Nevertheless, substantial gaps exist for certain population groups. The solution to meet the special needs of these population groups clearly is not readily apparent.

NOTES

1. Eugene Carter and Charles Fisher, "Health Insurance for the Aged: Hospital and Extended Care Admissions by State, Fiscal Year 1971," Social Security Administration, Health Insurance Statistics, HI-42, March 12, 1973.
2. U.S. Social Security Administration, Office of Research and Statistics, "Medicare: Health Insurance for the Aged, 1968, Section I: Summary," Washington, D.C., 1973, pp. 1–18, 19.
3. Evelyn Peel and Jack Scharff, "Impact of Cost-Sharing on Use of Ambulatory Services under Medicare, 1969," *Social Security Bulletin,* October 1973.

11

ROBERT G.
EVANS
University of British
Columbia

Beyond the Medical Marketplace: Expenditure, Utilization, and Pricing of Insured Health Care in Canada

THE ORGANIZATION OF NATIONAL HEALTH INSURANCE IN CANADA

To understand the structure of health care legislation in Canada, one must begin with federal-provincial relations. The division of powers between the federal government in Ottawa and the ten provincial governments is Canada's longest and most carefully defended border, and this division of powers (based on sections 91 and 92 of the British North America Act) clearly designates health

This paper owes a great deal to initial discussions with Uwe Reinhardt. At the conference, Herbert Klarman and Anne Scitovsky, the discussants, were both very helpful, as were Victor Fuchs, Lee Soderstrom, and other participants. Their improving influence should be obvious; the rest is mine.

Data used in the text are not separately referenced; a detailed discussion of sources is given in the appendix.

as a matter for provincial jurisdiction.[1] In a strict sense, there cannot be "national" health insurance in Canada; rather, there are ten separate "provincial" health insurance plans. Federal jurisdiction is limited to Indians, Eskimos, sick mariners, and the Armed Forces, and to a variety of specific services such as quarantine, immigration, food and drug control, and many other small areas.

And yet quite obviously there is a national health program covering hospital and medical care (with minimal specific exclusions) for almost all Canadian residents. It came about through a constitutional subterfuge whereby the federal government contributes a significant share of the total operating costs to any provincial plan meeting certain specified federal standards. The constitutional niceties thus are preserved, and indeed no province was forced to follow the federal lead and set up a conforming plan. Since the formulas for cost sharing cover roughly 50 per cent of each provincial plan's total operating costs, however, the financial pressures on the provinces to set up qualifying plans were irresistible.[2] The Hospital Insurance and Diagnostic Services Act of 1957 specified July 1, 1958, as the earliest date on which federal cost sharing for hospital care became available. Newfoundland, Saskatchewan, Alberta, and B.C. already had operating hospital plans that qualified for cost sharing and Manitoba initiated a plan on that date. The pressure on the remaining provinces brought in Prince Edward Island, Nova Scotia, New Brunswick, and Ontario in 1959, and finally Quebec in 1961. A similar scenario followed the passage of the Medical Care Act; B.C. and Saskatchewan had qualifying plans on July 1, 1968, and Manitoba, Nova Scotia, Newfoundland, Alberta, and Ontario initiated plans at various dates during 1969. Quebec and Prince Edward Island set up plans toward the end of 1970, and New Brunswick joined at the beginning of 1971. Thus 1971 is the first complete year of Canadian experience with both hospital and medical insurance. It is also the latest year for which expenditure data of all forms are currently available.[3]

The federal standards/shared funding/provincial administration structure that is required by the Canadian constitutional structure is very clearly a mixed blessing. On the positive side, national average-based cost sharing makes possible a more uniform level of service availability insofar as the federal contribution rises proportionately in the poorer provinces. Relating the federal contribution to national averages of expenditure brings it up over 60 per cent of hospital spending and over 80 per cent of medical spending in the poorest provinces,[4] thus permitting a national standard of health services that would have been quite out of reach of the provinces acting alone.[5] But the total effects of the minimum criteria for eligibility are much less clear.

In brief, these criteria are portability of coverage across provinces, universal access on equal terms and conditions to all, comprehensive coverage, and administration by a nonprofit public agency.[6] Portability clearly works to the general interest by preventing cost-conscious provincial agencies from finding ways of dropping migrants out of the system, while the requirement of public, nonprofit administration specified the initial form of organization believed most likely to achieve the other objectives with minimal overhead cost.[7] Universal access is becoming less relevant as provinces are recognizing that "premiums" represent a rather regressive poll tax and are shifting over time to total general revenue financing. But "equal terms and conditions" and "comprehensive coverage" do in fact impose significant limitations on the modifications that can be made on the supply side, insofar as they can be interpreted as prohibiting incentives directed at consumers to choose one form of delivery over another. A user of a closed panel plan, for example, could not receive a premium rebate if his plan were shown to use fewer hospital days, nor could one earn such a rebate by signing up with a well-baby clinic and agreeing not to use a pediatrician unless referred by the clinic.

Furthermore, cost sharing both distorts the structure of care delivery and dilutes incentives to economize. Provincial agencies are acutely aware of what services are or are not cost shareable; no provincial bureaucrat worthy of the name would allocate funds for a non-shareable program if the same result could be attained through a shareable route, even if the former were cheaper. This problem creates steady pressure to expand the coverage of the provincial plans—ambulatory care in hospitals must be insured since otherwise the insurance plan leads to excess hospitalization; extended care facilities should be covered in order to reduce acute care hospital use. Home care programs should also be subsidized with federal cost sharing. Thus, the open-ended nature of the federal commitment to currently covered services, combined with the steady pressure to "rationalize" utilization by expanding coverage, has stimulated interest in ways of dismantling the cost-sharing system and transferring full fiscal responsibility to the provincial governments. In return, the federal government would release to the provinces a larger share of personal income tax revenues, and/or revenues from other federal taxes (alcohol and tobacco). As yet, however, no package acceptable to both sides has been worked out.[8]

The provinces finance their share of the cost of hospital and medical care by a mix of taxes. Many provinces introduced retail sales taxes at the time the hospital plans were set up, and in some cases these were initially labeled hospital taxes. This revenue is not earmarked, however, and merely flows into general revenue. All provinces receive a share of the federal personal and corporate income tax collected from their residents. Quebec also levies its own personal income tax as well as an 0.8 per cent payroll tax introduced along with Medicare. The federal income tax was augmented by a "Social Development" surtax of 2 per cent ($100 maximum) when Medicare was introduced.

Revenue sources specifically associated with the hospital and medical insurance plans include "premiums" in some provinces and in a few, "utilization charges," but the universal access condition of federal participation restricts the role of such charges.[9] Thus the premium must not interfere with the requirement that 99 per cent of the population be insured—this requirement can be achieved by compulsion (making the premium a poll tax), by setting premiums well below expected cost per family (which would exclude nonpayers who have already paid most of the cost through other taxes), or by relatively high premiums combined with subsidies to low-income families (making the poll tax less regressive but more costly to administer). The regressiveness, expense of administration, and general pointlessness of the premium system is slowly leading provincial governments toward full general revenue financing of integrated medical and hospital "insurance." There are still a few voices raised arguing that premiums are desirable as a utilization control; if people are aware of the costs of the plans they may use less. No evidence for this argument has ever been adduced, however, any more than for the contrary position that visible premiums lead people to "get their money's worth." In any case, current premiums in no way reflect plan costs and could not be made to do so. They appear to be a transitional feature only.

A scattering of utilization charges persists, without clear rationale. Thus, B.C. charges $1.00 per day of hospital inpatient stay, and $2.00 per visit to a hospital outpatient department. Saskatchewan experimented with a $2.50 physician office visit fee and $2.50 per day hospital charge in 1968 but dropped both in 1971. It appears that the result of the medical charge was to reduce utilization on balance by lowering use by lower-income groups and raising use by upper-income groups.[10] In general, the purpose of the public plans is to reduce the inequality of access to services by income class.[11] And the "universal access on equal terms and conditions" principle is not consistent with utilization fees having a significant effect on use. Thus they are restricted to specific circumstances; it is proposed, for example, that elderly patients in B.C. extended care facilities should be charged a daily rate sufficient to mop up their monthly federal old age pensions rather than cumulating these payments for their heirs. But most utilization charges are said to cost as much to collect as they return in revenue, although of course the costing has never been done, so no one knows.

There is, however, a patchwork of arrangements, differing in each province, governing physician bills to the patient. When the plans were introduced, many provinces reimbursed physicians at a discount from the fee schedule (90 per cent or 85 per cent) to allow for the reduced uncollectable ratio. Treatment of the remaining 10 per cent or 15 per cent varied. In some provinces the physician was allowed to try to collect these amounts from the patient. Furthermore, some provinces permit physicians to bill the patient above the fee schedule—in Ontario physicians began after 1969 to bill the province for 90 per cent and then to bill the patient for whatever they might get. This practice was prohibited in 1971. Now if a physician submits a bill to the plan, he is not permitted to bill the patient as well. If he chooses, he may bill the patient directly and let the patient bill the plan. In Quebec, physicians may bill the plan or the patient at plan rates; in the latter case the patient is reimbursed. Only "nonparticipating" physicians may bill patients above plan rates, and their patients will not be reimbursed at all. In B.C. the physician may bill the patient directly, up to or above the fee schedule, if he has notified the patient in advance and obtained written consent. Otherwise the patient is not obligated to pay, and the B.C. Medical Association must disallow the bill if challenged. But the patient doesn't know this! It is not known how significant the practice of extra-billing direct to the patient is in those provinces where it is permitted, but informed opinion is that it is trivial. This would seem to agree with the public perception of Canadian medical care as "free."

If the economic relationships between third-party and consumer are relatively uninteresting in the Canadian insurance system, those between payment agency and provider are the heart of the whole system. Initially, it appears to have been the intent of the designers of both hospital and medical insurance plans to intervene as little as possible in the process of health service supply and merely to pay legitimate charges arising from an independent transaction between patient and provider. This may be an over-simplified view of the hospital insurance plan, since the federal requirements went beyond mere audit to ensure legitimacy of charges and included inspection and supervision to upgrade the quality of hospital services. However, the belief appears to have been that as long as hospitals and paying agencies were organized as not-for-profit entities, their economic behavior could safely be disregarded. In establishing the medical care plan, economic behavior of providers seems to have been ignored without even the safeguard of not-for-profit providers!

The implicit model of the delivery system underlying this approach was the naive medico-technical view of disease conditions arising independently in the population, requiring necessary care as defined by medical technology, and generating costs, again according to a fairly well-defined production technology and price structure. Expenditures for medical and hospital care were of course expected to rise insofar as it was believed that in the pre-insurance period patients were failing to seek "needed" care because they could not afford it, or providers were giving "charity" services on a volunteer basis. But nowhere in the legislation or procedures establishing either insurance plan was there any recognition that all three components of the delivery process—care seeking, choice of technique, and input costs—might shift in response to insurance coverage.

Care seeking in response to health status stimuli is likely to increase. This is the obvious response of demand to price, but appears to be a relatively small component of the Canadian insurance experience. Shifts also occur in definitions of best-practice health technology—more is performed at greater expense for any given disease state. And most difficult of all to deal with, health providers at all levels, from physicians down through hospital janitors, seem to have revised their income aspirations upward in response to the observation that the payment process was open-ended. If medical care payments were to be made according to fee schedules promulgated by medical associations alone, what besides adjustment lags limits physicians' fees and incomes? If hospital budgets are increased as required to cover wages negotiated by an increasingly unionized labor force, what besides the public spirit of trustees and administrators limits wage levels? And so it has turned out that the single most prominent influence of health insurance in Canada has been to increase the earnings of health providers.[12]

If one examines the net earnings of physicians, comparing their first full year of experience under insurance with their last year of earnings prior to insurance (a two-year span, except for New Brunswick, which began its plan on January 1, 1971), the following picture emerges.

Province	Time Period	Change in Net Physician Earnings	Change in Weekly Wages and Salaries	Relative Income Gain
Saskatchewan	1961–63	36.5%	6.6%	28.0%
B.C.	1967–69	14.5	13.0	1.3
Newfoundland	1968–70	36.3	18.7	14.8
Nova Scotia	1968–70	45.2	18.2	22.8
Ontario	1968–70	21.5	15.9	4.8
Manitoba	1968–70	48.1	15.3	28.4
Alberta	1968–70	19.4	18.6	0.7
Quebec	1969–71	51.0	15.6	30.6
P.E.I.	1969–71	70.1	11.2	53.0
New Brunswick	1969–71	34.6	17.1	14.9

SOURCES: Data appendix.

The final column adjusts for changes in the overall rate of inflation, which was accelerating in the late sixties, and brings out the dramatic gain in the relative income status of physicians that occurred in the insurance period. As will emerge below, the same pattern of dramatic income gains has also been true for hospital workers but over a longer time perspective.[13]

In fact, the peculiar federal-provincial structure of the Canadian insurance scheme militates against expenditure controls. In adopting a policy of "pay the bills," the federal government merely recognized its lack of constitutional authority to engage in regulatory activity with respect to the provincial plans. It could of course impose requirements to check fraud or raise quality standards as conditions for federal funding, and it went further to permit disallowance of claims for "medically unnecessary" procedures. But other than placing some limits on elective surgery, this provision has been empty. There is no payment limit for removal of healthy appendixes or for ritual tonsillectomies, for example.

The uniform standards of accounting for hospitals required by the federal participation agreement have, however, led to the generation of a formidable data base detailing the operations of each of the "budget review" hospitals in Canada whose services are reimbursed by the provincial agencies. This set of data is remarkable, not only for the vast amount of detailed information that it provides on the activities of hospitals, levels and patterns of output, utilization and cost of inputs, and so on, but also for the surprisingly weak management and control tool it has turned out to be. When the need arises to make estimates of the full costs of particular activities in Canadian hospitals, or the relative costs of hospitals engaged in similar activities, the data require vigorous massage to yield approximate answers. The reporting systems installed at the time hospital insurance was initiated are descriptive and epidemiological rather than managerial control systems—suitable for a strategy of minimal intervention by the public agency—in spite of their level of detail.

Standard hospital reports in Canada are of several types. Each hospital returns annually federal reports HS-1 and HS-2 providing information on facilities, services, and finances. In addition, each patient discharged generates a form documenting the episode for reimbursement purposes which is returned to the provincial agency. The basic content of these returns is standardized nationwide. Each provincial payment agency may impose its own budgetary returns, overlapping or extending the HS-1 and HS-2. Finally, hospitals may participate in a quarterly federal survey of major hospital indicators (partial HS-1 and HS-2) or return data to nonprofit agencies such as PAS or HMRI. But the federal statistical returns and the patient discharge forms, covering the whole population of hospitals and patients, respectively, form the backbone of the system.

The discharge forms report patient name, age, address, dates of admission and discharge, attending physician, discharge diagnosis (primary and secondary), and surgery and/or anesthesia if any. They provide a comprehensive picture of the in-hospital morbidity patterns of the Canadian population, as well as of the case-mix structure of each hospital. Unfortunately, none of this data can be directly linked either to ambulatory care or to the cost structures of specific hospitals. Much work can be done on the age and regional structure of morbidity, regional pattterns of patient flow, etc., but it is only within the past five years that provinces have seriously tackled the problems of machine processing these data. Within another five years most provinces will have established common patient and physician identifiers linking ambulatory and hospital records, but current ambulatory reporting is by fee schedule item and thus is procedural rather than diagnosis-specific.

The hospital statistical returns are institution-specific, keyed to line-item input budgets. They have been modified over time, but in their present form they divide all hospital expenditure into nursing services (wards, operating and recovery rooms, emergency, central supply, labor and delivery rooms, and nursery); special services (diagnostic and investigative units, special clinics, ambulatory services, and services such as pharmacy, physiotherapy, etc.); educational services (direct costs only of salaries or stipends to staff or students in medical, nursing, or other educational programs); and general services (administration, laundry, linen, records, physical plant, and all other nonclinical services). Each area reports direct expense for salaries and paid hours (medical and nonmedical) and supplies and other expenses. Separate totals for drugs and medical and surgical supplies are reported hospital-wide but are not allocated. Reports include not only cost and personnel input by area, but also a range of physical outputs—patient days (short and long term), admissions, discharges, deliveries, lab tests done (on a standard unit basis), radiological films taken, visits to each class of clinic, pounds of laundry processed, meal days produced, etc. (Not, however, stamps licked by administrative staff.)[14]

Compared to this vast array of data, much of which is tabulated and published and all of which is now on tape, the records of the medical plans are relatively sketchy. Medical data are generated by provider/patient contacts only, whereas hospital data report both contacts and annual descriptions of providers. The medical plans grew out of private, nonprofit, often physician-sponsored prepayment plans (see Shillington, 1972) in which participating physicians had agreed to accept payment according to uniform provincial fee schedules promulgated independently by the provincial medical association. These plans recorded only who did what to whom and paid accordingly.

These schedules vary from province to province, and definitions of procedures tend to shift both over time and across provinces. Thus one can be fairly sure about how many surgical operations of a particular type were performed; but, for example, the line between first and subsequent office visits (same condition), or general and partial examinations, is very blurred and seems to shift over time. Data are not generally collected on why procedures were carried out, although some provinces also request diagnostic data. And no data at all are collected on provider units (employees, capital, etc.) except for the information required by medical associations (name, age, residence, date and place of medical graduation, specialty)[15] and some additional data on billing (whether solo practice, grouped but billing separately, or grouped but billing jointly, whether or not eligible to bill as a specialist) required by the payment agency in reimbursing claims.

The weakness of both of these data collection systems is that they provide no link between costs and inputs, and any meaningful measure of output. Hospitals measure direct costs by department, but departmental services are not independently costed out or related back to patients and overhead cost is not allocated. Thus one can calculate direct laundry cost per pound of laundry processed for any hospital in the land, but in no hospital can one do more than estimate (rather crudely) the division of budget into inpatient, outpatient, and educational expense. Moreover, linkages between cost structure and patterns of patient output seem to have been examined only by academics; the public reimbursing agencies have not generally tried to relate cost to diagnostic mix in any systematic way in spite of the fact that they are consequently unable to make any but very crude cross-hospital or cross-time comparisons.[16] "Similarities" among hospitals for budget review purposes are assumed on the basis of indicators like size and location, rather than specific information on workload. Budgetary over-runs or requests for further funding are difficult to evaluate since changes in output patterns (diagnostic mix, length of stay or occupancy) are not related to changes in cost patterns. Thus when the initial relatively permissive attitude toward hospital expenditure began to harden in the mid-sixties, adequate informational tools to interpret and control cost escalation were simply not available.

A similar problem underlies medical care statistics. At first glance it might appear that fee schedules provide a firm price fixed to levels of output. Initially it was argued that fee schedules should remain the prerogative of medical associations, with government carrying on the "hands off" policy of its private, physician-sponsored predecessors.[17] The enormous increases in physician incomes and effective (though not list) prices before and during the introduction of Medicare eliminated that idea rather swiftly. In most provinces now, fee schedules are *de facto* negotiated with provincial governments although the process is often obscure to preserve the appearance of professional autonomy.[18]

The weakness in the process, of course, is that fee schedules price procedures, not care episodes. The mix and definition of procedures used during an episode can be and are varied at the discretion of the physician. Thus rates of payment to physicians tend to climb steadily over time, even given constant fee schedules; prior to Medicare this phenomenon could be explained by changing collection ratios but it has persisted since. Moreover, levels of procedures seem to depend on the available supply of physicians, as much as on the demographic structure of the population.[19] The profession and the paying agencies have responded in some provinces by developing "provider profiles" showing the patterns of procedures performed by individual physicians relative to groups of similar physicians (by region and specialty). These monitoring systems identify practitioners with unusual billing patterns (rates more than two standard deviations away from norm) and thus help to draw all providers toward uniform patterns. But they leave unanswered crucial questions such as: How well are procedures performed? Should they be performed at all? What is happening to patterns over time? Profile monitoring provides information neither on quality of care nor on the benefit from steady increases over time in procedural volume. It merely isolates a very few cases of apparent malfeasance. Like hospital audit, it is an instrument to detect fraud, not to manage performance.

The spectacular movements in hospital and medical expenditures in Canada, which we will now move to discuss in some detail, can thus be related, first, to a relatively naive initial policy of paying the legitimate bills and minimizing management intervention on the supply side,[20] and second, to an inadequate information structure on which to base efforts at management. The statistical record can be analyzed to try to observe what did (and did not) happen as national insurance was introduced; this will provide a backdrop for discussing the policy responses that have been attempted and that are now recommended.

THE QUANTITATIVE IMPACT OF NATIONAL HEALTH INSURANCE

Historical Patterns of Health Care Expenditure

The interpretation of patterns of use of and expenditure on health care in Canada, before, during, and after the introduction of the two national health insurance plans, is a complex problem that must be pursued at the level of particular classes of institutions and often of individual provinces. But an initial overview of the industry is provided by the data in tables 1 to 3, showing the distribution of personal health care spending from 1953 to 1971 in current dollars, current dollars per capita, and percentage of personal income. The effects of introducing first hospital and then medical insurance show up in the expenditure series for general and allied special

TABLE 1 Expenditure on Personal Health Care in Canada, 1953–1971 ($ million)

	General and Allied Special Hospitals	Other Hospitals	Physicians	Dentists	Prescription Drugs	Total
1953	280.4	123.6	176.6	60.5	48.8	689.9
1954	314.0	132.8	188.6	66.4	52.1	753.9
1955	342.4	137.6	206.5	68.6	59.5	814.6
1956	380.8	149.0	240.1	81.5	71.8	923.2
1957	422.9	164.5	271.8	85.0	103.2[a]	1047.4[a]
1958	462.3	178.3	301.3	90.5	112.4	1144.9
1959	543.7	191.9	325.7	99.0	130.2	1290.5
1960	640.6	204.4	355.0	109.6	132.6	1442.2
1961	722.1	226.9	388.3	116.7	135.8	1589.9
1962	811.8	242.3	406.1	121.5	144.4	1726.2
1963	909.8	265.1	453.4	136.9	161.7	1922.0
1964	1015.1	285.1	495.7	147.8	178.6	2122.3
1965	1144.5	317.4	545.1	160.1	211.5	2378.6
1966	1319.0	349.0	605.2	176.4	232.0	2682.3
1967	1523.0	393.3	686.2	187.2	265.5	3055.1
1968	1790.0	428.4	788.1	213.7	297.3	3517.5
1969	2024.7	476.6	901.4	239.7	318.5	3960.9
1970	2302.6	523.5	1028.9	262.1	360.4	4477.5
1971	2594.6	557.4	1236.2	298.8	422.5	5109.5
Annual % change						
1953–1959	11.7	7.6	10.7	8.6	12.3	11.0
1959–1965	13.2	8.7	9.0	8.3	8.4	10.7
1965–1971	14.6	9.8	14.6	11.0	12.2	13.6
1953–1971	13.2	8.7	11.4	9.3	10.6	12.0

[a]The definitions underlying the prescription drug expense series changed in this year. Annual average rates are from 1957 on.

hospitals and for physicians, which dominate personal health care spending. Personal health care spending in turn makes up about three-quarters of national health expenditures in Canada. The conceptual differences are discussed in the appendix.

The first thing that commands attention in the Canadian health care industry is the rapid growth in its level of expenditures. This increase is, of course, an international phenomenon, but in Canada the pattern of increase correlates well with extensions in insurance. The insured components—hospital and medical care—are the

TABLE 2 Per Capita Expenditure on Personal Health Care in Canada, 1953–1971 ($ million)

	General and Allied Special Hospitals	Other Hospitals	Physicians	Dentists	Prescription Drugs	Total
1953	18.89	8.32	11.90	4.08	3.29	46.47
1954	20.54	8.69	12.34	4.34	3.41	49.32
1955	21.81	8.77	13.15	4.37	3.79	51.90
1956	23.68	9.27	14.93	5.07	4.46	57.41
1957	25.46	9.90	16.36	5.12	6.21[a]	63.06[a]
1958	27.07	10.44	17.64	5.30	6.58	67.03
1959	31.09	10.98	18.63	5.66	7.45	73.81
1960	35.77	11.41	19.82	6.12	7.40	80.53
1961	39.52	12.42	21.25	6.39	7.43	87.02
1962	43.61	13.02	21.82	6.53	7.76	92.74
1963	47.97	13.98	23.91	7.22	8.53	101.61
1964	52.53	14.75	25.65	7.65	9.24	109.82
1965	58.16	16.12	27.70	8.13	10.75	120.87
1966	65.79	17.44	30.19	8.80	11.57	133.80
1967	74.61	19.27	33.62	9.17	13.01	149.67
1968	86.35	20.67	38.02	10.31	14.34	169.69
1969	96.29	22.66	42.87	11.40	15.15	188.36
1970	107.96	24.54	48.24	12.29	16.90	209.94
1971	120.15	25.82	57.24	13.84	19.56	236.61
Annual % change						
1953–1959	8.7	4.7	7.8	5.6	9.5	8.2
1959–1965	11.0	6.6	6.8	6.2	6.3	8.6
1965–1971	12.9	8.2	12.9	9.3	10.5	11.8
1953–1971	10.8	6.5	9.1	7.0	8.5	9.9

[a]See note to Table 1.

largest and fastest growing. Moreover, in each case the introduction of the national insurance plan is associated with significant increases in expenditure. In 1959 hospital insurance covered all provinces except Quebec—in 1959 and 1960 hospital expenditures were up nearly 18 per cent in each year. No other year in the period matches these. Medical care insurance was phased in province by province from 1968 to 1971—in 1969 and 1970 annual expenditure increases were over 14 per cent. In 1971 they jumped to 20 per cent. If we look only at these "leading sectors" and compute the

TABLE 3 Expenditure on Personal Health Care in Canada, 1953–1971 (as a percentage of personal income)

	General and Allied Special Hospitals	Other Hospitals	Physicians	Dentists	Prescription Drugs	Total
1953	1.43	0.63	0.90	0.31	0.25	3.53
1954	1.59	0.67	0.96	0.34	0.26	3.82
1955	1.61	0.65	0.97	0.32	0.28	3.83
1956	1.62	0.63	1.02	0.35	0.31	3.92
1957	1.68	0.65	1.08	0.34	0.41[a]	4.16[a]
1958	1.73	0.67	1.13	0.34	0.42	4.30
1959	1.93	0.68	1.16	0.35	0.46	4.59
1960	2.17	0.69	1.20	0.37	0.45	4.88
1961	2.40	0.75	1.29	0.39	0.45	5.29
1962	2.48	0.74	1.24	0.37	0.44	5.28
1963	2.62	0.76	1.30	0.39	0.47	5.54
1964	2.73	0.76	1.33	0.40	0.48	5.70
1965	2.79	0.77	1.33	0.39	0.52	5.80
1966	2.87	0.76	1.32	0.38	0.50	5.83
1967	3.02	0.78	1.36	0.37	0.53	6.05
1968	3.22	0.77	1.42	0.38	0.53	6.33
1969	3.28	0.77	1.46	0.39	0.52	6.42
1970	3.46	0.79	1.55	0.39	0.54	6.74
1971	3.54	0.76	1.68	0.41	0.58	6.96
Annual % change						
1953–1959	5.1	1.3	4.3	2.0	5.9	5.0
1959–1965	6.3	2.1	2.3	1.8	2.1	4.0
1965–1971	4.0	−0.2	4.0	0.8	1.8	3.1
1953–1971	5.2	1.0	3.5	1.6	2.5	3.7

[a]See note to Table 1.

share of total hospital and medical expenditures going to hospitals over this period, the movements in this share correlate precisely with the introduction of the two national plans. The hospital share drifted from 61.4 per cent in 1953 down to 60.5 per cent in 1958, then began a steady rise until 1968, when it peaked at 69.4 per cent. By 1971 it was down to 67.7 per cent.

The same coincidence of timing appears in Table 3. The total expenditure and expenditure per capita data are muddled by accelerating general inflation trends but the personal income share series corrects for this condition. Hospital spending increased its share of income fastest in the 1959–1965 period, whereas medical spending moved up fastest in the 1965–1971 period. From 1958 to 1961 the hospital share rose 38.7 per cent, or 11.5 per cent per year; from 1953 to 1958 and from 1961 to 1971 it rose about 4 per cent per year. The physician series is less dramatic, but it is clear that the upward trend accelerated after 1966. Clearly, public insurance has been closely associated with significant jumps in spending.[21]

But the *mechanism* is less obvious. Conventional economic explanations might focus on the pressure of increased demand on relatively inelastic supply, leading to a combination of utilization and price increase. There is reason to believe that demand-driven adjustments were not very important in the Canadian experience; this will emerge from the more detailed discussion below. A suggestion that supply-side factors may be of considerable importance emerges, however, if we point out that the relative availability of physicians and hospital beds also shifted over this period. General and allied special beds per fee-practice physician reached a peak of 7.18 in 1966, having drifted up slowly from 7.00 in 1958. From 1968 to 1971, however, they dropped over 10 per cent, from 7.12 to 6.38. The increase in physician share was associated with a rapid *increase* in the relative availability of physicians, far too rapid to be a response to insurance-induced demand. Noting also that the mid-1950s saw a rapid increase in the relative availability of hospital beds (Table 4 below), it rather looks as if plans were made to expand the supply of beds in the 1950s and of physicians in the 1960s (recalling that these are to a large degree policy variables in Canada) in anticipation of insurance. The mere observation of increased expenditure may be telling us more about supplier behavior than about increased demand, and we cannot resolve the issue without more detailed data.

The Response of the Hospital Industry—Administered Inflation

Expenditures on general and allied special hospitals dominate Canadian health spending. This sector is also the first to have been covered by universal health insurance. The dramatic increase in expenditures, from $280.4 million in 1953 to $2,594.6 million in 1971, or nearly 10 times, is the product of a combination of many factors that may or may not be associated with insurance coverage. It is thus of some interest to sort out the quantitative effects of population growth, utilization, general price inflation, sectoral

TABLE 4 Canadian Public Hospitals, Selected Operating Statistics, 1953–1971

	No. of Hospitals	No. of Beds	Beds per 000 Pop.	Expense per Patient Day	Patient Days per 000 Pop.	Admissions per 000 Pop.
1953	857	76224	5.13	12.47	1473.1	130.2
1954	870	79281	5.19	13.30	1532.7	132.0
1955	897	84761	5.40	14.05	1530.6	134.9
1956	909	86433	5.37	14.91	1578.1	141.4
1957	924	90154	5.43	16.11	1578.5	142.1
1958	955	94665	5.54	17.84	1624.1	143.0
1959	982	100059	5.72	18.88	1649.7	144.8
1960	972	101352	5.67	21.32	1643.2	146.1
1961	946	100506[a]	5.51[a]	23.10	1639.5	145.9
1962	964	106718	5.74	24.82	1721.0	149.7
1963	976	111165	5.87	26.87	1753.4	151.1
1964	996	114545	5.94	29.18	1762.4	152.8
1965	1011	117021	5.96	31.92	1778.3	152.2
1966	1027	122315	6.11	36.06	1793.9	152.0
1967	1036	126182	6.18	40.38	1806.2	151.6
1968	1043	129856	6.26	45.01	1850.8	155.1
1969	1040	132340	6.28	50.69	1854.9	156.4
1970	1039	135877	6.36	56.24	1880.2	161.1
1971	1043	138280	6.41	61.58	1896.6	164.9
% Change						
1953–1959	14.6	31.3	11.5	51.4	12.0	11.2
1959–1965	3.0	17.0	4.2	69.1	7.8	5.1
1965–1971	3.2	18.2	7.6	92.9	6.7	8.3
1953–1971	21.7	81.4	25.0	393.8	28.7	26.7

[a]The beds total for this year appears to be too low because of a classification error; neither beds nor beds per capita appears reliable.

price inflation, and changes in service mix over this period. It is not possible, owing to changes in the reporting procedures and reliability of data, to present a detailed picture of what happened, but several major trends are evident.

First of all, the 9.25 ratio of 1971 expenditures to 1953 is the outcome of a 45.3 per cent increase in population and an increase from $18.89 to $120.15 in expenditure per capita (Table 2). Moreover, patient days per thousand population rose from 1,473.1 in 1953 to 1,896.6 in 1971, or 28.7 per cent. Thus the expenditure per patient day implicit in these data increases from $12.82 to $63.35, or by 9.3 per cent per year. The reported data are $12.47 and $61.58 (Table 4; see also appendix), also yielding a 9.3 per cent increase annually. The increase of 13.2 per cent annually in hospital expenditure in Canada between 1953 and 1971 thus resolves into increases of 2.1 per cent in population, 1.4 per cent in patient day utilization, and 9.3 per cent in expenditure per patient day.

This increase has, of course, several sources. Ideally, one would like to trace out its shifts through the full accounting detail provided in present-day hospital statistics; but that would be a major paper in itself and in any case could not be carried back to 1953 because the detail is missing. Certain clear trends, however, emerge. In 1953 the cost per patient day of $12.47 was divided into $7.20 gross wages and salaries, 51¢ medical and surgical supplies, 53¢ drugs, and $4.23 other supplies and expense. By 1971 these components were $41.82, $1.93, $1.78, and $16.06, or had increased by 10.3 per cent, 7.7 per cent, 7.0 per cent, and 7.7 per cent annually. Wages and salaries rose from 57.7 per cent of the hospital budget to 67.9 per cent.[22]

The wage and salary component can be split into "price" and "quantity" components (if we assume that hours are a homogeneous commodity) since in 1953 9.18 hours were worked per patient day and in 1971 this figure had risen to 13.29 paid hours per patient day. A difficulty is that in 1953, 1.62 hours per patient day were worked by student nurses or interns who were then paid little or nothing. If these are treated as part of hours worked in both years, the increase in wages and salaries is made up of a 44.8 per cent increase in hours worked and a 303.8 per cent increase in wages and salaries per hour worked (from 78¢ to $3.14 at an average of 8.1 per cent per year).

Comparing these shifts with general trends in the Canadian economy, we find that over the period 1953–1971 the Consumer Price Index rose 2.2 per cent annually, the G.N.E. deflator rose 2.5

per cent, and average weekly wages and salaries (industrial composite) were up 5.0 per cent. Price indexes are not available for the various components of hospital expenditure, now or in 1953, but if we assumed that prices of hospital goods rose more or less in line with the rest of the economy, we would estimate quantity increases of 5.4 per cent annually for medical and surgical supplies, 4.7 per cent for drugs, 5.4 per cent for supplies and other expense, and about 2.1 per cent annually for labor input. These figures should not be taken too seriously, however, as no real price indexes exist. Still, they suggest a tendency for real resource use in hospitals to have increased fastest in supplies and drugs, less rapidly in labor input. The single largest component of the cost increase is clearly the change in levels of remuneration of hospital workers.

If we take the increase in average weekly wages of 139.2 per cent and assume that because of changes in hours worked per week a "true" hourly index might have increased 150 per cent, then assuming that hospital workers had merely moved up in line with workers generally, the wage bill in 1971 would have been $25.92 per patient day instead of $41.82. Out of expense per patient day of $61.58 in 1971, $15.90, or 25.8 per cent, is attributable to the increase in average hourly wages of hospital workers *relative* to all other workers. This observation, of course, says nothing at all about the division of this increase into differences in skill mix, "catch-up" effects left over from the period of charity hospitals, or pure inflation.

There are, of course, certain other effects that one can look for in the longer-term data. One might expect that changes in the pattern of the care episode, or in the mix of hospitals examined, might affect these results. Yet in fact such shifts in the relation between patient day and care episode have not had much effect. Average lengths of stay per separation and occupancy rates have both fluctuated somewhat, but stays were 10.9 days in 1953, 11.3 in 1971, and occupancy rates were 81.2 per cent and 81.3 per cent. Corresponding to these sluggish movements, admissions per bed fell from 26.3 to 25.7. Thus changes in patient day costs are clearly not explicable by changes in short-run capacity utilization.

Changes in hospital class of activity are a bit more complex. General and allied special hospitals include chronic and convalescent, specialty, and teaching hospitals, all of which exhibit relatively different activity patterns and cost experience. Chronic and convalescent hospitals are too small a portion of the total for shifts in their share to affect costs; for general (acute care) hospitals alone costs per day rose from $12.79 to $65.58, or 9.5 per cent annually. It is more difficult, however, to sort out the effects on patient day costs of growth in educational and outpatient expense since the departmental distribution of reported expenditure in 1953 was still relatively loose. Separate expenditures were reported for nursing schools; outpatients, emergency, and social service; laboratory; and radiology, the latter two departments having a significant proportion of outpatient work. These groups accounted for 1.76 per cent, 1.05 per cent, 2.49 per cent, and 3.34 per cent of total hospital expenditure. The difficulty is that 17.44 per cent of total expenditure is "unattributed" in 1953; if that component were equally spread over all departments, the above percentages become 2.13 per cent, 1.27 per cent, 3.02 per cent, and 4.05 per cent.

By 1971 nursing education had increased to 3.41 per cent of total budget, and total education was up to 6.48 per cent. If one assumed that education costs other than nursing were zero in 1953, the increase in direct educational costs per patient day would be from 27¢ to $3.99, or an increase of nearly 15 times. But in fact this is too small a budget component to matter, patient day expense net of education and special research projects is reported as $58.44 in 1971 compared with $12.20 expense net of nursing schools in 1953. Even assuming medical education and research at zero in 1953, the increase in expense net of education is 9.1 per cent annually. This line of argument, however, ignores the high indirect costs associated with education. Thus one could be underestimating the effects of expanding the educational sector.

In 1971, teaching hospitals of 500 beds or more had expenses per patient day of $83.70 if full teaching and $67.56 if partial teaching, whereas in 1953, all 500+bed hospitals had costs per patient day of $15.93. If we assume that 500-bed full-teaching hospitals in 1971 are roughly equivalent to 500+bed hospitals in 1953, it appears that costs have risen somewhat faster for this group—9.7 per cent annually compared with 9.3 per cent. But the difference is not large and is probably biased upward since not all 500+bed hospitals are full-teaching. Nor has there been any major shift in the numbers of hospitals with full or partial teaching programs, and the share of such hospitals in total patient activity has not expanded significantly. Hence we may tentatively conclude that although educational programs are undoubtedly much more expensive to operate than their direct costs would indicate, the *increase* in costs from 1953 to 1971 does not seem to be traceable to the expansion of educational programs.

Turning to outpatient clinics (which include short stay patients or day care surgery where relevant) we find that in 1971, outpatient clinics, emergency, and social service account for $1.82 per patient day. This compares with 16¢ per patient day in 1953, confirming the widespread view that such activity has increased in importance substantially faster than the regular inpatient service. These data also show clearly, however, that quantitatively the effects of this increase are trivial. Even after due allowance is made for indirect costs and overheads associated with an outpatient department, it appears that this sort of activity, like education, does not affect the conclusions reached above.

The above discussion suggests that the reported increases in expenditures per patient day really do reflect shifts in the cost of providing inpatient services, rather than being a result of shifts in the heterogeneous mix of hospital activities that are reflected in "per diems." To relate these increases to changes in insurance coverage, we must examine the behavior of expenses by subperiods and draw on some additional data on wages and hours worked. For this purpose we have divided the eighteen-year span into three equal subperiods: a pre-insurance phase 1953–1959, a "digestion" phase, 1959–1965, and a post-insurance phase, 1965–1971. The initial period is not really pre-insurance, since several provincial plans were in operation during that period; but the two largest provinces, Ontario and Quebec, began their plans in 1959 and 1961, respectively, so that 1959 rather than 1958 may be treated as a transitional year. This is supported by the observation that cost per day rose at an average rate of 7.2 per cent annually from 1953 to 1959 but only 5.8 per cent from 1958 to 1959. In 1960 it took off, to 12.9 per cent.

In these three subperiods, costs per day rose at average rates of 7.2 per cent, 9.2 per cent, and 11.6 per cent. Relative to the Consumer Price Index, these figures reduce to 5.6 per cent, 7.5 per cent, and 7.6 per cent. There is of course no particular rationale for using the CPI as a deflator, except that no hospital price index exists. This pattern suggests that the apparent cost surge after 1966 is in fact tied in with the general rate of inflation, but that a break in behavior did occur at the time national insurance was introduced. Hospital costs per day were rising substantially faster than general inflation rates prior to national health insurance, but their relative increase speeded up both during and after the period of introduction of the public plans. The fact that the share of personal income going to hospitals increased much faster in the 1959–1961 period than subsequently, in spite of the observations that both utilization and (price-adjusted) costs per day increases are relatively similar from 1959–1965 to 1965–1971, may be traced to the recession in

1961 that held down personal income growth. Whether national insurance served to insulate the hospital sector against this downturn, or whether hospital expenditures would have climbed through the recession without public insurance, we do not know.

What is fairly clear from Table 4 is that national insurance did not have any observable effect on utilization. Patient days and admissions per thousand population rose almost twice as fast annually in the pre-insurance period 1953–1959 and have generally been slowing down since the public plans were introduced. Increases continue, but are now less than 1 per cent per year. If not correlated with insurance, utilization does move very closely with bed availability. It seems in fact to be responding to new bed construction, partially stimulated by a federal building subsidy program started in 1948. This program provided a fixed dollar grant per bed, so was progressively eroded by inflation and finally terminated in 1970, although it had some effect in the 1950s.

More information emerges if we look at the components of cost per day by subperiods. The share of total expense accounted for by gross wages and salaries, and its relation to hours worked, is as follows:

| | Per Patient Day | | | | | | | |
	Gross Salaries and Wages	% Change	% of Total Budget	Hours Worked	% Change	Implicit Wage	% Change	Relative Wage Gain %
1953	$ 7.20		57.7	9.2		$0.78		
1959	11.72	62.8	62.1	10.6	15.2	1.11	42.3	11.4
1965	20.77	77.2	65.1	13.0	22.6	1.60	44.1	16.2
1971	41.82	101.3	67.9	13.3	2.2	3.14	96.3	29.9

Relative wage gain is the percentage increase in hospital wages relative to the average weekly wage (industrial composite); it measures the improvement in the relative income status of hospital workers.

This table suggests that there were some differences in behavior over these subperiods. The share of hospital budget going to wages and salaries has been rising but at a diminishing rate; the relative earnings of hospital workers have grown at an accelerating rate; and inputs of hours worked have first increased rapidly and then slowed down. In fact, hours worked per patient day rose after 1965 and then fell to its present level.

This suggests a behavior pattern of a rapidly expanding hospital sector in the 1950s, perhaps driven by the new funds made available through private and provincial insurance plans. Hospital workers were making income gains, labor inputs were rising, federal funds were adding new beds, and physicians were generating patients to fill them. Since the nonlabor budget share rose from $5.27 to $7.16 over this period, or 35.9 per cent, and prices generally rose only 9.5 per cent, it would appear that nonlabor inputs rose even faster than labor inputs. But our lack of any sort of hospital nonlabor price index is a hindrance here.

During the introduction of national insurance, all cost increases speeded up whereas utilization increases slowed down. Labor input increased 22.6 per cent compared with 15.2 per cent in the previous six years; relative hospital workers' wages rose 16.2 per cent faster than the general wage rate, and nonwage expense rose from $7.16 per day to $11.15, or 55.7 per cent, compared with general price increases of 9.7 per cent. It would appear that the initial impact of insurance was to increase substantially the real inputs to the hospital sector as well as to increase slightly the rate of increase in hospital workers' income status.

In the third phase, 1965–1971, increasing rates of cost increase have begun to generate official concern and reaction. Utilization increases are slowing down still more and labor inputs per patient day are nearly static. Nonlabor inputs have risen from $11.15 to $19.76, or 77.2 per cent; relative to the general price level increase of 24.2 per cent, this amounts to a 42.7 per cent increase (compared with 24.1 per cent, 1953–1959, and 41.9 per cent, 1959–1965), so it may be that nonlabor inputs are still accelerating. But it may also be that their prices have outstripped the CPI—we do not know. What is most striking about the 1965–1971 period is the dramatic increase in hospital workers' wages per paid hour—96.3 per cent, or 29.9 per cent faster than wages generally. This amounts to a rate of wage status gain of 4.5 per cent annually, sustained for six years. On a base of $20.77, 29.9 per cent yields $6.21; or 10 per cent of total hospital costs is attributable to the relative wage gains of hospital workers during the last six years. Over the whole span, if hospital wages had just kept pace with industry generally, they would have risen to $1.87 per hour.

Of course, whether this is attributable to national health insurance is another question. Relative wage gains did speed up during the period when insurance was being introduced but became much more rapid in the later period. One could argue that this is a delayed effect of insurance—it took time for employees to absorb the implications of cost-pass-through and unionization for them to apply the lesson. On the basis of this argument, insurance shifted the rate of expansion of hospital costs to a new higher trend, and workers learned to exploit this fact. But one could also argue that in an industry with inelastic demand and growing private insurance, cost-pass-through would have been discovered regardless of national insurance. Canadian experience alone cannot answer this question; some U.S. comparisons might be helpful. It is clear, however, that if future cost increases are to be moderated, some way of establishing appropriate relative incomes for hospital workers must be found. If they try to play catch-up with physicians, the cost inflation is only beginning!

It is, of course, true that the above line of argument still has not identified and pinned down the process of hospital expenditure increase in a fully satisfactory manner; there exists the major issue of shifts in labor force composition. It may well be that hospitals respond to insurance, not just by adding more personnel and machines, but by adding more complex and highly trained personnel. Thus the wage change series might include a significant increase in human capital input rather than merely input price change.

It turns out that this is a remarkably difficult proposition to test, not because of conceptual problems, but because numerous changes in reporting systems and a very detailed but constantly changing specification of the hospital labor force make the reconstruction of a set of consistent historical series a major research project in itself. This project is beyond the bounds of a survey paper such as this one. It cries out to be done as a federal research study.[23] However, a bit of indirect evidence can be brought to bear on the problem.

First of all, despite the attention given to complex diagnostic procedures and highly specialized forms of treatment, nursing services and general support staff (dietary, laundry, administrative) are still the backbone of the hospital. A series of longitudinal studies of particular classes of hospital manpower over the period 1961–1968 shows that the professional and technical classes of employees (radiologists, pathologists, radiology and laboratory technicians, psychologists, social workers, medical record librarians, pharmacists, dieticians, and physical and occupational therapists) increased their share of total hospital employment from 3.44 per cent to 4.68 per cent of total full-time employment in this field. The percentage increase is large (36 per cent increase in an expanding industry) but the absolute numbers are too small to affect total wage movements. Their share in part-time employment also rose, from 5.67 per cent to 6.32 per cent, but part-time employees are only about 10 per cent of the total.

In the same period, full-time graduate nurses and nursing assistants rose from 6.42 per cent and 19.00 per cent of total full-time employment to 8.90 per cent and 21.60 per cent, a smaller change (20 per cent) but a more significant quantitative shift. Thus, a picture emerges of a proportional increase in nursing and nursing assistant staff and a corresponding reduction in relative employment of the unskilled "other" category. It is thus plausible to argue that in fact the human capital input per hour worked did rise somewhat over the period under consideration.

But this change, it turns out, does not appear to explain the wage shift. The reason is that average wages for nursing personnel generally (graduates and assistants) are not markedly different from those of other staff. In the first half of 1971, nurses on short-term units averaged $3.11 per hour and on long-term, $2.86 per hour. These made up 80 per cent of all nursing hours in public hospitals. By comparison, averages in general services were: administration $3.28, dietary $3.36, medical records $2.76, housekeeping $2.21, plant operation and security $3.28, and laundry and linen $2.19. Thus the pattern of wage differentials is simply not large enough to explain a major shift in the average from a change of 10 per cent or even 20 per cent. We may conclude that shifting personnel mix has had very little to do with the overall pattern of wage inflation.

Two other points deserve comment before leaving this issue. Part of the wage increase has clearly been attributable to the phasing out of the unpaid or almost unpaid workforce of student nurses. In 1953, student nurses, nursing assistants, and interns accounted for 1.62 out of 9.18 hours worked per patient day. Yet even if we pulled *all* of these out of the base for computing wage and salary cost in 1953, we divide wage and salary cost per patient day of $7.20 by 7.56 to arrive at an average wage of 95¢ and an increase in average wages from 1953 to 1971 of 232 per cent. Although substantially below 304 per cent, this figure is also well above the approximately 140 per cent increase in general wage levels—on the *maximum* possible allowance for the effects of eliminating unpaid or low-paid student labor. And of course student labor is not yet fully phased out.

Finally, one should note that the elimination of student labor has been associated in the latter part of the period with the closing of hospital nursing schools. Thus the relative constancy of hours per patient day masks a reduction in education hours and a continued rise in patient care hours. The hospitals have responded to budgetary pressures by shedding functions; thus the experience of stable hours input during this period may be only a temporary trend break.

A report recently prepared by the Health Economics and Statistics Branch of the Department of National Health and Welfare (*Sources of Increase in Budget Review Hospital Expenditures in Canada, 1961 to 1971*, Ottawa: December, 1973), essentially confirms this picture in the post-insurance period. From this report we see that from 1961 to 1971 total hospital expenditures rose 13.7 per cent annually, patient days rising 3.0 per cent and costs per day rising 10.3 per cent. The authors of the report also conclude that outpatient workload shifts were not large enough to affect the pattern of expenditures and that morbidity shifts in patient diagnostic mix may be important but cannot be identified.

Sources of expenditure increase are identified by department, but unfortunately only expenditure on supplies and other nonlabor expense is so allocated. Gross salaries and wages, drugs, and medical and surgical supplies are each treated as aggregates. But the labor cost per patient day is shown to have increased over the period 1961–1971 substantially faster than the nonlabor cost (11.2 per cent annually against 8.5 per cent) and to account for roughly three-quarters of the increase in cost per patient day compared with one-quarter for nonlabor cost. During this period, paid hours of work per patient day rose 2.1 per cent annually and labor cost per paid hour rose 8.7 per cent. Thus wage increase accounts for about seven-eighths of labor cost increase per patient day. This source is shown to have accounted for over 50 per cent of total expenditure increase in budget-review hospitals, even including effects of population growth and higher utilization. The possible effects of shifts in labor force composition in this process are touched on, and shifts are described in general terms, but the quantitative effects of such shifts are unknown. The relative significance of labor cost per hour as a source of expenditure increase over the period is accelerating, but much of this can be accounted for by general inflation in the economy. The rate of *relative* wage gain is, however, somewhat faster in the later period; hospital hourly wages as reported in *Sources of Increase* rose 8.1 per cent faster than general industry wages, 1961–1965, and 21.3 per cent faster, 1965–1971. This may be partly a result of the timing of the phase out of nursing education—the impact of the shift away from hospital nursing education and toward more medical education on hospital total costs and average hourly wages has not yet been analyzed. In analyzing the response of hospital expenditure to insurance, however, the message of the report parallels that of this paper—wage inflation in the hospital sector is the main source of increase and the timing does not particularly correspond to the extension of insurance, the expansion of utilization, or even the expansion of employment. The most rapid *relative* wage increases have come in the late 1960s, when paid hours per patient day have been static and both population and utilization increase have slowed down.

Summing up, a picture seems to emerge of rapid increases in hospital capacity and utilization as a precursor to national health insurance. During the pre-insurance period hospital inputs, wages, and costs were rising rapidly, and hospital relative wages also were moving up. Private insurance may have fed this process, but government insurance was more likely a result of it. This would follow insofar as expenditure increases prior to the national plan increased burdens on the uninsured and further restricted their access. Moreover, provincial and private insurance plans came under increasing fiscal strain. Most of the discussion surrounding the national hospital plan focused on its role as a vehicle for moving more resources into the hospital sector (it worked!) and thus was a response to increasing expenditure burdens. The initial insurance period saw a jump in hospital expenses, as hospitals appear to have accelerated their expansion of paid hours per patient day. Hospital wages rose at about the same rate as prior to insurance, although their relative status improved faster. The picture does not suggest a strong demand-induced wage inflation resulting from expanded employment. Finally, the very rapid expansion in hospital expenditures in the mid-sixties triggered a bureaucratic response that has been fairly successful in containing increases in labor inputs. But the problem of relative hospital wages continues unaffected, as hospital employees seem to be improving their wage status at an accelerating rate. In the absence of a detailed job breakdown in the industry, of course, it is not possible to say whether they are still "catching-up"; the industrial composite weekly wage of $137.64 in 1971 divided by 40 yields an "average" hourly wage of $3.44, which is still above the hospital average of $3.14. But neither wage rate is skill adjusted or experience adjusted. In any case, it is clear that present bargaining and budget-setting procedures in hospitals do not approximate a competitive market process! Thus it is far from clear that continuation or completion of catch-up would have any relevance to future trends. The problem of hospital wage determination is still unresolved.

Policy Responses to Hospital Cost Inflation

This subject leads into the issues surrounding hospital reimbursement and budgetary control. We have argued that the problems of hospital cost inflation in Canada have little to do with utilization, insurance-induced or otherwise, but rather a lot to do with increases in earnings of hospital workers and secondarily with increases in real resource use per patient day (whether "quality" upgrading by managers, pressure for more hands to lighten the load from employees, or demands for further services by physicians). The process of budgetary control has not been particularly successful in promoting efficiency and/or containing costs.

As mentioned above, the initial intention of the Canadian hospital insurance system was to provide a method of paying whatever expenses the hospital system generated. Insofar as a policy toward appropriate levels of expenditure existed, it seemed to involve encouraging increase; the point of a federal program was to mobilize more resources, to lower financial barriers to utilization, and to maintain or increase standards of care. Consequently, the process of budget review did not initially emphasize efficiency or cost control; and when it became apparent in the late 1960s that hospital expenditures were taking an accelerating share of national resources and that "something" should be done, neither the review and reimbursement process nor the statistical framework that surrounded it proved adequate for the task. After more than five years of discussion and study, they still are not.

The budget review process varies in detail from province to province, and in fact from year to year in a given province, depending on the state of the provincial treasury. For most of the first decade of insurance, provinces employed some variant of a line-item budget approval prior to the budget year, combined with a review and settlement at year's end.[24] The prospective budget is based on an expected patient day load, and the ratio of total budget to forecast load creates a synthetic per diem that is used as a basis for distributing the hospital's budget over the year but is not an independent price in the sense that if actual load is above or below forecast, the total budget will not be adjusted proportionately. If there are significant deviations from forecast, partial adjustments may be made at year's end. But both agency and hospital are well aware of the difference between average and marginal costs per day, at least in this context.[25]

The patient day forecast is generally based on the preceding year's experience adjusted for any known special factors in or outside each hospital. It tends to be quite accurate. It is not defined in terms of diagnostic mix, although certain special subpopulations (such as renal dialysis cases) would be forecast separately. For each hospital, expected procedure workloads and input requirements by category are then developed from this forecast; the particular procedure forecasts thus implicitly embody some judgement about diagnostic and severity mix based on the past experience of the hospital. But the judgement never becomes explicit. Once physical requirements, personnel, supplies, and equipment by category are approved, the final budget will then depend on negotiated wage scales for the positions in each hospital's approved establishment. Formally, these negotiations take place between hospital managements (on a provincial basis) and provincial unions or associations. But since wage costs are usually passed directly to the provincial reimbursing agency, it is not entirely clear what besides public interest stiffens the negotiators for management.[26] This may be one explanation for the unusually rapid wage increases in hospitals.

The review process has required provincial reimbursing agencies to accumulate a great deal of detailed information about each hospital, much of it informal. In Ontario, the Hospital Services Commission appoints financial representatives, each responsible for several hospitals, whose task is to work within the hospital as the Commission's agent during the preparation of a budget but to act as the hospital's representative in steering the budget through the Commission. In B.C., the Hospital Insurance Service maintains a budget "model" of each hospital (which is *not* revealed to that hospital!) which it uses in evaluating the annual submissions. Thus the reimbursement process is very information-intensive.

The problem, however, is that none of this information is organized in a way linking expenditure with output. Neither hospital nor reimburser knows total costs of inpatient care in a given hospital (except for hospitals with no outpatient or educational activity) since all data is based on inputs. Direct laundry costs per pound processed, or nursing ward costs per patient day, can be calculated, but no allocation of overhead or indirect costs is carried out. If a hospital's diagnostic mix shifts, or if its patient day load and/or length of stay changes, the reimbursing agency may know in which direction the budget should shift, but never by how much. Thus hospitals are exhorted to lower length of stay. They reply that this would raise their per diem, and that the paying agency would not approve all the necessary increase. The paying agency says that it will approve the *necessary* increase, but no more. Yet no one knows what is necessary. The same problem arises if patient day forecasts are over- or under-run; no one knows by how much a marginal patient day costs less than average. Arbitrary rules of thumb are used. Nor can comparisons across hospitals be made with any confidence, because "similarity" embodies no adjustment for differences in diagnostic mix. Everyone knows this is important; and this has been shown analytically,[27] but no one is sure what the appropriate adjustment should be. Thus similarity is judged on proxies such as size, location, or educational role. The process of negotiation and budget determination for the largest hospitals in each province is one of the financial responsibilities of senior financial and health officials in the provincial government and is given appropriate attention and weight; but the data from which the province might determine what it is buying simply do not exist. As long as budgets are based on levels of inputs, and inputs cannot be associated in any comprehensive way with outputs (in terms of cases treated by type or students trained), budgeters fall back on incrementalism (last year plus X per cent) and add in the special requests generated by medical technology and the relatively loose wage negotiation process. Hence the statistical outcomes mentioned above.

As the inability of budget review to limit cost escalation has become more apparent, public policy has responded along two main lines. Efforts have been made to encourage greater efficiency in hospitals and to reduce the size of the inpatient hospital sector by substituting other forms of care. Both policies have tended to move the problem out of the hospital sphere and into the realm of medical practice organization; neither has come to grips with the ballooning incomes of hospital workers.

The "management" orientation is reflected in Volume II of the 1969 *Task Force Report* dealing with hospital services. Much was made of the poor management practices in hospitals, and the recommendations covered the range of training (and even licencing!) better hospital managers, giving them more scope, and creating incentives for efficiency. Hospital reimbursement has correspondingly moved toward global budgeting, using line-item input reports as a guide to setting global amounts but giving administrators more discretion in allocating expenditures within total budgets. Experiments have been tried with fixing annual target budgets and allowing managers to share under-runs and use their share for capital expansion or other projects—the incentive reimbursement approach. It seems fair to say, however, that the managerial approach has been relatively unsuccessful for several reasons.

First, the limited possibilities of comparison across hospitals with existing data make reliable identification of "good" and "bad" management impossible. Moreover, detailed analysis suggests that there is very little variance across hospitals in *relative* efficiency within each province; the style of medical practice and the pattern of reimbursement jointly determine most of hospital behavior.[28] The administrator may not have much discretion. Even if one could identify desirable behavior and if the administrator had enough control over style of care delivery to do what the reimburser desired, creation of incentives is almost impossible. Reimbursement incentives work only if a dollar of "profit" (shared cost under-runs) is worth more to management than a dollar of operational expense. In a nonprofit industry whose capital expansion needs are met out of a separate budget on the basis of regional and political needs, this is not so. Direct incentives to managers themselves are likewise ruled out as long as hospitals are nominally controlled by independent boards of trustees—the careers of administrators and/or their levels of remuneration are only indirectly influenced by payment agencies. Rewarding efficiency by "promotion" to a larger hospital is not possible. And finally, everyone knows that hospitals cannot be allowed to go bankrupt. The penalties for inadequate performance can never be absolute; at worst one can fire the administrator. But this weakens any ability he might have to run a tight ship even if he wanted to—the organization itself is never at risk. The focus on improved management has not been abandoned—it is still obviously true that better management can yield more health care for a given budget—but as a technique for overall cost containment it is of less interest.[29]

Attention thus shifts to ways of reducing hospital utilization—by providing institutional alternatives such as convalescent care, day care surgery, home care; by shifting medical practice away from fee-for-service practice and toward salaried group practice or other arrangements; or by simply closing beds. All of these efforts are currently underway; and although it is too early to make any final judgement about their success, certain patterns have become apparent.

The institutional alternatives approach has the advantage of being supported by medical as well as economic opinion; the deleterious effects of excessive hospitalization on the patient are well recognized and are often more important than economic objectives in initiating new programs. Particularly in the pediatric area, it has been demonstrated that significant medical improvements as well as economic savings can be achieved through day care surgery units or ambulatory medical treatment facilities.[30] The main problems with this approach are twofold. First, the tendency for utilization to rise to match supply ensures that unless new facilities are balanced by withdrawal of old, total costs rise. If a home care program or convalescent beds move less severely ill patients out of acute hospitals, new acute care patients flow in. Moreover, discharge from lower intensity facilities is more difficult. Canadian experience parallels Feldstein's judgement in the U.S.;[31] provinces with well-developed convalescent care systems, like Alberta, have relatively higher hospital costs per capita.

A further problem arises because of the structure of reimbursement. Ambulatory alternatives to inpatient care have tended to be based in hospitals. But hospitals' budgets are geared to inpatient care; and administrators tend to view reduced days of care as threatening reimbursements. Thus a day surgery unit that eliminates a two-day stay minor surgery case is perceived as "costing" the hospital two per diems. The unit price or reimbursement received for an ambulatory case is less than would have been received for a corresponding inpatient. As the hospital's inpatient base shrinks, and its ambulatory load expands, it must negotiate (legitimately) ever higher per diems, and this is not easy to do. Reimbursing agencies see the problem differently. They see *total* inpatient utilization failing to fall as ambulatory care expands and they are less willing to negotiate higher rates. The crucial aspects of the problem are the responsiveness of utilization to facilities and the inability of either agency or hospital to quantify the full unit costs associated with either inpatient or ambulatory episodes. If episodes could be accurately priced and reimbursed independently of treatment mode, the process of moving patients out of inpatient care would be strongly encouraged.

The utilization response, in Canada as in the U.S., has been traced to the mode of organization of medical practice. Evidence exists that physician groups paid on a salary basis use substantially less hospital care for their patients than does the fee-for-service sector.[32] This has led numerous observers and some government study groups to recommend reorganization of medical practice into community health centers (now a very elastic term with features parallelling HMO's) as ways of moderating hospital costs.[33] But there is general agreement that this is a long, slow process. Several provincial governments are committed to the idea in principle, but organized medicine is strongly opposed to modification of the present system.

As for the most simple-minded approach, closing beds, this has been adopted as official or unofficial policy in several provinces. "Standards" of numbers of "needed" acute care beds per thousand population, which never were based on anything very much, are being revised downward; and provincial governments are mounting increased resistance to providing capital for new hospitals or hospital expansion. This tactic is of course easiest in provinces with rapidly growing populations such as Ontario and B.C., but actual closure of hospitals is politically extremely difficult. (The first province to adopt bed limitation as an official tactic was, however, Quebec, after the Castonguay Report stated that at least a third of the province's beds were unnecessary.) This approach probably holds the greatest promise of cost moderation in the near term, whereas long-run efforts at control will probably depend on reorganization of medical practice and some improved method of hospital wage determination.

Medical Insurance and Medical Expenditures—Cause or Effect

The question of reorganizing medical practice leads directly into consideration of the impact of Medicare on service supply. Statistical evaluation of this impact is hampered by the fact that the program is so recent, 1971 being the first full year of national coverage for which complete data are available. Moreover, in each of the provinces private nonprofit plans pre-dated the public program and provided a significant degree of insurance coverage.[34] The introduction of insurance is not a clear-cut, point-in-time phenomenon.

Table 5 shows, however, that when data are examined at the provincial level the timing of the public plans is quite apparent. The proportion of personal income in each province spent on physicians' services takes an abrupt jump away from its previous pattern in each province either in the year the public plan was introduced (underlined) or immediately after. The Saskatchewan picture is of course muddled by the physician strike of 1962 and its aftermath and Alberta physicians seem to show a degree of anticipation, but elsewhere the change is very systematic. Whether this is a new plateau share of personal income or a new upward trend is too soon to tell (total Canadian personal income was up 10.4 per cent in 1971, so the apparent leveling off of the "physician share" may be exogenous). But it is clear that in each province public insurance was associated with significant increases in the share of personal

TABLE 5 **Physician Expenditures as a Percentage of Personal Income, Canada and Provinces, 1957-1971**

	B.C.	Alta.	Sask.	Man.	Ont.	Que.	N.B.	N.S.	P.E.I.	Nfld.	Can.
1957	1.25	1.17	1.40	1.37	1.10	.96	1.10	1.20	1.33	.79	1.11
1958	1.36	1.16	1.35	1.36	1.16	1.04	1.16	1.18	1.44	.86	1.16
1959	1.44	1.18	1.35	1.46	1.18	1.05	1.08	1.22	1.33	.86	1.18
1960	1.48	1.25	1.35	1.33	1.19	1.05	1.19	1.26	1.40	.97	1.20
1961	1.52	1.30	1.69	1.60	1.27	1.15	1.27	1.30	1.34	.95	1.20
1962	1.48	1.31	1.03	1.47	1.23	1.16	1.20	1.29	1.19	.93	1.24
1963	1.43	1.27	1.45	1.47	1.31	1.23	1.27	1.25	1.42	1.00	1.30
1964	1.49	1.32	1.65	1.41	1.35	1.21	1.26	1.31	1.29	1.04	1.33
1965	1.44	1.31	1.48	1.46	1.36	1.22	1.25	1.31	1.35	.97	1.33
1966	1.49	1.27	1.41	1.46	1.33	1.23	1.17	1.33	1.29	.95	1.32
1967	1.48	1.45	1.57	1.43	1.39	1.23	1.30	1.27	1.29	.96	1.36
1968	1.56	1.67	1.45	1.43	1.45	1.26	1.29	1.41	1.33	1.12	1.42
1969	1.63	1.62	1.52	1.67	1.48	1.28	1.31	1.51	1.49	1.46	1.46
1970	1.73	1.76	1.75	1.90	1.60	1.24	1.31	1.75	1.33	1.56	1.55
1971	1.67	1.82	1.58	1.78	1.66	1.71	1.48	1.75	1.86	1.51	1.68
% Change											
1957–1964	19.2	12.8	17.9	2.9	22.7	26.0	14.6	9.2	−3.0	31.7	19.8
1964–1971	12.1	37.9	−4.2	26.2	23.0	41.3	17.5	33.6	44.2	45.2	26.3
1957–1971	33.6	55.6	12.9	29.9	50.9	78.1	34.6	45.8	39.9	91.1	51.4

NOTE: Data of entry to Medicare underlined.

income received by physicians. (Table 5 also shows that this increase was superimposed on a general uptrend which may have been leveling off in the mid-sixties.)

Why this was so is less clear. In conventional economics, of course, the answer is obvious—lower prices to consumers, greater demand, greater utilization, and higher prices charged by suppliers. And undoubtedly some of these changes occurred. But tracing them down is not all that easy. First of all, list prices of physician services did not particularly respond to public insurance. Table 6 contains provincial fee schedule indexes (after Medicare the index reports benefits paid by the provincial agency) compiled by the Department of National Health and Welfare since December 1963 and compares these indexes with total expenditure and total expenditure per capita.[35] Expenditure data are standardized to the same base as prices in 1964; no average fee level for 1963 is available. This table shows, first, that both total expenditure and

TABLE 6 Indexes of Fee/Benefit Schedules (annual averages), and Corresponding Indexes of Total Expenditure and Total Expenditure per Capita on Physicians' Services, Canada and Provinces, 1963–1973

	B.C.	Alta.	Sask.	Man.	Ont.	N.B.	N.S.	P.E.I.	Nfld.	Can. (Ex. Que.)[a]
Dec. 1963										
FB	100	100	100	100	100	100	100	100	100	100
1964										
FB	103.7	101.8	100.0	100.0	100.0	100.0	100.0	112.1	100.0	100.6
TX	103.7	101.8	100.0	100.0	100.0	100.0	100.0	112.1	100.0	100.6
TXPC	103.7	101.8	100.0	100.0	100.0	100.0	100.0	112.1	100.0	100.6
1965										
FB	103.7	104.2	100.0	100.0	105.9	100.0	100.0	112.1	100.0	103.6
TX	111.6	112.5	104.4	110.9	110.9	108.0	107.2	125.6	106.0	109.0
TXPC	108.3	111.0	103.4	110.4	108.5	107.4	107.0	125.6	105.1	107.2
1966										
FB	103.7	107.6	100.0	100.0	107.8	112.7	100.0	112.6	100.0	105.4
TX	130.3	124.8	113.9	119.3	121.8	112.4	120.0	132.5	116.1	120.7
TXPC	121.3	121.9	112.2	119.0	116.2	111.4	119.6	132.5	113.8	116.4
1967										
FB	114.0	116.6	100.9	111.0	117.0	125.4	105.7	112.7	105.5	114.0
TX	143.9	155.0	119.2	130.3	140.9	135.8	126.5	146.8	131.3	137.8
TXPC	129.2	148.5	117.2	129.9	131.2	133.7	125.4	146.8	127.1	130.2

1968										
FB	114.0	124.3	113.1	133.1	120.0	125.4	122.7	129.1	116.7	120.1
TX	165.8	199.2	124.7	144.1	163.0	149.7	153.4	171.1	169.7	160.1
TXPC	144.6	186.7	122.2	142.5	149.0	146.2	150.6	169.5	162.0	148.7
1969										
FB	121.1	127.2	124.1	133.1	128.2	138.5	122.7	129.1	116.7	126.6
TX	196.9	217.0	136.4	180.8	186.2	167.7	183.0	207.0	243.9	184.7
TXPC	166.8	198.8	134.1	177.5	167.5	163.4	177.7	203.3	229.2	168.8
1970										
FB	121.1	131.2	128.1	133.1	130.8	138.5	122.7	147.3	116.7	128.7
TX	225.5	254.5	146.3	216.9	219.6	182.4	230.4	206.6	290.1	216.1
TXPC	184.9	228.1	146.6	212.1	193.1	177.7	220.9	204.7	271.0	194.0
1971										
FB	121.1	135.2	133.9	133.1	134.7	138.5	122.7	147.3	115.1	131.3
TX	247.2	294.0	159.8	226.3	249.8	228.1	248.4	310.1	314.0	243.1
TXPC	197.7	258.3	162.3	219.9	215.4	219.7	237.2	301.7	290.5	214.8
1972										
FB	126.3	135.4	137.8	133.1	136.7	138.5	130.0	151.2	115.3	133.7
1973										
FB	134.6	138.0	143.0	133.1	136.7	138.5	136.2	152.5	124.9	136.9
Dec.1973										
FB	137.5	143.1	143.0	133.1	136.7	138.5	137.4	152.5	127.3	137.2

NOTE: Data of entry to Medicare underlined.

aQuebec had no fee schedule for general practitioners prior to Medicare.

total expenditure per capita rose steadily year by year in each province whether or not list fees rose. Fee increases accelerated the process; their absence did not inhibit it. Of course, much of this is attributable to improving collections ratios over the period, and probably also greater adherence to fee schedules. But this pattern of behavior persists after Medicare is introduced. The mechanism that drives expenditure clearly does not operate through listed fees alone (or even primarily), and since listed fees are now pegged to actual fees it does not seem to operate through actual fees either. Unfortunately we have no data at all to adjust collections ratios and approximate actual fee movements prior to Medicare.

In Table 7 the same point emerges at the aggregate level. Here the nine-province fee benefit index (weighted by 1964 provincial populations) has been linked to the Consumer Price Index Medical Care Component for earlier years. It shows physicians' fees rising at about the same rate as all prices from 1957 to 1971, faster than the general price level before Medicare, but substantially slower since. Recalling that actual prices probably moved faster than list in the pre-Medicare years, but not since, it follows that relative price increases in the medical care industry have *slowed down* since insurance went into effect. Yet expenditures go on climbing. If list prices really reflected actual prices over this period, one could derive an apparent quantity increase for 1957–1971 by dividing expenditure change by price change—this "quantity" estimate increases by 8.0 per cent per year. Adjusting for population change brings this rate down to 5.9 per cent per year, still a very healthy rate of "real" service input.[36]

These rapid increases in expenditure, whether "quantity" or hidden price change, should show up either as increases in average gross receipts per physician or as increases in the number of physicians available per capita. These data are displayed in tables 8 and 9. As pointed out in the appendix, they apply to fee-practice physicians only; although this represents only about two-thirds of the total physician stock, the remainder are not included in physician expenditure data and neither set nor collect fees. The increase of 28.7 per cent in physician stock per capita combines with an increase of 173.1 per cent in gross receipts per physician to yield an increase of 251.5 per cent in physician expenditures per capita, and a 29.9 per cent increase in population yields the 350 per cent increase in physician expenditures of Table 7.[37] Annualizing, population rose 1.9 per cent per year; physicians per capita, 1.8 per cent, and gross receipts per physician, 7.4 per cent, for a total of 11.4 per cent.

TABLE 7 Physician "Price" Movements in Canada, 1957–1973 and Implicit "Quantity" Changes (1961 = 100)

	Physician Services[a] (list price)	Consumer Price Index	Physician Services Expenditure[b]	Apparent "Quantity" Index[c]	"Quantity" per Capita
1957	89.5	94.4	70.0	78.2	85.9
1958	94.4	96.8	77.6	82.2	87.8
1959	97.1	97.9	83.9	86.4	90.1
1960	98.4	99.1	91.4	92.9	94.8
1961	100.0	100.0	100.0	100.0	100.0
1962	103.0	101.2	104.6	101.6	99.7
1963	104.9	102.9	116.8	111.3	107.2
1964	107.1	104.8	127.6	119.1	112.6
1965	110.3	107.4	140.4	127.3	118.2
1966	112.2	111.4	155.9	138.9	126.6
1967	121.4	115.3	176.7	145.6	130.3
1968	127.9	120.1	203.0	158.7	139.8
1969	134.8	125.5	232.1	172.2	149.5
1970	137.0	129.7	265.0	193.4	165.6
1971	139.6	133.4	318.4	228.0	192.8
1972	142.3	139.8			
1973	145.7	150.4			
% Change					
1957–1971			354.9%	191.6%	124.4%
1957–1973	62.8%	59.3%			
Per annum	3.1%	3.0%	11.4%	8.0%	5.9%

[a] Average value of the C.P.I. physicians' fees component, 1957–1964, linked in 1965 to the N.H.W. Fee Benefit Index (Table 6).
[b] Expenditure on physician services (Table 1), indexed on 1961 = 100.
[c] Physician services expenditure ÷ list price.

Several interesting points emerge from these data. First of all, the rise in physician stock has been twice as rapid as that of the population, and has been accelerating. The introduction of Medicare coincides with a significant increase in the rate of additions to the physician stock. Furthermore, gross receipts per physician have gone ahead much more rapidly than list prices. If one accepted the Table 7 list price increase of 56.0 per cent from 1957 to 1971, the implicit average increase in real output per physician would be 4.1 per cent per year. Yet physician practices are not adding new inputs rapidly; physician practice expenses rose at 5.8 per cent per year from 1957 to 1971 compared with general price level increases of

TABLE 8 Indexes of Average Gross Receipts per Active Fee-Practice Physician, Canada and Provinces, 1957–1971, Canada Average 1957 ($20,804) = 100

	B.C.	Alta.	Sask.	Man.	Ont.	Que.	N.B.	N.S.	P.E.I.	Nfld.	Can.	Can.[a]	Can.[b]
1957	114.1	112.3	109.1	113.8	105.8	81.2	88.5	94.4	74.6	109.6	100.0	100.0	3.78
1958	119.7	119.3	113.0	120.3	112.6	87.8	93.9	94.5	85.6	117.0	106.2	107.2	3.91
1959	128.0	121.4	113.9	132.5	116.1	90.0	90.9	102.6	90.6	118.6	110.1	113.5	3.87
1960	134.9	134.7	130.1	123.9	122.7	94.5	108.3	109.6	97.0	137.4	116.7	122.4	4.15
1961	133.9	140.5	130.3	139.7	130.8	106.3	116.4	111.7	96.1	130.7	124.3	128.2	4.21
1962	132.2	149.9	111.7	139.4	133.5	112.6	115.3	112.0	94.6	119.3	126.5	132.0	4.21
1963	133.0	148.6	171.4	138.9	147.3	123.8	126.8	112.7	112.5	134.1	137.9	145.4	4.37
1964	146.7	157.1	175.4	139.9	159.6	128.9	133.6	123.7	111.3	147.2	147.0	159.4	4.73
1965	152.3	170.1	180.1	153.4	171.9	139.4	142.4	132.1	123.0	152.0	157.7	171.7	4.85
1966	173.3	182.0	193.0	161.5	183.9	148.5	145.5	144.0	126.3	161.9	169.3	181.0	4.83
1967	185.6	210.6	193.0	176.2	205.3	160.8	172.5	146.1	138.1	175.5	185.9	203.0	5.08
1968	201.2	249.4	199.7	192.7	228.0	173.9	187.1	172.2	156.6	207.9	205.6	222.7	5.21
1969	214.9	251.8	216.4	236.8	246.0	187.7	203.6	197.6	180.3	249.8	222.7	240.1	5.25
1970	235.0	285.8	236.4	280.4	278.1	186.9	223.0	234.5	181.5	276.5	244.3	267.4	5.42
1971	239.7	298.9	244.7	271.7	296.4	259.5	260.5	234.9	246.4	264.8	273.1	305.0	5.70
% Change	110.1	166.2	124.3	138.8	180.2	219.6	194.4	148.8	230.3	141.6	173.1	205.0	50.79
Per annum	5.4	7.2	5.9	6.4	7.6	8.7	8.0	6.7	8.9	6.5	7.4	8.3	3.0

NOTE: Date of entry to Medicare underlined.
[a] Canada net receipts (100 = $12,852).
[b] Canada net relative to average wage (average weekly wage × 50).

Changes in Canada:	1957–1964	1964–1971
Average gross	47.0%	85.8%
Average net	59.4	91.3
Relative net	25.1	20.5

TABLE 9 Active Fee-Practice Physicians (per 100,000 pop.), Canada and Provinces, 1975–1971

	B.C.	Alta.	Sask.	Man.[a]	Ont.	Que.	N.B.	N.S.	P.E.I.	Nfld.[a]	Can.[a]
1957	94.5	73.3	71.4	72.9	88.1	73.6	58.0	66.8	66.7	22.9	78.0
1958	95.6	73.7	72.8	74.4	89.2	74.8	59.0	67.4	66.0	23.6	79.1
1959	98.4	74.2	73.9	75.6	90.8	76.2	59.8	67.9	66.3	24.0	80.5
1960	100.6	73.7	73.3	76.9	90.8	76.6	59.4	69.9	65.0	26.1	81.0
1961	103.3	73.5	72.9	78.1	91.0	77.0	58.9	71.6	64.8	27.7	81.5
1962	105.8	73.6	72.6	79.5	91.4	77.5	58.5	73.5	64.5	29.5	82.2
1963	106.2	74.1	73.1	80.2	91.8	77.9	59.1	74.0	65.8	30.0	82.7
1964	106.8	74.6	73.7	80.6	92.2	78.4	59.7	74.3	65.1	30.6	83.2
1965	107.5	75.1	74.2	81.0 (86.9)	92.7	78.9	60.2	74.5	66.1	30.9 (50.4)	83.8 (84.6)
1966	105.9	77.2	75.3	83.4 (89.5)	92.9	81.8	61.1	76.6	67.9	31.8 (51.5)	85.1 (85.9)
1967	105.0	81.3	78.5	83.5 (89.8)	93.6	82.5	61.9	79.4	68.8	32.2 (52.2)	86.2 (86.7)
1968	108.2	86.3	79.2	83.9 (90.0)	95.4	83.3	62.5	81.3	70.0	33.9 (54.4)	87.9 (88.7)
1969	117.0	91.0	80.1	85.1 (91.7)	99.1	84.9	64.3	84.2	73.6	38.5 (59.7)	91.4 (92.3)
1970	120.3	94.3	82.6	84.4 (95.3)	102.6	88.4	63.6	87.2	74.5	40.4 (63.8)	94.8 (95.6)
1971	125.8	101.8	88.3	89.7 (101.2)	107.4	95.4	67.2	93.0	81.3	44.3 (69.3)	100.4 (101.5)
% Change	33.1	38.9	23.7	23.0	21.9	29.6	15.9	39.2	21.9	93.4	28.7

[a]Numbers in parentheses include salaried practitioners, which are aggregated in other provinces.

3.2 per cent and wage increases of 5.2 per cent. Physician net incomes rose steadily relative to the average weekly wage, as shown in the last column of Table 8. What is striking is that average earnings of physicians relative to this industrial composite rose *faster* in the period 1957–1964 than in the Medicare period 1964–1971. The difference is not great, but it is enough to suggest that the introduction of Medicare did not bring about a change in the longer-run forces that drive the relative incomes of physicians.

Thus we are left with the observations that Medicare was associated with rapid increases in the numbers of physicians and rates of expenditure on their services, but not with major changes in physician list prices. Physician relative income continued to climb rapidly, but no faster than before Medicare; actual prices and real outputs per physician are unknown. We have, however, some fragmentary data on real outputs. The before-and-after Medicare study of physician utilization in Montreal reports that aggregate visit rates did not rise in response to insurance and that physician hours of work did not increase. Instead, physicians reorganized their practice patterns and generated more income from a given number of initial patient contacts.[38] This is supported by data from Trans-Canada Medical Plans showing that in insured populations, rates of physician-generated services per capita tend to rise faster over time and to be more closely associated with physician availability than are rates of patient-generated services.[39] Aggregate data from Quebec for 1971 and 1972, the first two years of insurance, show the same phenomenon, incredible quarter-to-quarter rates of increase of certain specific physician-generated services as well as a shift across fee schedule items from, for example, "ordinary" to "complete" office examinations.[40]

Rather than a linkage from demand through price and quantity to physician expense driven by independent shifts in demand, we seem to be observing a linkage from supply of physicians through quantity of services as determined by the physician to total expense. What we observe, and what generates expense, is not demand in the economist's sense but utilization, and utilization is the outcome of patient demand and physician behavior. This behavior is at least partially dependent on the relation between desired and actual physician incomes. The role of national health insurance may simply have been to relax further any market constraints on how physicians manipulate utilization to generate income. Table 8 suggests, however, that these constraints were not very significant before Medicare. Undoubtedly there was also a once-for-all increase in the ratio of actual to list prices as the plans drove uncollectables to zero in one year, but the primary force driving up physician expenditures in the late 1960s is the increase in physician stock and the changes in physician practice patterns.

This creates a rather puzzling inconsistency. In the time series data, each province shows a clear jump in share of income devoted to medical services when public insurance is introduced; and as pointed out above, in most provinces physician incomes rose rapidly in the years spanning the introduction. Yet over the longer period, physician incomes relative to wages and salaries generally have moved up about 3 per cent per year, and this increase did not accelerate in the 1968–1971 period. Of course, wages and salaries do not move with personal income; over this period they have tended to lag behind. But the key question is the difference made by insurance. In the absence of the public plan, would the rapid increase in physicians per capita from 1968 to 1971 (14.2 per cent in three years) have driven down average physician incomes? Or would it merely have given rise to price and quantity adjustments in the private market that would have pushed up costs anyway? There is some evidence cross-sectionally in Canada that although *absolute numbers* of physicians per capita have little systematic effect on relative physician income, *rapid rates of growth* of the stock push down relative incomes (Evans, 1972, Ch. 3). The evidence is not worth much, but we might tentatively suggest that national insurance speeded up physician reactions to an increase in numbers and affected the timing of their income-maintaining responses. Had Medicare not been introduced, the influx of physicians to the market might have held down income increases in the short run and generated pressure for increases in list prices and changes in individual billing practices. Medicare speeded up the process by shifting actual prices relative to list (hence the slower movement of list prices post-Medicare) and by enabling billing practices to shift rapidly without patient backlash (the Enterline findings). Physician influence over the private market seemed to be strong enough, however, that over the long haul they would have been able to absorb the influx and restore their incomes to the long-term upward trend. Of course, this is all hypothetical; we have very little post-Medicare data yet and political variables have now superseded whatever market forces were previously operative.[41]

Table 10 merely provides some corroborative evidence on the role of physician pricing behavior. It shows the variation across provinces in fee levels: B.C., Manitoba, Alberta, and Ontario tend to be high priced whereas the eastern provinces are lower. Highest of all is B.C. Yet these are also the provinces with the largest

TABLE 10 Relative "Prices" of Medical Services across Provinces, Various Years (Ontario = 100)

	1968 All Services Fee Schedule (Sept. 1)	1969 ———— All Services ———— Fee Schedule (Sept. 1)	Benefits Paid (Oct. 1)	1973 ———— All Services ———— Benefits Paid All Services [b]	Visits Only
		General Practitioners			
B.C.	110.9	106.5	106.5	117.25	122.19
Alta.	99.4	106.6	113.2	115.53	121.28
Sask.	104.7	95.2	89.9	92.25	95.14
Man.	127.3	115.5	109.1	103.95	103.30
Ont.	100.0	100.0	100.0	100.00	100.00
Que.[a]	—	—	—	—	92.72
N.B.	98.3	97.9	92.5	—	86.07
N.S.	110.2	99.1	93.6	—	96.38
P.E.I.	98.7	89.0	98.9	—	85.66
Nfld.	96.6	86.8	86.8	—	85.65
		Specialists			
B.C.	108.9	112.7	112.7	103.64	124.20
Alta.	99.9	99.0	97.4	101.75	104.31
Sask.	103.4	95.4	90.1	87.44	90.34
Man.	112.9	106.1	100.2	92.05	93.02
Ont.	100.0	100.0	100.0	100.00	100.00
Que.	108.1	101.2	101.2	—	91.80
N.B.	95.6	101.4	95.8	—	89.38
N.S.	109.5	101.9	96.2	—	98.14
P.E.I.	104.9	96.5	107.2	—	101.78
Nfld.	100.0	94.1	94.1	—	91.90
		All Physicians			
B.C.	109.6	110.8	110.8	110.33	122.84
Alta.	99.7	102.1	103.4	108.53	115.78
Sask.	103.9	95.3	90.0	89.80	93.58
Man.	118.6	108.7	102.7	97.90	99.96
Ont.	100.0	100.0	100.0	100.00	100.00
Que.[a]	—	—	—	—	92.42
N.B.	96.2	98.7	93.2	—	87.15
N.S.	109.9	99.2	93.7	—	96.95
P.E.I.	99.8	92.0	102.2	—	90.88
Nfld.	97.8	89.2	89.2	—	87.67

[a] Quebec general practitioners had no fee schedule in 1968 or 1969.
[b] Payments for laboratory services in eastern provinces are not on a unit basis.

number of physicians per capita. B.C. is the most prominent example—always at or near the top of all provinces in prices, yet far ahead of the others in numbers of physicians (Table 9) and near bottom in physician incomes (Table 8). The inference is that as increases in physician stock spread the patient load more thinly, incomes per physician fall. The response is to try to drive *up* prices and/or to generate more output. Neither tactic has been fully successful in B.C., but then the physician stock is abnormally large there and probably includes a relatively larger number of semi-retired practitioners.[42]

If in fact physician behavior is the key to utilization and expenditure behavior, as Canadian insurance experience suggests,[43] it follows that efforts to modify patterns of expenditure by incentives directed at the consumer of care cannot hope to influence overall cost trends. Copayment is pretty much a dead issue in Canada, both because of its distributional effects and because it cannot come to grips with the real problems.[44] Public policy has instead been directed at two approaches—control within the existing structure of medical practice, and modification of that structure.

Control in the existing structure includes negotiation of list fees and could be extended to unilateral determination of such fees by government (although this has not been suggested out loud). The evidence now seems fairly clear that this will not work because billings can be expanded almost indefinitely on a given schedule. Moreover, procedural multiplication can be harmful to the patient's health and can generate substantial external costs in the hospital sector and elsewhere. The "provider profiles" mentioned above merely identify very unusual practitioners; they give no leverage to government over changes in general practice standards over time. A variety of gimmicks have been suggested or tried—absolute limits on physician earnings (Newfoundland) merely lead to more physician leisure. Prorationing of billings against a fixed pool of reimbursement has been suggested as a short-run measure, but in the long run it seems to accentuate the pressures on physicians to multiply procedures by penalizing the "non-multipliers" for the excesses of their colleagues.[45] So far the only sure-fire method of cost containment appears to be the current suggestion by the Council of Health Ministers that physician immigration be restricted. Fewer doctors, like fewer hospital beds, surely does mean lower costs. Combined with "physician-extender" programs, it may not mean fewer services. Thus the escalation of medical costs could be limited to that generated by the income aspirations of current physicians and future Canadian graduates.

Income aspirations of physicians seem to be somewhat muted at present, partly because of large gains in the 1960s, but also because the last five years have seen an outpouring of public and private opinion that "something" should be done about the private practice, fee-for-service mode of medical care delivery. Just as this form of medical care delivery seems to make rationalization of hospital use almost impossible, so it stands in the way of achieving limitations on medical costs. The root of the problem is that although fee-for-service creates incentives for unnecessary care, private practice blocks any information channel that would enable a regulatory agency to determine necessity (or even the accuracy of the billing). The best that can be done is to identify "unusual" patient or provider patterns. As much as 50, or 90, per cent of tonsillectomies may be unnecessary, but which ones? And who has authority or ability to decide? Thus, attempts to achieve public accountability for medical care delivery fail before the enormous information advantage possessed by the physician, exactly the same problem that made the private market useless as a regulatory device.

The recommended solution in Canada is some form of public organization, owning facilities and hiring physicians, tied into a much more complete network of patient information. The label attached is usually "Community Health Center," although the name means something different to almost everyone using it. The primary features of the C.H.C. are, however, that it combines conventional medical practice with a more general social and public health concern, that it is not dependent on fee for service, and that unlike a medical practice it is nonprofit. It is also quite far down the road as a system of medical care delivery, and the road itself is far from clear. Nevertheless, almost every group that has studied the Canadian health insurance system agrees that we cannot stay where we are. Insurance changes only the demand side of health care—the supply side is crucial. The hardest part of the job lies ahead.

APPENDIX

Data Sources for Text Tables

The most comprehensive data on health care costs in Canada are prepared by the Health Economics and Statistics Directorate of the

Department of National Health and Welfare, Government of Canada. Their personal health care concept, generally speaking, covers all health care expenditures that are, or prior to the public medical and hospital plans were, made by persons from family budgets, payments to hospitals, physicians, dentists, and for prescription drugs. It excludes public health, research, and educational expenditures on health care, but does include governmental expenditures on special-category hospitals. Research charged to a hospital budget is included in PHC, which also includes hospital operating costs but not capital expenditures.

The personal health care concept also excludes health expenditures that are not directed by the health care provider "establishment," such as nonprescription drugs, eyeglasses and appliances, services of health professionals outside hospitals other than physicians and dentists, and nursing home care. The line between nursing homes (excluded) and private convalescent hospitals (included) becomes a little fuzzy but is drawn on the basis of administrative arrangements. Private hospitals contracting with the provincial agency and providing insured care for all or part of their patients are included with respect to their expenditure on insured patients. The amounts involved are trivial.

Annual PHC data for Canada and the provinces are published irregularly, the latest being Canada, Department of National Health and Welfare, *Expenditure on Personal Health Care in Canada, 1960–1971*, Ottawa, n.d. This is the basis for Table 1; pre-1960 data are from Canada, Department of National Health and Welfare, *Expenditures on Personal Health Care in Canada, 1953–1961*, Health Care Series Memorandum #16, Ottawa, March 1963. In 1960 and earlier, expenditure in hospitals run by the Department of National Defense (like private hospitals, a very small part of the Canadian hospital industry) are excluded. The earlier prescription drug series also fails to include prescribed drugs sold outside retail pharmacies. The inclusive series can be pushed back to 1957 by earlier "occasional memoranda" from Health and Welfare but the series breaks there.

A more inclusive definition of the health care industry is the basis for a new data series, recently released as Canada, Department of National Health and Welfare, *National Health Expenditures in Canada, 1960–1971*, Ottawa, October 1973 (including comparative U.S. data). It adds to PHC nursing home care, nonprescription drugs, eyeglasses and other appliances, services of other health professionals outside institutions, costs of prepayment administration, voluntary organizations, research, new-facility construction, and public health activity. Some specific exclusions are made (such as government of Canada hospital facility construction) but these are quantitatively trivial. This comprehensive series indicates that total health expenditures per capita in Canada rose from $113.50 in 1960 to $306.11 in 1971, compared with $80.53 and $236.61 for PHC. Thus the PHC percentage has risen from 71.0 per cent to 77.3 per cent, indicating the faster growth of the hospital and physician sectors.

Data on the physician stock and physician incomes are generated along with the health care expenditure series and are reported in Canada, Department of National Health and Welfare, *Earnings of Physicians in Canada, 1961–1971*, Health Care Series #30, Ottawa, n.d. Earlier data are from *Earnings of Physicians in Canada 1957–1965*, Health Care Series #21, Ottawa, April 1967. This series covers "active fee practice" physicians, those "whose main employment is in the provision of personal medical care services" and "whose professional income is mainly in the form of fees for services rendered." It thus excludes all salaried physicians providing medical care, whether in a private group practice, on a hospital staff, or in public service. In fact, however, prior to 1970 a small number of salaried physicians working in group practices were included; only those in Manitoba and Newfoundland where salaried service was quantitatively important were excluded. In 1970 all salaried group practitioners were excluded, so that the reported increase in manpower in 1971 over 1970 is remarkably low. In this paper we have added back-salaried physicians outside Manitoba and Newfoundland for 1970 and 1971 to keep the series consistent. Bracketed figures in the text tables show the effects of adding back-salaried practitioners in those two provinces as well.

As a measure of the availability of physician services, the fee practice physician is somewhat unsatisfactory. To compare, for example, service availability in Newfoundland with the national average by looking at fee practitioners only is grossly inaccurate. Similarly, it appears that some of the discrepancy between Quebec and Ontario in physicians *per capita* is made up by larger teaching programs in Quebec with more hospital staff, interns, and residents supplying medical services but appearing in hospital budgets. (Quebec, Commission d'enquête sur la santé et le bien-être social, *Analyse comparative des coûts de l'hospitalisation au Québec et en Ontario*, Annexe I du rapport, Gouvernement de Québec, September 1967.) Total active civilian physicians in Canada in 1971 are reported as 32,625 (Canada, Department of National Health and Welfare, *Health Manpower Inventory, 1972*, Ottawa, October 1972) but this includes administration, teaching, part-time practitioners, etc. This source, which also includes stock estimates back to 1963, merely references the Canadian Medical Directory, but another federal publication, *Health Services in Canada, 1973*, produces the same figure and refers to it as prepared by the Ministry of National Health and Welfare, based on data from Medical Marketing Systems, Ltd. (Seccombe House, formerly Canadian Mailings Ltd.), which maintain records for the drug detail men and other medical suppliers. The Health Manpower Inventory divides this total of 32,625 into 12,566 general practitioners, 13,616 specialists, 1,257 "not in private practice," and 5,186 interns and residents. Yet this breakdown implies 26,182 active practitioners, or 20 per cent more than the 21,895 active fee-practice physicians in 1971 reported in *Earnings of Physicians* (see above) when all reporting salaried practitioners are added in. No "reconciliation statement" is prepared. Moreover, no documentation is provided about the methodology employed in the tabulation, so the primary official source of data on the physician stock is effectively undocumented (in contrast, for example, to the detailed methodology available in *Earnings of Physicians*). For further discussion of alternative estimates prior to the manpower inventory, see R. G. Evans, *Price Formation in the Market for Physician Services in Canada, 1957–1969*, Ottawa, 1973, especially Chapter III and Appendix III-3.

The active fee-practice series is, however, preferable as a basis for analyzing market behavior since this group sets fees and receives them and is the provider of almost all insured care under the Medicare plan. The income series associated with this group and reported in the text has certain problems as well. It includes part-time physicians who are semi-retired, or who entered practice part way through the year. This is partly corrected by focusing on the physicians with net incomes above some arbitrary minimum— in 1971 this minimum is $15,000. Any self-employed practitioner netting less than $15,000 *cannot* be fully employed! In 1971 average gross and net incomes for this group were $61,516 and $42,624 compared with $56,824 and $39,203 for all fee-practice physicians. Thus, $42,624 would be a better estimate of the net earnings of a "representative" fully employed practitioner. Unfortunately, a time series of this sort is not very meaningful since it would move with the (arbitrary) choice of full-time cutoff. There are also problems in the gross income and expenses of practice data as a result of disentangling group practices with salaried physicians; and the investment earnings component of nonprofessional income is almost certainly understated since all data are drawn from tax returns that do not include capital gains prior to 1972. Physicians tend to invest in assets (such as medical arts buildings) yielding high capital gain but low income, and it is hard to believe that the average physician in fee practice earned only $798 from all nonfee sources in 1971, including incidental wages and salaries, given one's fragmentary knowledge of physician-owned real estate holding companies! Some of this may be picked up in 1972 and after, as half of capital gain must now be reported as income (when realized). The same sort of problem arises with expenses of practice, some of which of course reemerge as investment income. Still, it is doubtful if these factors influence trends over time to any great degree.

The physician price series for earlier years is the Consumer Price Index, physicians' fees component, prepared by the Dominion Bureau of Statistics and reported in Canada, Department of National Health and Welfare, Research and Statistics Memo, *Health Care Price Movements*, Ottawa, April 1968. The overall CPI is from Canada, Dominion Bureau of Statistics, *Canadian Statistical Review: Historical Summary 1970*, Ottawa, August 1972. Updating of statistics in this issue was from the February 1974 issue of the *Canadian Statistical Review* (monthly). All population data (June 1st annual data) and average weekly and hourly wage data are drawn from these sources.

The CPI index was relatively limited—fees for office visits, home visits, an obstetrical confinement, and an appendectomy as reported by six general practitioners in each metropolitan area to a semi-annual telephone survey. It was phased out city by city as Medicare spread across the provinces. The Department of National Health and Welfare also prepares an index of provincial fee schedules, starting in December 1963. In earlier years this index might differ substantially from fees charged to uninsured patients. As each province entered Medicare, this index was shifted from a listed-fees to a benefits-paid basis (since many provinces pay less than 100 per cent of the schedule or impose administrative limitations). These data are unpublished but were generously supplied by the Health Economics and Statistics Division, Health Programs Branch, National Health and Welfare. A compound index was constructed using the CPI index to 1964, the N.H.W. fee schedule index to 1968 or whenever each province entered Medicare, and the N.H.W. benefits paid index thereafter. The 1965 overlap between CPI and N.H.W. was used to link these two series (the CPI is Laspeyres, the N.H.W. Paasche) and the second point of linkage was implicit in the N.H.W. procedure that reports only month, year, and size of percentage increase in fee or benefit schedule from December 1963 to the present by province. Until 1970, however, when Quebec entered Medicare, Quebec general practitioners had no fee schedule. Thus the Canadian average fee benefit schedule (FB) is a weighted average of the nine other provinces. An index of total expenditure on physicians' services can then be derived from the personal health care data and compared to changes in listed prices or benefits to indicate the extent to which listed fees account for changes in total expenditure. A similar sort of comparison can be made between list prices and physician gross receipts.

The primary source of hospital data is the set of *Hospital Statistics* volumes published annually by the Dominion Bureau of Statistics. Hospital reporting by D.B.S. began in 1932 but in 1952 a new and more extensive reporting system was introduced and the reports expanded to two volumes. Since then, the structure and content of the reports have changed from time to time but the volume of data collected has steadily expanded until now seven volumes are published annually in addition to Mental and Tuberculosis Hospital statistics and numerous occasional studies on manpower and salaries.

In dealing with the text data, a number of points must be kept in mind. First of all, "general and allied special hospitals" in the D.B.S. data excludes all private hospitals since these do not report the same detailed federal returns. In the total personal health care expenditure, however, national health and welfare includes any private hospital providing care under contract with a provincial agency. The discrepancy is not large, but is just enough to keep the numbers inconsistent! Data on number of hospitals and number of beds in the text are taken from Canada, D.B.S., *Hospital Statistics, Vol. I—Hospital Beds, 1971*, Ottawa, November 1973, historical data, pp. 46–50. Patient days are adult and child only and include chronic, convalescent, rehabilitation, and other specialties. Patient days per thousand population were calculated by taking the reported average daily number of patients for each year, multiplying by 365 (or 366), and dividing by national population. Admissions per thousand population were calculated by dividing reported total admissions by population. The ratio of the two does not equal reported mean stay per separation (discharge or death) presumably because in an expanding hospital sector, admissions systematically outran separations in every year.

This may not be the whole explanation; a number of small arithmetic discrepancies turn up in this vast array of data, particularly in earlier years. As mentioned in the text, total hospital beds in general and allied special hospitals seem to be undercounted in 1961. Data on p. 33 of *Hospital Beds, 1971* suggest that in 1961 about 1,800 chronic, convalescent, and rehabilitation beds were shifted to mental and "restored" the following year.

Costs per patient day in the text always refer to total expenditures per adult and child patient day, excluding new-borns. Earlier data sources often include new-borns, whole or part-weighted. Cost per day back to 1956 is reported on pp. 28–30 of Canada, D.B.S., *Hospital Statistics, Vol. VI: Hospital Expenditures, 1971*, Ottawa, October 1973. For the earlier years, data were taken from *Hospital Statistics, Vol. II, Expenditures* for each year. Reconstructing these data, however, it must be noted that prior to 1956 *net* expenditure per patient day was reported, excluding courtesy rebates to staff and revenue from nurses' board. Reported patient day costs from p. 89, Col. 5, of the 1953 publication ($11.95) have, for example, been adjusted upward by the ratio of gross to net (p. 105), and similarly in 1954 and 1955. The 1953 total was then allocated by class of expenditure using the proportions in *Hospital Statistics, Vol. II*, p. 88 (wages and salaries, drugs, etc.). No allocation by department was possible since throughout the 1950s reporting procedures permitted a very high "undistributed expenditure" component that was nearly a fifth of the total. The breakdown in 1971 used data reported in tables 30–33 of Canada, D.B.S., *Hospital Statistics, Vol. VII: Hospital Indicators, 1971*, Ottawa, August 1973; Table 18 provided paid hours data to compare with the hours data in Table 31 of *Hospital Statistics, Vol. I, 1953*. Historical length of stay and occupancy data came from *Hospital Statistics, Vol. I, 1971*, and all 1953 and 1971 disaggregated expenditure data came from *Hospital Statistics, Vol. VI, 1971*, and *Vol. II, 1953*.

Data for the subperiods between 1953 and 1971 are much less comprehensive than one would like, because reporting categories and definitions kept changing so as to make the construction of long and consistent series on the internal expenditure components of hospitals rather difficult. Gross salaries and wages and paid hours are drawn from the 1953 *Hospital Statistics, Vol. II*. Gross salaries and wages for 1959, 1965, and 1971 are drawn from *Hospital Statistics, Vol. VI*. Expenditures and paid hours are from *Hospital Statistics, Vol. VII, Indicators*. Data on numbers and wages of professional and technical employees over the period 1961–1968 are taken from a series of twelve occasional papers published by D.B.S., *Health Manpower in Hospitals, 1961–1968*, the first *general* and each following paper covering eleven specific occupations and reporting *inter alia* the share of total hospital budgets made up by their wages. Wages per paid hour by occupation in 1971 are from Canada, Dominion Bureau of Statistics, *Hospital Indicators, January–June 1971*, Ottawa, October 1971, which was based on the quarterly survey but not reproduced in the annual volume.

The general principles followed in data preparation were, first, to emphasize construction of consistent series over time, and, second, to choose data concepts as closely as possible related to potential insurance responses or behavior. There is a huge quantity of statistical data on hospitals that could be used to show the responses of detailed hospital budgets wherein shifts occurred after the insurance programs were introduced; but such a project was well beyond the resources available for this paper. The Department of National Health and Welfare has made a good beginning with its *Sources of Increase in Budget Review Hospital Expenditures in Canada, 1961 to 1971*, Ottawa, December 1973. It is to be hoped that this project will be pushed back to pre-insurance days and expanded in detail. It would also be helpful if federal statisticians could spend some time on indicating the appropriate reconciliation of sources, where possible! So far, number generation has tended to outrun either documentation or reconciliation, but the trends appear favorable.

NOTES

1. Thus, the federal publication *Health Services in Canada 1973* (Ottawa: Department of National Health and Welfare, 1973), which summarizes the national programs, opens its first sentence by referring to the B.N.A. Act. This publication, issued annually in previous years as *Health and Welfare Services in Canada*, is a good overview of the general provisions of the provincial hospital and medical programs as well as the direct service programs of the federal government. In earlier years it also provides a statistical sketch of the hospital system at a point in time, amplifying material in the annual Canada Year Book published by the Dominion Bureau of Statistics.
2. The federal government pays 25 per cent of each province's own per capita cost for covered hospital services, plus 25 per cent of the national average per capita cost of such services, plus 50 per cent of the national average per capita cost of covered medical services, all multiplied by the provincial population.
3. A brief history of the development of health insurance in Canada is provided by Malcolm G. Taylor, "The Canadian Health Insurance Program," *Public Administration Review*, 33 (January–February 1973). Other brief descriptions are J.E.F. Hastings, "Federal-Provincial Insurance for Hospital and Physician's Care in Canada," *International Journal of Health Services*, 1 (1971); R. Kohn, "Medical Care in Canada," in J. Fry and W.A.J. Farndale (editors), *International Medical Care* (Oxford: Medical and Technical Publishing Co., 1972) and

A. P. Ruderman, "The Organization and Financing of Medical Care in Canada," in British Medical Association, *Health Services Financing* (London, 1970). Hastings tends to focus relatively more on current administrative questions and on the impact of health insurance on other health and social services and the organization of health personnel; Kohn provides a current snapshot description of health services, insured or uninsured, which tends to cover the "official" features with limited analysis; Ruderman in his description discusses the relatively limited role of price and income effects in the Canadian system and argues that the private market economy approach is not and never was particularly relevant. A more extensive history of the pre-Medicare nonprofit comprehensive insurance plans from which Medicare evolved is C. H. Shillington, *The Road to Medicare in Canada* (Toronto: Del Graphics, 1972). Symposia on the hospital system include the September 16, 1962 issue of *Hospitals: J.A.H.A.*, Vol. 35, No. 18, and *Medical Care*, Vol. 7, No. 6, Supplement (November–December 1969). The cornerstones of description in this field are, of course, the *Report of the Royal Commission on Health Services* (Hall Commission) (Ottawa: The Queen's Printer, 1964); and supporting studies: the Report of the Commission d'enquête sur la santé et le bien-être social (Castonguay-Nepveu Commission) (Quebec: Gouvernement de Québec, 1970); and *The Report of the Ontario Committee on the Healing Arts* (Toronto: The Queen's Printer, 1969). Someone, somewhere, may have read all this. John Evans suggests that Canadians spend more time and effort studying health care than most other countries do delivering it; see "Physicians in a Public Enterprise," *Journal of Medical Education*, 48 (November 1973). The present author strives to uphold that tradition.

4. Taylor, op. cit.

5. It must be recalled, of course, that standards of services cannot be measured only by expenditure. The dramatic increase in provider incomes, physicians, and hospital workers (see below), which have been the principal quantitative effect of health insurance, have tended to even out provincial differentials. Thus, health providers have moved faster up the wage structure in poorer provinces, without any observable associated improvement in health status. In medical care, however, much of this behavior pre-dated the federal legislation—see R. G. Evans, *Price Formation in the Market for Physician Services 1957–1969* (Ottawa: The Queen's Printer, 1972), Ch. 3.

6. These terms are spelled out in more detail in the annual *Health Services in Canada*. The hospital program required participating provinces to sign an agreement with the federal government detailing licensing, inspection, and supervision requirements and federal audit. These requirements were not imposed in the medical care plan, either as Taylor suggests because of provincial objections to federal intervention, or because public regulation of physicians is a much more contentious issue than regulation of hospitals!

7. Administrative costs have certainly been held down—in 1971 prepayment and administration of health plans cost Canadians $5.54 per capita compared with $12.83 in the U.S.; total health expenditures per capita are $306.11 and $386.92. Canada, Department of National Health and Welfare, *National Health Expenditures in Canada, 1960–1971* (Ottawa: 1973). (Both countries, of course, bury compliance costs in provider budgets, but it seems likely that compliance costs are also lower given a uniform national system.) The bargain looks a little different, of course, when one discovers that the existing system of administration does not generate data sufficient to understand or control operating expense! But at least the U.S. is no better off.

8. The nub of the problem appears to be the desire of the federal government to turn over tax revenues that will initially yield revenues higher than current health costs but that will grow less rapidly (alcohol and tobacco levies). The provinces prefer a larger income tax share, since the income elasticity of this tax will keep pace with past rates of cost increase. The federal authorities note that their plan provides incentives to rationalize delivery at the provincial level, as well as initial resources to support change. The provinces argue that this scheme imposes all the risks of cost containment on them (as well as the political unpopularity).

9. Moreover, revenues thus collected are subtracted from shareable costs, making them "50¢ dollar" revenues from a provincial standpoint.

10. R. G. Beck, *The Demand for Physicians' Services in Saskatchewan*, Ph.D. dissertation, University of Alberta, 1971. The charge also lowered use among large families and aged-head families, and was politically unpopular. The Liberal government that imposed it was defeated in 1971 and the charge removed by the incoming N.D.P.

11. This is not solidly established but emerges in several studies—e.g., Beck, *The Demand for Physicians' Services in Saskatchewan*, shows a steady weakening in the relation between income and utilization after Medicare. P. E. Enterline *et al.*, "The Distribution of Medical Services Before and After 'Free' Medical Care—The Quebec Experience," *New England Journal of Medicine*, 289 (November 29, 1973), report a shift in number of visits—up for lower-income families, down for upper-income families, zero net change. R. E. Badgley *et al.*, "The Impact of Medicare in Wheatville, Sasketchewan, 1960–1965," *Canadian Journal of Public Health*, 58 (March 1967), show evidence of a similar shift, although less concrete in the absence of visit data.

12. Anne Scitovsky has correctly pointed out that although this paper identifies sources of expenditure increase in insured health care and relates them to increased provider incomes, it does not establish that these developments are a result of national health insurance. In some sense one could never establish this. Who knows what would have happened? But it is true that although a short-run expenditure response to national insurance is identifiable in both hospital and medical care, the response of provider incomes are less clear-cut. The hospital response, if it is that, has a long lag, whereas the physician response, on the contrary, may be merely a speeding up of long-run trends that would have happened anyway. If this all sounds a little *ad hoc*, it is. I've also changed some of the hospital wage numbers and their explanation. I regret undercutting Anne's comments but it made a better paper!

13. It is, of course, true that relative earnings of health care providers rose prior to the public insurance plans as well. To what extent this was attributable to the spread of private insurance no one knows.

14. A detailed description of the reporting is available in a pair of booklets published annually by the Dominion Bureau of Statistics and the Department of National Health and Welfare, *Instructions and Definitions for the Annual Return of Hospitals Form HS-1, Facilities and Services* and *Form HS-2, Financial*.

15. In Quebec the medical association collects additional data from each practitioner on auxiliary personnel employed, hours of work, and distribution of activity of hours of work. Analysis of the relationships among practice characteristics, physician characteristics, and pattern of workload is now being carried out by A. P. Contandriopoulos and J. M. Lance, "Modèle de Prévision de la Main-D'Oeuvre Medicale," Document de Travail No. 8, McGill University,

May 1974. The authors express some reservations about the quality of the practice characteristics data.

16. Some efforts have been made to carry out such estimates—e.g., R. G. Evans, "Behavioural Cost Functions for Hospitals," *Canadian Journal of Economics*, 4 (May 1971); and R. G. Evans and H. D. Walker, "Information Theory and the Analysis of Hospital Cost Structure," *Canadian Journal of Economics*, 5 (August 1972).

17. This view was still being urged in 1969; see Canada, Department of National Health and Welfare, *Task Force Reports on the Costs of Health Services in Canada*, Vol. III, pp. 170–182. That particular report, on medical prices, seems more concerned with physician autonomy.

18. Thus in 1970 the B.C. Medical Association promulgated a new fee schedule. The province declared it too high, and said that the plan would not pay it. The profession replied that its members would collect the increase from patients. The government advised patients not to pay, and published (by name) each physician's gross receipts from the plan in the newspapers. The profession thereupon lowered its schedule and a compromise was adopted; but it worked to defeat the government at the next election. In most provinces the process is less open.

19. This is an implication of empirical research in B.C. See R. G. Evans *et al.*, "Medical Productivity, Scale Effects, and Demand Generation," *Canadian Journal of Economics*, 4 (August 1973). It has also been commented on by informed observers. (John Evans, "Physicians in a Public Enterprise.")

20. This was expressed as a positive goal in the Hall Commission Health Charter for Canada. "BASED on freedom of choice, and upon free and self-governing professions. . . ." Report of the Royal Commission, pp. 11–12.

21. These comparisons also illustrate the dangers of interpreting share movements. In 1961, a recession year, personal income was down and the jump in hospital share was accentuated. The long boom of the early sixties held the physician share nearly constant from 1961 to 1966; only when the growth of the economy slowed did physicians' share move up again.

22. Canadian hospital accounts do not include employee benefits in gross salaries and wages but classify these as "supplies and other expense." These amount to about 9 per cent of the total budget in recent years. (Notice that hospital budgets include little or no capital expense.) In 1969, radiologist and pathologist remuneration was transferred from "supplies and expense" to "gross salaries and wages"; this amounts to about 2.5 per cent of total budget and has been transferred back to supplies and expense in this paper for consistency. The 1971 data also reflect an exclusion from hours worked of intern and resident time and classroom hours, thus biasing downward the change in hours per patient day from 1965 to 1971. The effect appears, however, to be quantitatively insignificant (of the order of 0.2 to 0.3 hours per patient day).

23. One study has been conducted that attempts to examine wage change by employment category within the hospital labor force and relate such changes to wages in similar occupations elsewhere in the economy: Canada, Department of National Health and Welfare Research and Statistics Memo, *Salaries and Wages in Canadian Hospitals 1962 to 1970*, Ottawa, n.d. (1971). This source draws on data from the Department of Labour as well as D.B.S. and N.H.W. Unfortunately, the longest data span assembled is 1962 to 1969, and in this case the 1969 data are contaminated by failure to include a major subsequent retroactive agreement in Quebec in 1970. The report is carefully documented

and extremely honest about its limitations; it does show that by 1969 hospital employees in such service trade occupations as cooks, laundry workers, maids, and seamstresses were paid well above their private industry counterparts. But its coverage, both cross-sectionally and over time, is far too limited to support any general conclusions.

24. Saskatchewan, typically, tried out a variety of innovative approaches in the 1940s, long before anyone else had considered the problem. See B. Roth *et al.*, "The Saskatchewan Experience in Payment for Hospital Care," *American Journal of Public Health*, 43 (June 1953).

25. Although in calculating savings to be achieved by reduced utilization of acute inpatient facilities, for example, this distinction may be forgotten by exponents of alternative programs.

26. On one occasion, however, the Minister of Health in B.C. simply refused to pay all of the negotiated wage increases and forced hospitals to find the differential by cutting staff or using their own revenue sources (e.g., the preferred accommodation differential). The policy was monumentally unpopular, and it is asserted that hospitals merely ran up their lengths of stay; but there is some evidence that it slowed cost trends. In Quebec the provincial government has participated directly in wage negotiations since 1966.

27. Evans, "Behavioural Cost Functions for Hospitals," and Evans and Walker, "Information Theory and the Analysis of Hospital Cost Structure."

28. *Ibid*. These findings relate to aggregate hospital budgets. Some provinces, particularly Quebec, are using cross-hospital subindexes, such as dollars per pound of laundry processed, as control devices to identify and place administrative pressure on hospitals that are above average on these direct departmental costs. This may simply lead back to standardizing the internal structure of hospital budgets—uniform inefficiency again.

29. A cynic might fear that better managers in the existing structure might make the problem worse; they'll simply negotiate better for more money!

30. R. G. Evans and G. C. Robinson, *An Evaluation of the Economic Implications of a Day Care Surgery Unit*, Final Report, N.H.W. Grant #610-21-14, Vancouver, October 1973.

31. M. Feldstein, in "An Econometric Model of the Medicare System," *Quarterly Journal of Economics*, 85 (February 1971), reports that extended care facilities raise costs per hospital *episode*—what is saved on lower acute care stays is lost in long extended care stays.

32. J. L. McPhee, *Community Health Association Clinics* (Regina: Saskatchewan Department of Public Health, August 1973); and J. E. F. Hastings *et al.*, "Prepaid Group Practice in Sault Ste. Marie, Ontario: Part I," *Medical Care*, (March–April 1973).

33. The *locus classicus* is the report of the Commission d'enquête (Castonguay Commission). The federal equivalent was the Community Health Centre Project, directed by J. E. F. Hastings, which reported to the Council of Health Ministers in July of 1972 and supported the C.H.C. concept strongly. More recently the Report of the British Columbia Health Security Programme Project (Victoria: December 1973) also endorsed the C.H.C. idea.

34. The nonprofits on which the national program was modeled, provincially based but affiliated as Trans Canada Medical Plans, covered 30 per cent of the population in 1967 (adding in the population of Saskatchewan, which had a universal public plan since 1962). Coverage was, however, proportionally much higher in the western provinces. Moreover, most of the population had *some* medical coverage, although private insurance plans were more likely to

limit coverage to in-hospital care and/or impose copayment features. With reference to the role of insurance in expanding demand for care, the TCMP plans had an average cost per insured of $34.95 in 1967, compared with a national average of $33.63 for medical expenditures of all Canadians. Moreover, TCMP subscribers were concentrated in high-cost provinces. See Evans, *Price Formation in the Market for Physician Services*, Ch. 2; or Trans-Canada Medical Plans, *Annual Enrollment Experience and Annual Financial and Statistical Experience Report, 1967 Year* (mimeo.), July 1968.

35. The indexes are current-weighted composites derived from a sample of key items in each provincial fee schedule, with the size of the sample growing over time. By contrast, the C.P.I. Component (discontinued after Medicare) was a base-weighted index of prices of four procedures performed by general practitioners in urban areas, measured by telephone survey. For further discussion, see R. G. Evans, *Price Formation in the Market for Physician Services*, Ch. 1 and Appendix 1–2, where it is also shown that although the proportion of specialists in Canada rose from 35 per cent in 1957 to just over 50 per cent, the impact of this change on measured prices is almost certainly less than 10 per cent overall.

36. The table suggests that this "quantity" increase has accelerated since Medicare, but the 1971 increase is distorted by the massive effects of the introduction of the Quebec program. In that province average gross incomes of physicians jumped 38.9 per cent, 1971 over 1970, and net incomes were up 50.1 per cent. Expenses of practice rose 8.6 per cent on average. This leads to the suspicion that there was substantial under-reporting of income in Quebec prior to 1971.

37. There are a few conceptual discrepancies in moving from physicians to physician services. See *Earnings of Physicians in Canada, 1961–1971*.

38. Enterline *et al.*, "The Distribution of Medical Services Before and After 'Free' Medical Care"; and A. D. MacDonald *et al.*, "Physician Service in Montreal Before Universal Health Insurance," *Medical Care*, 11 (July–August 1973).

39. Evans, *Price Formation in the Market for Physician Services*, Ch. 4.

40. Regie de l'Assurance-Maladie du Quebec, *Annual Statistics 1972*, Quebec, n.d.

41. This whole paragraph is in response to Anne Scitovsky's comment that this paper really says more about the forces driving expenditure increase than about the role of health insurance, and that its treatment of the impact of insurance on physician incomes was inconsistent. I have attempted to rationalize the inconsistency, but I confess I do not know the answer.

42. Within B.C., however, the effects of differing physician density across regions on regional provider incomes seem to have been almost entirely (about 85 per cent) wiped out by variations in practice patterns; Evans *et al.*, "Medical Productivity, Scale Effects, and Demand Generation."

43. This is, of course, a growing view in the U.S., V. Fuchs and M. Kramer, *Determinants of Expenditures for Physicians' Services in the United States 1948–1968* (New York: National Bureau of Economic Research, Occasional Paper No. 117, 1972) being perhaps its leading exponents. The discretionary behavior of the physician and his influence over demand emerges also in the work of M. Feldstein, U. Reinhardt, and J. Newhouse, often by default.

44. Moreover, if copayment were to become large enough to reduce demand and utilization, private insurance would return for the good risks.

45. J. Y. Rivard, *La Rémuneration du corps médical*, Annexe 13 to the Castonguay Report; also Ch. 5 of Evans, *Price Formation in the Market for Physician Services*.

11 ‖ COMMENTS

Herbert E. Klarman
New York University

Evans' paper is really a short monograph that might just as well be entitled "What Every Interested American Ought to Know about Canadian Health Insurance." The Canadian experience with health insurance is important to this country because (1) it has coupled public financing with continued private production of health services; (2) variation among its provinces in approach and in timing has produced evidence from several significant social laboratories; and (3) a good many Canadian institutions, including the federal structure of government and relationships between physicians and hospitals, resemble our own. In chronological time, Canadian actions with respect to health insurance have preceded ours, so that they may provide us with a leading indicator.

In preparing this paper, Evans has intentionally cast a wide net. To continue the metaphor, he has achieved a substantial catch. The quality of the catch is variable, however. The paper could benefit from more work; it affords rewarding reading even now.

Beginning with an elegant introduction to the Canadian Constitution (the British North America Act), Evans relates how a central government that apparently lacks authority in the health field has managed to establish a roughly uniform nationwide system of nearly universal hospital and medical insurance by wielding the instrument of federal-provincial cost sharing. The hospital plan went into operation in the provinces in the period 1958–1961; the medical plan, in 1968–1970. Evans describes the two insurance plans in considerable detail—their respective benefits, sources of financing, methods of paying providers, and the basic data systems. Both structure and function are depicted with a broad brush, but also with a sense of the degree of diversity that characterizes the several Canadian provinces. (Under the circumstances, the latter aspect is not quite systematic.)

Ten numbered tables plus four more text tables, supported by an appendix on the data sources and on the splicing of time series, constitute a gold mine of trend data on personal health expenditures in Canada by object, on health care prices, and on health services utilization. Several tables also furnish detail by province. At almost every point the data beg for comparison with the United States; in small measure I shall try to respond to this need. Throughout, the paper invites more detailed description or more refined analysis; for this a discussant can only encourage the author to continue his good work and to amplify it.

POLICY PROPOSITIONS

Owing to time limitations in preparing the paper, Evans' policy propositions are not so well supported by the analyses developed in the paper at hand as they might be. Nevertheless, Evans is both a scholar and a man of experience, and his views on policy are worthy of respect for themselves. More important for this context, however, his policy views help the reader to understand why certain problems were selected for study and others were neglected.

I trust that what follows is a fair presentation of Evans' policy propositions stemming from his interpretation of the Canadian experience with health insurance:

1. Copayment by consumers is beside the point, for physician behavior is dominant. (In a footnote Evans adds: if copayment turned out to be important enough, private health insurance would sell policies to cover it.)
2. It is difficult to discover incentives toward greater managerial efficiency if managers are not allowed to do anything much with the savings they achieve or to apply them toward doing a better job.
3. Profiles and audits of providers are of limited value. They can only detect fraud.
4. It follows that it is necessary to try to control the flow of funds. The question, which is not answered, is how.
5. It comes down to this: Health insurance is a limited device. Complementary instruments are required.
6. As a practical matter, it is important to take steps to curtail the supply of hospital beds.
7. Canada will move toward a policy of restricting the number of physicians.

None of these propositions strikes me as unreasonable or implausible. Indeed, I incline to put even greater emphasis on a reduction in the supply of hospital beds in the long run. With respect to physicians, it is essential to explore the implications of their relationship with hospitals.

THIRD PARTIES AND CONSUMERS

Evans concludes that the economic relationships between third parties and consumers in Canada are relatively uninteresting. Why? He gives these reasons.

1. The existing system of health insurance premiums is pointless.
2. There is a scattering of utilization charges among the provinces, without rationale.
3. Utilization charges are probably costly to collect.
4. Extra billing by physicians is trivial (in contrast to the United States experience under Medicare).

Evans' conclusion on this score is important not only for policy purposes, but also because it leads him to emphasize a different set of economic relationships, those between third parties and providers. It would be highly useful, therefore, to document this conclusion. Of special interest are case materials that attempt to describe which policies have been tried and what ensued. Such materials serve administrators of health plans; they also shed light on the inferences drawn from quantitative studies.

THIRD PARTIES AND PROVIDERS' EARNINGS

For Evans, the economic relationships between payment agencies and providers of health services are at the heart of the Canadian health insurance system. How can this be, given the original lack of intention and desire on the part of government to intervene in the provision of services?

His answer is that certain consequences of health insurance were not foreseen. Utilization of services has increased somewhat; more expensive techniques are being adopted; and, in an open-ended payment system, providers revise their income aspirations upward.

Indeed, for Evans, the most prominent effect of health insurance in Canada has been the increase of earnings by health providers, both physicians and hospitals. Two factors are involved: (1) the policy adopted at the outset to pay all legitimate bills and to minimize interference with management; and (2) the inadequacy of the information structure on which intervention on the supply side might be based.

PHYSICIANS

Closer examination of the Canadian data, as well as comparison with data for the United States in the same intervals, suggests that in the case of physician services, health insurance must have been only one of the factors involved, for it appeared rather late. Table 1 presents annual rates of increase in expenditures in both countries; to show the component factors as well and to save space, panel A is for Canada and panel B is for the United States.

Early in the 1960s expenditures for physician services rose at the same rates in the two countries—7 to 8 per cent a year. The figure rose in both countries to 10 per cent a year by 1965. After that the Canadian rate of increase was higher, 13 vs. 10 per cent by 1968, and still higher in the next interval, 16 vs. 11 per cent.

However, the Canadian data indicate an increase in the per capita use of services of 11 per cent in the last interval. The figure is dubious on several grounds: It is considerably higher than any past figure; it is accompanied by a low—indeed, lower—rate of price increase; and it departs appreciably from the United States experience. It is not unreasonable to postulate some spillover between the United States and Canada.

TABLE 1   Physician Services: Annual Rates of Increase in Expenditures, Population, Price, and per Capita Use, Canada and the United States, Selected Intervals

Interval	Expenditures	Population	Price	Per Capita Use
A. Canada				
1953–1956	10.8%	3.0%	N/A	N/A
1956–1959	10.7	3.1	N/A	N/A
1959–1962	7.7	2.3	2.0%	3.4%
1962–1965	10.3	2.1	2.3	5.8
1965–1968	13.1	2.0	5.0	5.7
1968–1971	16.2	1.5	3.0	11.3
B. United States				
1950–1955	6.0%	1.7%	3.4%	0.9%
1955–1960	9.1	1.7	3.3	4.1
1960–1962	7.0	1.6	2.6	2.8
1962–1965	10.4	1.4	2.6	6.4
1965–1968	9.8	1.1	6.2	2.5
1968–1971	10.9	0.9	7.1	2.9

SOURCES: *Canada*—Evans' paper provides basic data for my computations.
United States—Herbert E. Klarman, Dorothy P. Rice, Barbara L. Cooper, and H. Louis Stettler, *Sources of Increase in Selected Medical Care Expenditures, 1929–1969* (Washington, D.C., Social Security Administration, 1970); for subsequent years, Social Security Administration, unpublished data.

One can only surmise about plausible explanations. Is it possible that medical insurance in Canada, by establishing a single source of payment within a province, led simultaneously to a more correct reporting of earnings by physicians? If so, there would be a one-time shift in the data base. Utilization changes would be overstated, if price increases were understated for whatever reason. An improved ratio of collections to charges would serve to increase earnings while official prices remained the same. In the United States there is good reason to believe that after 1965 the fractionation of fees became widespread, thereby understating the official rise in fees; has Canada had a similar experience?

Certainly the fact of an appreciable increase in physician earnings is not contestable. However, because of the high increase in per capita utilization reported in his data, Evans may be neglecting prices unduly over the long run. Evans appropriately emphasizes the discretion of the physician in prescribing additional visits and services. In the United States Rappleye[1] and Ginzberg[2] have long made this the core of their policy positions on health manpower. Fuchs and Kramer offer this ability of physicians to generate more services as their preferred explanation of the statistical significance of the physician supply variable in their demand equation.[3] Adam Smith does not distinguish between influence on quantity of service and on price when he recognizes that the reward of physicians must be such "as may give them that rank in society which so important a trust requires."[4] To have better judgment on the Canadian fee data, more needs to be known than is reported in this paper about how physicians are actually paid. May I add that Evans is uniquely able to furnish such information.[5]

There is a wealth of provincial data that Evans does not explore and that I am unable to handle. Take Saskatchewan, for example. Table 6 shows it to have been successful in keeping down physician services expenditures. How? Not by keeping down the number of physicians; its supply rose at the overall Canadian rate, according to Table 9. What about its fee level? Well, it rose at a rate slightly higher than for Canada, according to Table 6; or it may have risen at a lower rate in recent years, according to Table 10. A reconciliation of the fee data, which are undoubtedly ambiguous in spots, would be a useful endeavor.

HOSPITALS

In Canada, average earnings of hospital employees have increased by 8 per cent a year. For a similar period, earnings of hospital employees in the United States rose by 5 per cent a year.

Evans asks whether the increase in average employee earnings reflects in part a higher personnel mix. Data bearing directly on the question are not available to him, but on balance he concludes that a change in personnel mix probably had nothing to do with it. For the United States, Feldstein reports a reduction in the average skill level of hospital workers. This trend was

TABLE 2 Hospitals: Annual Rates of Increase in Cost Components, Canada, 1953–1971, and the United States, 1955–1968

Cost Component	Canada	United States
Average Cost/Patient Day	9.3%	7.8%
Labor Cost/Patient Day	10.5	7.5
Personnel/Patient Day	2.1	2.3
Average Annual Earnings	8.3	5.1
Nonlabor Cost/Patient Day	7.2	8.2
Proportion Labor to Total:		
Initial Year	57.7	61.7
Terminal Year	70.3	59.6

SOURCES: *Canada*—Computed from basic data in Evans' paper.
United States—Martin S. Feldstein, *The Rising Cost of Hospital Care* (Washington, D.C.: Information Resources Press, 1971), p. 17.

coupled with increases in wages for some hospital occupations that brought them to levels above those in other industries.[6]

Although staffing ratios are lower in Canada than in the United States (and appropriately so, given the longer average duration of stay in the former—13.3 hours per patient day vs. 14.9 hours), the rate of increase in the former still lags—2.1 vs. 2.3 per cent a year (Table 2). However, labor cost per patient day has increased at a higher rate in Canada, owing to the higher rate of increase in average earnings. The result, which is not easy to understand, is that in Canada labor costs have risen to 70 per cent of total cost from a base year figure of 58 per cent, whereas in the United States the trend was gradually downward, from 62 to 60 per cent (Table 2).

A possible approach to reconciling some of these divergent tendencies is to examine differences in the definition of accounts. In the United States fringe benefits are classified as nonlabor expenses; are they so classified in Canada? In the United States nonlabor expenses incorporate increasing amounts of depreciation, which used to be neglected; does the situation differ in Canada?

Evans concludes that wage inflation is the main source of increase in hospital expenditures in Canada. The timing of the wage inflation does not correspond to the extension of health insurance, nor to the increase in hospital use, nor even to the expansion of hospital employment. Indeed, the increase in use was small, and corresponded to the increase in hospital beds. It is not clear what led to the increase in wages. From the experience of the United States after Medicare, either of two explanations is tenable: the extension and then operation of universal hospital insurance; or the method employed to pay hospitals. Can the experience in Canada help one choose between them?

REGULATION OR CONTROL THROUGH REIMBURSEMENT

For both types of provider, Evans stresses the importance of negotiated earnings and sees no obvious basis for the exercise of restraint.

He mentions the accumulation of a formidable hospital data base and regrets the failure hitherto to apply it. He looks forward to better coding and machine processing of the data. Furthermore, he would employ the data to explain differences in cost among hospitals and to set prices for inpatient and outpatient services. For these purposes direct departmental expenses, without any allocation of overhead, are useless, in Evans' opinion.

Here I differ. The fact is that economists do not yet know how to explain cost differences among hospitals. Moreover, for a multiproduct firm, it is not possible to calculate the average cost of each product; only the marginal cost is calculable.[7] If so, what is the use of allocating overhead expenses? At least direct departmental expenses can help in making comparisons within a hospital over time and among institutions, preferably also over time.

Evans is doubtful about the efficacy of close monitoring of institutions to achieve greater efficiency. Believing that he is right, I should still like to see some documentation from the Canadian experience.

Evans concludes from his study of Canadian health insurance that the supply side is crucial. Again I tend to agree; the study of demand has preoccupied us unduly. It is salubrious to hear a call for increased concentration on supply factors at a conference devoted exclusively to the economics of health insurance.

NOTES

1. Willard E. Rappleye, *Personnel—The Key to Effective Health Programs* (New York: Josiah Macy, Jr. Foundation, 1950).
2. Eli Ginzberg, *Men, Money and Medicine* (New York: Columbia University Press, 1969).
3. Victor R. Fuchs and Marcia J. Kramer, *Determinants of Expenditures for Physicians' Services in the United States, 1948–1968* (New York: National Bureau of Economic Research, Occasional Paper No. 117, 1972), p. 36.
4. Adam Smith, *The Wealth of Nations* (New York: Random House, 1937), p. 105.
5. Robert Evans, *Price Formation in the Market for Physician Services in Canada, 1957–1969* (Ottawa: Information Canada, 1973).
6. Martin S. Feldstein, *The Rising Cost of Hospital Care* (Washington, D.C.: Information Resources Press, 1971), pp. 56, 61.
7. George Stigler, *The Theory of Price* (New York: Macmillan, 1946), p. 307.

Anne A. Scitovsky

Palo Alto Medical Research Foundation

Like Professor Klarman, I am much impressed by Professor Evans' paper. He has tackled a formidable problem and really combined three if not four different papers in one. There is, to begin with, a historical-descriptive section on the organization of national health insurance in Canada. This is followed, first, by a detailed analysis of the rise in hospital expenditures in the period 1953–1971, and then by a somewhat less detailed analysis of the increase in physician expenditures in the period 1957–1971. Finally, the sections on hospital and physician expenditures contain a discussion and evaluation of government policy responses to hospital cost inflation as well as Professor Evans' own recommendations on how to solve the problem of medical care cost inflation in Canada. He has assembled and analyzed a vast body of data that I am sure future researchers will heavily draw from. Let me therefore preface my comments by saying that any criticisms I have are minor compared to the job he has done.

My main comment is that Professor Evans' paper is not so much a study of the effects of national health insurance in Canada as an analysis of the increase in hospital expenditures in the period 1953–1971 and in physician expenditures in the period 1957–1971. Early in his introductory section, he *does* say: ". . . the single most prominent influence of health insurance in Canada has been to increase the earnings of health providers." The earnings of health providers, both in the hospital sector and in the physician sector, did indeed rise very substantially during these periods. But his data do not really show that this was the result of national health insurance.

For example, he shows that hospital workers' wage rates as well as gross wages and salaries per patient day actually rose *less* in the period 1959–1965 (the immediate post-hospital insurance period) than in either the preceding or the subsequent six-year periods. He himself seems to change his mind about what exactly health insurance had to do with the inflation of costs as he proceeds to analyze the data in detail. In the section on hospital costs, he refers to a Canadian government report on hospital expenditures over the period 1961–1971 and says: "In analyzing the response of hospital expenditure to insurance . . . the message of the report parallels that of this paper—wage inflation in the hospital sector is the main source of increase and *the timing does not particularly correspond to the extension of insurance*, the expansion of utilization, or even the expansion of employment" (italics mine). Actually, let me add that what increase in utilization there has been also does not seem to correspond to the extension of insurance. As Table 4 shows, the rate of increase in utilization, in terms of both admissions and patient days per 1,000 population, was slower in the post-insurance than in the pre-insurance period. Only employment as measured by hours worked per patient day shows some relation to the extension of insurance. As the table on p. 457 shows, it rose at a somewhat faster rate in the post-insurance period—22.6 per cent between 1959 and 1965 as against 15.2 per cent between 1953 and 1959; however, this increase accounts for only a very small part of the increase in average labor costs per patient day between 1959 and 1965. Thus, the role of national health insurance is a relatively minor factor in explaining the increase in hospital costs, and we have to look to other factors for an explanation.

This Professor Evans does very thoroughly and, I think, successfully, in the hospital sector of the paper, and more superficially in the physician sector. To begin with the hospital part of his paper, his data bear out his thesis that it was supplier behavior—the rapid and considerable increase in hospital workers' wages and in labor costs per patient day—that was the major factor underlying the increase. However, although he shows that the rise in wage rates cannot be explained as demand-induced wage inflation resulting from expanded employment, he does not really come up with a satisfactory explanation. He explores various possible explanations. For example, he considers that there may have been a shift in the mix of hospital personnel from less-skilled to more-skilled workers, but concludes that this was not the case, although here his data are not entirely satisfactory. He also explores the possibility that the phasing out of unpaid or almost unpaid workers (student nurses, nursing assistants, and interns), which in 1953 accounted for about 17–18 per cent of hours worked per patient day, may have been a factor. But even when he adjusts for this change he finds that it explains only a small part of the increase in hospital wage rates (about 24 per cent). He mentions the possibility that hospital workers' wages were still catching up from the period of very low wages during the period of charity hospitals, and he shows that in 1971, the average hourly hospital wage was still somewhat below that of the average industrial hourly wage—$3.26 compared to $3.44. Unfortunately, lack of data on the mix of skills in both the hospital and the industrial sectors prevent him from pursuing this possible explanation. The reason for the increase in hospital wages is therefore left largely unexplained.

I also want to raise a question that bothers me. According to Professor Evans, 70 per cent of the average cost per patient day in Canada in 1971 was labor cost; in the United States in the same year, it was about 58 per cent. Yet in Canada, hours worked per patient day in 1971 were 13.29, or 1.66 hospital workers per day, assuming an eight-hour work day, whereas in the United States it was 3.01 workers per day. What is the explanation? Do the U.S. figures for cost per patient day include some costs that are not included in the Canadian figures? Or do the Canadian figures for labor cost per patient day include something not included in the U.S. figures? Or do Canadian hospitals employ a higher proportion of highly skilled employees? The explanation may lie in the longer average length of stay in Canada than in the U.S. (11.3 days in 1971 in Canada as against 8.03 days in the U.S.). Since shorter stays result in higher average costs per day because the first few days of any hospital stay are the most expensive, involving a high percentage of nonlabor costs (operating room, x-rays, lab tests, etc.), this seems one possible explanation. I don't want to belabor this point, but it does intrigue me.

To turn to the physician expenditures part of Professor Evans' paper, as I already said, his analysis here is less thorough. He compares the period 1957–1964 with the period 1964–1971. His choice of 1964 as the dividing point between the pre- and post-Medicare periods puzzles me since Medicare was enacted only in 1966, and all but one of the ten provinces have introduced programs only quite recently—one in 1968, five in 1969, two in 1970, and one in 1971. In addition, I have some questions about his analysis of the changes in expenditures that occurred in the period 1957–1971.

Any analysis of physician expenditures hinges on the adequacy of the index used to deflate expenditures. Professor Evans does not tell us what exactly is included in the new N.H.W. benefits paid index nor what the implications of linking the old CPI physician fee index to the new index are. He himself seems to have some doubts about the index since he says: "*If* list prices really reflected actual prices over this period, one would derive an apparent quantity increase for 1957–1971 by dividing expenditure change by price change—this quantity estimate increases by 8.0 per cent per year." Again, a bit later, he says: "*If* one accepted the Table 7 list price increase of 56 per cent from 1957 to 1971, the implicit average increase in real output per physician would be 4.1 per cent per year (italics mine in both quotations). A more detailed explanation of the index, and Professor Evans' reasons for being so tentative about it, would therefore seem to be called for in a paper of this kind.

Not knowing what exactly the fee/benefit index reflects leaves it to the reader to speculate about what some of the causes of the increased "real" output might be, especially since Professor Evans does not make much of an attempt to explain it. He does state that the stock of physicians rose twice as fast as population in the period 1957–1971. But this does not explain the increase in "real" output *per physician*. On the basis of some fragmentary evidence, he doubts that physician visit rates have increased. He concludes, therefore, that the increase in "real" output is attributable to the fact that physicians to a large extent are able to determine the demand for their services and, as he puts it, "manipulate utilization to generate income." I am the first to agree that the physician can and does play an important role in determining the demand for his services, and have argued so for a long time. Undoubtedly this explains a good part of the increased "real" output. But another possible contributory factor that Professor Evans does not mention is the possible increase in the percentage of specialists as against general practitioners. This may, of course, be accounted for in the index but, as I said, I have no way of knowing. If it is not, and there was such a shift in Canada, this could explain at least part of the increased "real" output since specialists not only charge higher fees than GP's but also generate more ancillary services such as lab tests and x-rays per visit. It would be interesting to know, therefore, if and in what way the distribution of Canadian physicians by field of specialty changed in the period 1957–1971.

Just one more point on this subject. Many physicians undoubtedly "manipulate" demand to increase their income by ordering too many lab tests or x-rays or by performing marginal or even unnecessary surgery; or, as Professor Evans points out, they may "shift across fee schedule items from, for example, 'ordinary' to 'complete' office examinations." But there are also other changes in practice patterns that increase physician income and are not quite in the same "manipulative" category. Take, for example, a fairly recent study of "The Effects of 'Free' Medical Care on Medical Practice—the Quebec Experience," reported by Philip Enterline in the *New England Journal of Medicine* (May 31, 1973). He interviewed a random sample of Montreal physicians before and after the Province of Quebec put Medicare in effect in November 1970 (the surveys were done October 1969–May 1970 and October 1971–May 1972). He found that the total number of *all* patient contacts declined by almost 10 per cent in the post-Medicare period. However, when you look at the change by type of contact, you find that total face-to-face contacts increased by 4.8 per cent. Telephone contacts declined by 41 per cent, office visits increased by 32 per cent, hospital inpatient visits dropped by 16 per cent, hospital clinic visits stayed about the same, and home visits dropped by 63 per cent. This change in practice patterns undoubtedly raised physicians' incomes, since telephone calls are probably rarely charged for and since home visits (at least in the U.S.) are relatively underpriced in relation to other types of visits (a doctor can see several patients in his office—at a fee not much lower than that for a home visit—for every one home visit he makes and thus make more money). If this type of change in practice patterns occurred in other parts of Canada, either as a result of Medicare or because of a long-term trend (in the

U.S., for example, there has been a steady decline in home visits), this also would explain some of the increase in "real" output.

In conclusion, let me say that I am in full agreement with Professor Evans that copayment on the part of patients is not the answer to stemming the rise in medical care costs, or rather not the *sole* answer. I do not think that copayment is as ineffective as Professor Evans seems to think, and I believe that some copayment on the part of patients is desirable. But I feel very strongly, and have argued so in a recent paper, that some forms of restraints on suppliers of medical services have to be devised—primarily on physicians since they to a large extent determine not only the demand for their own services but the demand for hospital services. The hospitals, as somebody said recently, don't have patients—they only have doctors. I am not sure that I agroo with Professor Evans' recommended solution, but I have to admit that I have no counter-proposal.

12

MARTIN FELDSTEIN
Harvard University

and

BERNARD FRIEDMAN
Northwestern University

The Effect of National Health Insurance on the Price and Quantity of Medical Care

The study reported in this paper uses a microsimulation model to estimate the effects of alternative national health insurance policies. Unlike previous microsimulation studies, the current analysis uses an explicit model of the supply and price response in the markets for hospital care and physicians' services. Indeed, two quite different models of supply and price response are examined and their implications are contrasted.

A *microsimulation* model of household demand is necessary if the analysis is to provide useful results in the comparison of specific health insurance proposals. The effects of alternative national health insurance policies depend crucially on the stochastic character of health care demand. More specifically, the effects of

The methods and programs used in this paper were developed in a project supported by the Department of Health, Education, and Welfare. The model in Section 1 was described in an unpublished technical report, "National Health Insurance Simulation Model" (August 1972), and the methods in Sections 2 and 4 were described in "Supply and Price Response in National Health Insurance Analysis" (September 1972). We are grateful to the Department of Health, Education, and Welfare for its support of this research and to B. Mitchell, G. Moyer, and D. Schenker for useful discussions.

different sets of deductibles, coinsurance rates, and other parameters of insurance policies depend on particular stochastic distributions of health expenditures. *Aggregate* specification of demand behavior cannot capture the subtle differences in the response of demand to different types of insurance policies. The current investigation uses a stochastic simulation model of demand based on the actual experience of more than 300,000 families. The basic demand model, described in detail in Section 1, is an extension of the simple aggregate health care demand model used in Feldstein, Friedman, and Luft (1972).

A serious weakness of all previous microsimulation studies of national health insurance, including our own (1972), has been the neglect of the supply and price response to national health insurance. The current analysis shows how an aggregate model of supply and price response can be combined with a microsimulation model of demand. Although there are no explicit *aggregate* demand equations, the complete model is solved for prices that equate supply and demand. The supply model and the method of finding the equilibrium are described in Section 2. Some illustrative results are then presented in Section 3.

The supply and price response of sections 2 and 3 is based on the simplest model of aggregate supply and the assumption of market clearing equilibrium. The markets for hospital care and for physicians' services may not behave in this way. Hospital prices may rise in response to increases in demand because hospitals change the nature of their product and not because it is more expensive to produce a larger quantity of the old product. Physicians may increase prices in response to greater demand or increased insurance without setting a market clearing price. Section 4 develops a model with these characteristics, describes the simultaneous interaction of demand with this supply behavior, and presents some illustrative results.

Most of the debate about the effects of national health insurance has focused on the uncertainty about the responsiveness of household demand. The current study shows that our uncertainty about supply response may be even more important.

1. A MICROSIMULATION MODEL OF DEMAND

The annual health care expenditures of a group of families with the same demographic composition, income, and insurance coverage can be described by a joint frequency distribution of expenditures on hospital services and medical services. Each such distribution is conditional on the gross prices charged for hospital and physician services. Let $F^i(E_h, E_m | P_h, P_m)$ be such a distribution for insurance coverage i with:

E_h = family's total expenditure for hospital services
E_m = family's total expenditure for medical services
P_h = gross price per unit of hospital services
P_m = gross price per unit of medical services

There is an associated distribution of net out-of-pocket expense $G^i(N | P_h, P_m)$ that is related to F^i by the insurance reimbursement formula.

The expenditure distribution associated with any particular insurance structure and prices is derived from a "baseline" *quantity* distribution that would prevail in the absence of any insurance and with prices equal to unity: $F^0(X_h, X_m | P_h = 1, P_m = 1)$. There is, of course, a different baseline expenditure distribution for each family type. A specific national health insurance proposal can be described in terms of the deductibles, coinsurance rates, and maximum net out-of-pocket expenditure for each type of family. D_h and D_m will be used to denote the deductibles, C_h and C_m the coinsurance rates, and MAX the maximum net out-of-pocket expenditure.

The equations relating expenditure in the presence of insurance to the baseline distribution and the prevailing gross prices is an extension of a traditional constant elasticity demand model. The most appropriate way to extend a constant elasticity specification to deal with deductibles and a maximum net spending limit is uncertain. One approach, offered as a tentative specification until better empirical evidence is available, assumes a constant elasticity of the quantity demanded with respect to the *net price* paid for expenditures over the deductible. The net price of an additional unit of hospital care depends on the family's current level of expenditure. More generally, the net price paid by the family depends on (1) the gross price charged by the hospital (P_h), (2) the effective coinsurance rate (1 for expenditures below the deductible, (C_h) between the deductible and the maximum net expenditure limit, and 0 above that limit) and (3) a parameter, λ, representing the nonmonetary costs (Acton, 1972; Phelps and Newhouse, 1972) to the consumer of health services.

If there were no deductibles ($D_h = D_m = 0$) and no maximum net expenditure (MAX $= \infty$), the two expenditure equations would be:

(1)
$$E_h = P_h \cdot X_h \left[\frac{P_h(C_h + \lambda)}{1 + \lambda} \right]^{\alpha_h} \left[\frac{P_m(C_m + \lambda)}{1 + \lambda} \right]^{\alpha_m}$$

(2)
$$E_m = P_m \cdot X_m \left[\frac{P_h(C_h + \lambda)}{1 + \lambda} \right]^{\beta_h} \left[\frac{P_m(C_m + \lambda)}{1 + \lambda} \right]^{\beta_m}$$

Notice that if there is no insurance, $C_h = C_m = 1$ and the equation is the usual constant elasticity demand equation. With complete insurance, $C_h = C_m = 0$ but demand remains finite because $\lambda > 0$ implies a positive nonmonetary cost.

To allow for deductibles and for the maximum net expenditure limit, it is necessary to distinguish four separate cases. Let $\hat{E}_h = X_h P_h^{1+\alpha_h} P_m^{\alpha_m}$ and $\hat{E}_m = X_m P_h^{\beta_h} P_m^{1+\beta_m}$, the expenditures that would occur at prices P_h, P_m if there were no insurance.

Case i If $\hat{E}_h < D_h$ and $\hat{E}_m < D_m$, then $E_h = \hat{E}_h$ and $E_m = \hat{E}_m$. Here the insurance is irrelevant because the deductibles exceed the expenditure that would be made in the absence of insurance. The total net out-of-pocket expenditure is $N = E_h + E_m$.

Case ii If $\hat{E}_h > D_h$ and $\hat{E}_m > D_m$, then

(a)
$$E_h = D_h + P_h(X_h - D_h P_h^{-1}) \left[\frac{P_h(C_h + \lambda)}{1 + \lambda} \right]^{\alpha_h} \left[\frac{P_m(C_m + \lambda)}{1 + \lambda} \right]^{\alpha_m}$$

$$E_m = D_m + P_m(X_m - D_m P_m^{-1}) \left[\frac{P_h(C_h + \lambda)}{1 + \lambda} \right]^{\beta_h} \left[\frac{P_m(C_m + \lambda)}{1 + \lambda} \right]^{\beta_m}$$

and

$$N = D_h + D_m + C_h(E_h - D_h) + C_m(E_m - D_m) < \text{MAX}$$

or

(b)
$$E_h = D_h + P_h(X_h - D_h P_h^{-1}) \left[\frac{P_h \lambda}{1 + \lambda} \right]^{\alpha_h} \left[\frac{P_m \lambda}{1 + \lambda} \right]^{\alpha_m}$$

$$E_m = D_m + P_m(X_m - D_m P_m^{-1}) \left[\frac{P_h \lambda}{1 + \lambda} \right]^{\beta_h} \left[\frac{P_m \lambda}{1 + \lambda} \right]^{\beta_m}$$

and

$$N = \text{MAX}$$

Case iii If $E_h > D_h$ and $\hat{E}_m < D_m$ then either:[1]

(a) $E_h = D_h + P_h(X_h - D_h P_h^{-1}) \left[\dfrac{P_h(C_h + \lambda)}{1 + \lambda} \right]^{\alpha_h} \left[\dfrac{P_m(C_m + \lambda)}{1 + \lambda} \right]^{\alpha_m}$

$E_m = \hat{E}_m$

$N = D_h + C_h(E_h - D_h) + \hat{E}_m < \text{MAX}$

or

(b) $E_h = D_h + P_h(X_h - D_h P_h^{-1}) \left[\dfrac{P_h\lambda}{1 + \lambda} \right]^{\alpha_h} \left[\dfrac{P_m\lambda}{1 + \lambda} \right]^{\alpha_m}$

$E_m = P_m X_m \left[\dfrac{P_h\lambda}{1 + \lambda} \right]^{\rho_h} \left[\dfrac{P_m\lambda}{1 + \lambda} \right]^{\rho_m}$

$N = \text{MAX}.$

Case iv If $\hat{E}_h < D_h$ and $\hat{E}_m > D_m$, the results bear an obvious analogy to Case iii.

These four sets of demand equations can be used to generate the distribution F^i corresponding to any gross prices, insurance characteristics, and demand parameters. More specifically, given a baseline distribution $F^0(X_h, X_m)$ we can draw values (X_h, X_m) with the appropriate probability and calculate the corresponding E_h, E_m. Average gross and net expenditures $(\bar{E}_h, \bar{E}_m,$ and $\bar{N})$ are then readily computed. This procedure is done separately for each family type. These calculations and the aggregates produced by combining the averages for different family types could be used to assess the effects of alternative national health insurance proposals if supplies were infinitely elastic at fixed values of P_h and P_m. This was essentially the procedure used in Feldstein, Friedman, and Luft (1972) with a simpler model that did not distinguish hospital and medical services. The more general use of the demand simulation model when prices are endogenous is discussed in the next section. The remainder of this section describes our data sources, the derivation of the family baseline distributions, and the calibration of the model to 1970 aggregate experience.

The primary data are the individual insurance claims for more than 300,000 federal government employees and their dependents in 1970. All of these persons had the very comprehensive Aetna "High Option" coverage. A tabulation of the joint frequency distribution of hospital and medical services (a 24-by-24 matrix of relative frequencies with an associated matrix of cell means) was derived for all male employees. Similar tabulations were derived separately for female employees, dependent spouses, and children. The Aetna coverage uses a $50 deductible per individual (except that the first $1,000 of hospital room and board is fully reimbursed) and a coinsurance rate of 20 per cent for both hospital and medical services. For each category of individual, the observed bivariate frequency distribution was used to infer the baseline distribution corresponding to each of several alternative sets of demand parameters (α's, β's, and λ). This procedure uses the inverse of the demand function with $D_h = 0$, $D_m = 50$, $C_h = C_m = 0.20$, and MAX $= \infty$. The prices were both normalized to be 1.

Family baseline distributions for sixteen different family compositions (e.g., husband and wife; husband, wife, and three children; etc.) were produced by convoluting the baseline distributions for individuals.[2] Persons over 65 were assumed to be excluded from the basic national health insurance plan and were therefore ignored in calculating family distributions. For each of the sixteen family compositions, twelve income categories were defined in order to implement national health insurance specifications that are income related and to assess the tax burdens that balance the new government expenditures.

The demand simulation model provides average gross and net expenditures for each of the 192 family types. These are also aggregated to national averages and subaverages by using population counts computed from the Current Population Survey of 1971.

Although the experience of the federal employees with Aetna High Option coverage is an extremely rich and valuable source of data, these employees are not a representative sample of all U.S. families, particularly in regard to geographic distribution, employment status, and occupation. For each set of demand parameter assumptions (α_n, α_m, β_n, β_m, λ) the following additional steps are taken to calibrate the baseline distributions to known national aggregates for 1970. The typical family insurance coverage in 1970 was assumed to be $D_h = 100$, $D_m = 100$, $C_h = 0.25$, $C_m = 0.40$, and MAX $= \infty$.[3] This typical coverage is used for a preliminary simulation to estimate the national aggregate expenditures corresponding to each set of demand parameters. Suppose that the estimated expenditures for some set of demand parameters are E_h^* and E_m^* and that the actual expenditures are E_h^0 and E_m^0. The ratios E_h^*/E_h^0 and E_m^*/E_m^0 are then used to deflate the expenditure units of the corresponding baseline distributions. With this calibration completed, the implications of various national health insurance plans may be compared for the given set of demand parameters.

2. A SUPPLY RESPONSE MODEL AND THE EQUILIBRIUM SOLUTION

In the supply response model, the usual interaction of supply and demand provides a market clearing reaction of quantities and prices to a change in insurance coverage. The computational problems and novelty of the model occur because there are no aggregate demand equations but only individual demand equations and a microsimulation model.

The basic idea and computational procedure for the supply response model can be described most easily by ignoring the distinction between hospital and medical services. The solution for the more general case will be discussed below. Let Q be the aggregate quantity of health services consumed by all households, P the price level, and E the expenditure ($E = Q \cdot P$). Since there are no natural units in which to measure Q, we take the current price prevailing in the absence of national health insurance (P_0) to have the value 1 and thus define the quantity in the absence of national health insurance (Q_0) to be equal to the expenditure (E_0).

An aggregate supply function with constant price elasticity can be written:

(3) $\quad \ln Q = \ln Q_0 + \gamma \ln P$

If an *aggregate* market demand function could be written in terms of the gross market price and the features of the national health insurance program, the two equations could be solved for the changes in P and Q that would accompany alternative NHI plans. However, such an aggregate demand function is the outcome of a very complex and stochastic set of individual demand functions that cannot be given an aggregate parametric summary. Only by operating the demand simulation model described in Section 1 can points on the demand curve be calculated. The market equilibrium is found by combining the aggregate supply function of Equation (3) with demand generated by the simulation model.

The process of convergence to an equilibrium solution of this iterative simulation process is best described with the aid of a diagram. Figure 1 shows the change in the price-quality equilibrium that results from the introduction of national health insurance. More specifically, in the absence of NHI the market is in equilibrium at point A. The demand curve ($D1$) relates the quantity demanded to the *gross* price for the structure of private health insurance prevailing before NHI. The $D1$ curve is not actually known but points on it can be found by using the demand simulation model. The supply function S corresponds to Equation

FIGURE 1

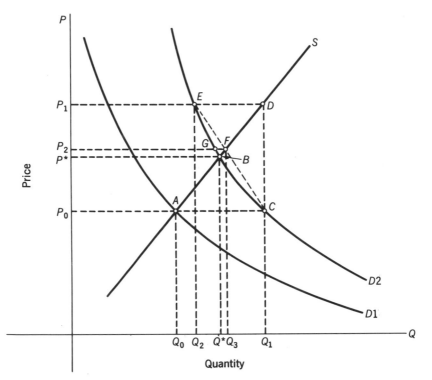

(3). The introduction of NIII shifts the demand function to $D2$ and the equilibrium to B. The computational problem is to determine the coordinates of the point B even though the two demand curves are not directly observable.

The following feasible and efficient procedure is used. First, the demand simulation model is used to find the aggregate quantity that would be purchased under NHI if price were unchanged—i.e., it locates the point C and the quantity Q_1. Second, the supply function is used to solve for the price P_1 at which the quantity Q_1 would be supplied. Third, the demand simulation model is used again to find the aggregate quantity demanded in the presence of NHI but with the gross market price P_1; this is Q_2 at point E. It is clear from Figure 1 that (if the aggregate demand function is well behaved) the equilibrium price after NHI (P^*) lies between P_0 and P_1. Similarly, the new equilibrium quantity (Q^*) lies between Q_1 and Q_2. The fourth step in the analysis is to approximate the unknown demand curve ($D2$) in the relevant range by the straight line connecting points C and E. This is shown as a broken line in the figure. For computational purposes it is defined by the equation

(4) $$Q = Q_2 - \frac{Q_1 - Q_2}{P_1 - P_0} (P_1 - P)$$

Equations (3) and (4) may now be combined and solved for equilibrium price quantity point. This corresponds to point F and thus to P_2 and Q_3.

The next step checks on the closeness of the approximations of F to the true new equilibrium B. Since, by construction, F is on the supply function, the test of closeness depends on the gap between the trial solution (point F) and the demand curve. To assess this, the demand simulation model is again used. Simulating with gross price P_2 yields the point G. If the quantities at G and F are sufficiently close, the analysis is complete. If they differ by more than some prespecified amount, the iterative procedure can be continued in order to achieve greater accuracy.

The method of increasing accuracy is illustrated in Figure 2, with

FIGURE 2

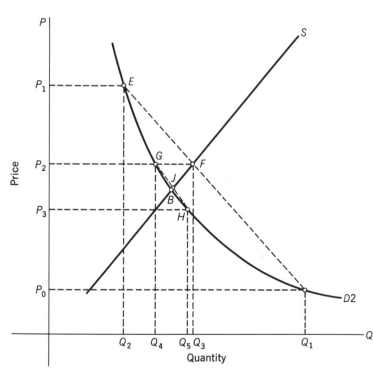

notation carried over from Figure 1. If Q_3 is greater than Q_4, the curve $D2$ is convex toward the origin in the relevant range; this is the case that will now be described. If the inequality is reversed, the curve is concave and the calculations are modified accordingly. Since the equation for the supply curve is given, it is possible to solve for the price P_3 at which the quantity Q_4 would be supplied. Demand simulation then identifies the point H and the quantity Q_5 that would be demanded at price P_3. The points G and H are analogous to the old points E and C. The equation of the line joining G and H is found and used as a local approximation to the demand curve. The intersection of this approximation and the supply curve identifies the point J, which is much closer to B than F was. This is verified and the accuracy evaluated by a further simulation at the price corresponding to J.

This iterative simulation method of finding the post-NHI market equilibrium is easily extended to separate markets for hospital care and medical services. The procedure begins by using the demand simulation model described in Section 1 to calculate the hospital and medical expenditures, E_h and E_m, that would prevail with NHI if the prices remained unchanged.[4] Since the pre-NHI prices are normalized at 1, these expenditures are also equivalent to quantities. This yields quantities that may be denoted QH_1 and QM_1, corresponding to point C of Figure 1.

The two aggregate constant elasticity supply functions are:

(5) $\ln QH = \ln QH_0 + \gamma_H \ln PH$

$\ln QM = \ln QM_0 + \gamma_M \ln PM$

where QH_0 and QM_0 are the aggregate quantities before NHI, PH and PM are prices of hospital and medical care $(PH_0 = PM_0 = 1)$, and γ_H and γ_M are supply elasticities. Substituting the values QH_1 and QM_1 into QH and QM yields the prices PH_1 and PM_1 at which these quantities would be supplied; these prices correspond to point D of Figure 1. The demand simulation model is then repeated using PH_1 and PM_1 and the deductibles, coinsurance rates, and values of MAX provided for by the NHI plan. The aggregate quantities demanded at these prices, QH_2 and QM_2, correspond to point E of Figure 2.

Although the coordinates of two points like C and E were sufficient to define a linear demand equation when hospital and medical services were not distinguished, a third point is now needed if the cross-price effects are to be taken into account. A new price corresponding to the average of PH_1 and the pre-NHI price $(PH_0 = 1)$ is selected for hospital care. A similar value is selected for medical care. At these prices $(PH_2$ and $PM_2)$, a new set of quantities

$(QH_3$ and $QM_3)$ is obtained by simulation. The coordinates of the three quantity-price points $(QH_1, QM_1, 1, 1)$, (QH_2, QM_2, PH_1, PM_1), and (QH_3, QM_3, PH_2, PM_2) can be used to evaluate the parameters of the two linear equations that approximate the demand function in the presence of NHI. More specifically, we take the aggregate demand equations to be:

(6) $QH = a_1 + a_2PH + a_3PM$

and

$QM = b_1 + b_2PH + b_3PM$

The three parameters of each equation can be obtained by substituting the values of the variables for each of the three price quantity points. The two supply equations (5) and the two demand equations (6) are then solved simultaneously to obtain trial equilibrium values (QH_4, QM_4, PH_3, PM_3) that correspond to point F of Figure 1. This set of values corresponds to a point on the supply functions. To check the accuracy of the approximation to the demand, the demand simulation is recomputed for prices PH_3 and PM_3. This yields a point that is analogous to G of Figure 1. If this is not sufficiently accurate, a further iteration is computed as described above for Figure 2.

3. AN ANALYSIS OF TWO NHI PLANS

This section calculates the equilibrium quantities and prices associated with two alternative NHI options. The analysis emphasizes the substantial sensitivity of the results to the elasticities of supply as well as to the demand parameters.

The first NHI plan (NHI-1) has low annual deductibles of $50 for hospital care and $50 for medical services and very low coinsurance rates of 10 per cent for both types of services. There is no limit, however, to the family's maximum net expenditure (MAX = ∞). These characteristics of the NHI plan are the same for all income levels and all family demographic compositions. The second NHI plan (NHI-2) has the same $50 deductibles but a coinsurance rate of 20 per cent for both types of expenditure. Each family's net expenditure is limited to 10 per cent of family income. This is a substantial reduction in risk, especially for lower- and middle-income families.

The individual demand equations are simplified by assuming no cross-price elasticities (i.e., $\alpha_m = \beta_h = 0$ in the demand equations of Section 1). Although hospital services and other services are substitutes for some purposes, they are also complements in other contexts. The assumption of zero cross-elasticity may therefore be a reasonable starting point for a preliminary analysis.[5] Two different sets of price elasticities have been used. The "moderate" price elasticities assume that the own-price of hospital care (α_h) is 0.5 and the own-price elasticity of medical care (β_m) is 0.4. The "low" elasticity pair assumes that $\alpha_h = 0.25$ and $\beta_m = 0.20$. The relative nonmonetary cost parameter, λ, is assumed to be 0.10 in all the calculations. The same baseline distributions are used in all income classes; this implicitly assumes that there is zero income elasticity of demand.

Table 1 analyzes the first NHI plan. Column 1 presents baseline figures for 1970 with no NHI program. Total expenditure on covered services for the population under age 65 is $23.3 billion. This corresponds to hospital services of $12.9 billion and other medical care expenditure of $10.4 billion.[6] Because the pre-NHI prices are normalized to be unity, these expenditures can also serve as measures of quantities for comparison with the post-NHI quantities.

Column 2 shows the impact that NHI-1 would have if prices remained unchanged. Total national expenditures on the covered health services would increase 38 per cent to $32.2 billion. The quantity of hospital services rises 38 per cent to 17.8, and the quantity of other medical services rises 38 per cent to 14.4. The effective coinsurance rates are 17 per cent for hospital care and 25 per cent for other medical care. The cost to the government is therefore $25.6 billion.

An analysis with supply elasticities of 0.8 for both hospital care and other services is presented in column 3. The results are substantially different from the "pure demand case" of column 2. Prices rise by approximately 30 per cent. Total expenditure of $37 billion is 15 per cent higher than the estimate that ignored the endogenous price increase. The higher gross prices also imply a smaller increase in the quantities of care. The quantity of hospital services is 15.7, indicating that the rise from the pre-NHI value of 12.9 is only 22 per cent, or about half of the estimated increase when the price response was ignored. The comparison is similar for medical services. It is interesting that national spending increases $13.7 billion, but the extra volume of services is worth only $5.3 billion at the pre-NHI prices. Column 4 shows comparable

TABLE 1 Effects of NHI Plan 1

	Baseline Simulation (no NHI) (1)	"Moderate" Demand Elasticities				Supply ∞ (6)	"Low" Demand Elasticities		
		Supply ∞ (2)	Elasticities 0.8 (3)	Elasticities 0.2 (4)	Price Response Model (5)		Elasticities 0.8 (7)	Elasticities 0.2 (8)	Price Response Model (9)
National health expenditure[a]	23.3	32.2	37.0	42.3	38.1	27.2	30.5	35.9	35.0
Cost to government[a]	N.A.	25.7	29.9	34.5	30.8	21.0	23.9	28.6	27.8
Quantity of hospital care[a]	12.9	17.8	15.7	14.1	14.3	15.0	14.5	13.8	13.7
Quantity of medical care[a]	10.4	14.4	12.9	11.6	10.4	12.2	11.8	11.3	10.4
Price of hospital care	1.00	1.00	1.28	1.58	1.55	1.00	1.15	1.40	1.44
Price of medical care	1.00	1.00	1.31	1.72	1.54	1.00	1.17	1.48	1.47
Effective coinsurance rate, hospital care	N.A.	0.17	0.16	0.16	0.16	0.19	0.19	0.18	0.18
Effective coinsurance rate, medical care	N.A.	0.25	0.23	0.21	0.23	0.27	0.25	0.23	0.24

NOTE: The "moderate" demand elasticities are $\alpha_n = 0.5$ and $\beta_m = 0.4$; the "low" elasticities are $\alpha_n = 0.25$ and $\beta_m = 0.20$.
[a]Billions of 1970 dollars.

results for lower supply elasticities of $\gamma_H = \gamma_M = 0.2$. The total spending increases are greater but the quantity increases are smaller.

Columns 6, 7, and 8 present the same comparison of supply elasticities but with a lower pair of demand elasticities.[7] Although the effects of the NHI plan are now smaller, the implications of different supply elasticities are still very important. It is clear, moreover, that plausible differences in supply elasticities are at least as important as a source of uncertainty in total expenditure and in the cost to the government as the plausible differences in demand elasticities.

Table 2 presents a corresponding analysis for the second national health insurance option. The higher coinsurance rates $(C_H = C_M = 0.2)$ decrease total expenditure but the maximum out-of-pocket expenditure of 10 per cent of income increases total expenditure. If prices remained constant, the net effect of these two changes in the NHI program would be a small reduction in total cost; with the moderate demand elasticities, total expenditure is $31.9 billion under plan NHI-2 in contrast to $32.2 billion under plan NHI-1. The effect of less elastic supply is to increase prices under both plans. The higher price substantially increases the probability that each family's expenditure will exceed 10 per cent of income. At this point, the MAX limit becomes effective and the coinsurance rate ends. Although demand is limited by the non-monetary price $[\lambda/(1 + \lambda)]$, there is a substantial increase in demand. The result is that NHI-2 becomes more expensive than NHI-1. The government's cost is generally lower under the second plan because the higher coinsurance rate on relatively small expenditures more than outweighs the extra cost of providing complete protection for expenditures above 10 per cent. Only if the supply elasticities are very low would prices rise enough to reverse this situation and make NHI-2 more expensive; this happens here with $\gamma_H = \gamma_M = 0.2$. Notice that with the lower demand elasticities the rise in expenditure is always sufficiently small so that NHI-2 entails lower total expenditure and lower cost to the government.

The supply elasticity can also affect the distributional impact of a national health insurance plan. Because the current simulations assume a zero income elasticity of demand for health services, the first NHI plan provides the same expected benefits at all income levels to families with any fixed demographic composition. NHI-2, on the other hand, limits each family's net expenditure to no more than 10 per cent of family income. For low-income families, this is a substantial reduction in the net price of health services, whereas for

TABLE 2 Effects of NHI Plan 2

	Baseline Simulation (no NHI) (1)	"Moderate" Demand Elasticities				"Low" Demand Elasticities			
		Supply ∞ (2)	Elasticities 0.8 (3)	0.2 (4)	Price Response Model (5)	Supply ∞ (6)	Elasticities 0.8 (7)	0.2 (8)	Price Response Model (9)
National health expenditure[a]	23.3	31.9	37.3	43.8	36.5	26.5	29.5	34.9	31.7
Cost to government[a]	N.A.	24.2	28.9	34.6	28.3	19.0	21.4	25.9	23.2
Quantity of hospital care[a]	12.9	18.4	16.3	14.5	15.4	14.8	14.4	13.8	14.1
Quantity of medical care[a]	10.4	13.4	12.4	11.4	10.4	11.7	11.5	11.1	10.4
Price of hospital care	1.00	1.00	1.34	1.77	1.45	1.00	1.15	1.42	1.28
Price of medical care	1.00	1.00	1.25	1.59	1.37	1.00	1.13	1.37	1.31
Effective coinsurance rate, hospital care	N.A.	0.19	0.18	0.17	0.18	0.24	0.23	0.22	0.23
Effective coinsurance rate, medical care	N.A.	0.31	0.29	0.27	0.30	0.34	0.33	0.31	0.32

NOTE: The "moderate" demand elasticities are $\alpha_n = 0.50$ and $\beta_m = 0.40$; the "low" demand elasticities are $\alpha_n = 0.25$ and $\beta_m = 0.20$.
[a]Billions of 1970 dollars.

higher-income families the effect on price is much smaller. The result is a more substantial increase in spending at lower incomes.

These distributional effects are presented in Table 3. The analysis refers to the second NHI plan and to the moderate price elasticities. Columns 1 through 3 describe the impact on families of two adults and two children in the case in which prices are unchanged—i.e., infinitely elastic supplies of hospital and medical services at the original prices. Column 1 presents the average net benefit received by families at each income level—i.e., the average cost to the government as insurer. These net benefits fall rapidly for the first few income classes and then fall more slowly, reflecting the highly skewed distribution of health spending. Similarly, the average direct out-of-pocket payments by the family (column 2) increase rapidly for the first few income classes and then more slowly. The total quantity of care received is, with prices fixed at unity, the sum of the net benefits and direct payments; these quantities are shown in column 3. The quantity of care consumed also falls rather rapidly at first and then more slowly.

All three columns show that substantial progression is introduced by the single feature of a 10 per cent maximum limit on direct payments, even when there is a relatively low 20 per cent coinsurance rate. It is convenient to have a summary measure of the distributional impact and a method of combining the benefits (or payments or quantities) in different income classes into a single measure that reflects a constant value judgement about distributional equity. The "uniformly distributed dollar" (UDD) measure is useful for this purpose. For example, the UDD value of benefits is a weighted sum of the average benefits per family in each income class:

$$(7) \qquad B_{\text{UDD}} = \frac{\sum_i B_i W_i N_i}{\sum_i W_i N_i}$$

where B_i is the benefit per family in income class i, W_i is the weight given to a marginal dollar of a family in income class i, and N_i is the number of families in class i. Notice that if $B_i = 1$, $B_{\text{UDD}} = 1$; thus one unit in the B_{UDD} measure is the social value of $1.00 given to each family—i.e., the social value of a uniformly distributed dollar. It is convenient to relate the W_i's to income by a simple functional relation. The constant elasticity function $W_i = Y_i^{-\alpha}$ is both familiar and convenient. For $\alpha = 1$ it implies that the weight given to a marginal dollar of income varies inversely with the income of the recipient family. The higher the value of α, the more egalitarian the implied preferences.

TABLE 3 Distributional Aspects of NHI Plan 2: Supply Response Model

Income Class	2 Adults and 2 Children						All Families		
	$\gamma_H = \gamma_M = \infty$			$\gamma_H = \gamma_M = 0.8$			$\gamma_H = \gamma_M = \infty$		
	Net Benefits	Direct Payments	Quantity	Net Benefits	Direct Payments	Quantity	Net Benefits	Direct Payments	Quantity
	(1)	(2)	(3)	(4)	(5)	(6)	(7)	(8)	(9)
<$ 2,000	$823	$ 87	910	$968	$ 90	814	$201	$ 28	229
$ 2,000–	700	132	832	830	140	745	202	42	245
$ 3,000–	647	143	790	770	154	709	261	62	323
$ 4,000–	620	151	771	735	163	689	297	77	374
$ 5,000–	589	157	746	709	170	675	346	95	441
$ 6,000–	564	162	726	678	176	656	365	107	473
$ 7,000–	536	165	701	651	180	638	387	120	507
$ 8,000–	513	169	682	617	185	617	409	134	543
$10,000–	487	172	659	586	189	596	424	148	572
$12,000–	465	175	640	551	192	576	429	158	586
$15,000–	434	178	612	520	197	552	424	168	592
$25,000+	413	179	592	484	199	527	395	167	562
UDD Values									
$\alpha = 0.0$	497	169	667	596	186	602	351	112	462
$\alpha = 0.5$	522	165	687	626	180	620	307	86	393
$\alpha = 1.0$	562	156	718	672	170	647	262	62	324
$\alpha = 1.5$	623	141	765	742	153	688	231	45	276
$\alpha = 2.0$	696	122	819	825	131	735	214	36	250

NOTE: All calculations use "moderate" demand elasticities, $\alpha_n = 0.5$ and $\beta_m = 0.4$.

Table 3 shows the B_{UDD} values corresponding to values of α between zero and 2. The value of $\alpha = 0$ corresponds to the simple average of benefits with no weighting for distribution. The average benefit (cost to the government) per family with two adults and two children is thus $497. For someone whose distributional preferences correspond to $\alpha = 1$, these benefits are equivalent to $562 distributed uniformly to all such families. With more egalitarian preferences ($\alpha = 2$), the benefits are equivalent to $696 distributed uniformly. Conversely, the average value of direct out-of-pocket payments is $169 per family of two adults and two children, but this amount is equivalent to a smaller uniformly distributed payment of $156 for $\alpha = 1$ and $122 for $\alpha = 2$. Finally, the average quantity of services is $667 per family. Applying the same UDD evaluation to these benefits implies that for $\alpha = 1$, they are equivalent to a constant $718 per family.

The effect of introducing supply elasticities of 0.8 for hospital and medical services is to increase prices and therefore expenditures at all income levels. The equilibrium quantities are now smaller than before. Benefits rise by about 18 per cent in the lower-income classes and about 14 per cent in the higher-income classes. Direct costs rise by about 7 per cent in the lower-income classes and about 11 per cent in the higher-income classes. Thus in both of these ways the NHI-2 plan is slightly more redistributive when the supply response is explicitly recognized. But the relatively greater direct payments by higher-income families just about offset the relatively lower benefits from the insurer and make the proportional change in the quantity of services approximately equal at all income levels; the quantities shown in column 6 are almost exactly 90 per cent of the quantities in column 3.

Although the NHI-2 plan is very progressive with respect to income when attention is focused on families with a single demographic composition, this characteristic is disguised when all family types are combined. Average family size increases with family income; there are fewer single-person families and larger average numbers of children. Columns 7 through 9 show that this has striking effects on the distribution of average benefits, direct payments, and quantities of care. Average benefits rise with income until $15,000 and then fall only slightly. Average direct payments rise much more sharply with income. The net effect is that quantity increases with family income up to $25,000, despite the income-related limit on direct payments. It is clear from this comparison that it is important to take demographic structure into account in evaluating the distributional impact of alternative NHI plans.

4. A PRICE RESPONSE MODEL

Neither hospitals nor physicians are like the typical economic agents to which the traditional theory of price and quantity determination applies. These differences—the nonprofit nature of hospitals, the special expertise of physicians, and the physicians' professional interest—may not be enough to vitiate the applicability of the traditional theory in sections 2 and 3. Nevertheless, it seems useful to provide an alternative response model that contains special features of the health care sector. The "price response model" presented in this section incorporates ideas about the markets for physicians' services and hospital care that were previously developed by Feldstein (1970, 1971a, 1971b, 1974). An important characteristic of this alternative model is that the price-quantity equilibrium need not be market clearing; excess demand and nonprice rationing may prevail in equilibrium.

Consider first the model of physicians' behavior. The price response model specifies that the effect of NHI is to raise the gross price of physicians' services by an amount that depends on the increased insurance coverage of physicians' services. More complete insurance raises the physicians' price not only because it increases demand, but also because physicians take into account the financial impact of their fees on their patients. Moreover, physicians may seek to maintain excess demand in order to have the opportunity to select the types of patients and diagnoses that they like to treat; an increase in insurance permits gross prices to be raised without reducing the desired degree of excess demand.[8]

More specifically, the change from the pre-NHI price, PM_0, to the post-NHI price, PM_1, is given by the function:

$$(8) \quad \frac{PM_1}{PM_0} = \left[\frac{NPM_1}{NPM_0}\right]^{-\delta_M}$$

where NPM_0 is the average *net* price of physicians' services prevailing before NHI (i.e., the product of PM_0 and the effective coinsurance rate before NHI) and NPM_1 is the average *net* price that would prevail after NHI if physicians did not alter their gross price.[9] The computational procedure for deriving PM_1 is straightforward. The demand simulation model is used to calculate NPM_0 as the ratio of aggregate *direct* patient expenditure on physicians' services to aggregate *total* expenditure on those services. The insurance coverage is then changed to the NHI plan and the calculation is repeated to obtain NPM_1. Since NPM_1 depends on the gross price PM_0, no iterative procedure is necessary. Applying Equation (8) then yields the new price that prevails under NHI.

The supply function of the physician now indicates the *desired* supply at each price. The same constant elasticity function will be used:

(9) $\ln QM_1 = \ln QM_0 + \gamma_M \ln PM_1$

If the aggregate demand at price PM_1 (and corresponding hospital price PH_1) is less than or equal to the desired supply QM_1, the equilibrium quantity is "demand-determined"; i.e., each family gets the quantity of physicians' services that it wants at the new prevailing price. If, however, as is probably more likely, the aggregate demand exceeds supply, the new equilibrium is "supply-determined." Each family obtains only some fraction of the services that it would like to purchase with the new prices and insurance coverage. In the absence of better information about nonprice rationing, the current model specifies that each family receives the same fraction of the quantity that it demands regardless of income, demographic composition, or desired expenditure. More specifically, the "rationing constant" for physicians' services is defined as:

(10) $RM = \dfrac{QM_1}{QMD}$

where QMD is the aggregate quantity of physicians' services demanded at prices PM_1 and PH_1 under the NHI plan, and QM_1 is the desired aggregate supply defined in Equation (9). Each individual family then obtains RM times the quantity that it demands according to the basic demand equations in Section 1, with $P_h = PH_1$ and $P_m = PM_1$.

Notice that the use of nonprice rationing increases the likelihood that some families would receive less care than in the absence of NHI even if NHI improves everyone's coverage. This will clearly happen when the supply elasticity is zero but the demand elasticity is non-zero. NHI then increases demand and results in a rationing parameter RM less than 1. Unless all families' demands are increased in exactly the same proportion, the NHI would reduce the quantity of care received by some families.

Although the hospital services section of the price response model has the same formal structure as the model of physicians' services, the interpretation of this behavior is quite different. An analysis of hospitals' response to the growth of private insurance in the 1960s and to the introduction of Medicare and Medicaid suggests that hospitals respond to insurance by increasing the cost per patient day through more sophisticated care and higher staff wages. Prices rise in response to additional insurance not because of a greater unit cost of providing more of the same type of care (i.e., a rising supply curve in the traditional sense) but because hospitals produce a different product and choose to pay higher wages. To analyze this as a response to NHI, the price response model with a demand-determined equilibrium would be used. The price of hospital services after the introduction of NHI is given by

$$
(11) \qquad \frac{PH_1}{PH_0} = \left[\frac{NPH_1}{NPH_0} \right]^{-\delta_H}
$$

where NPH_0 is the average *net* price of hospital services prevailing before NHI and NPH_1 is the average *net* price that would prevail after NHI if hospitals did not alter their gross price. The analysis in Feldstein (1971a) suggests this type of behavior with $0 < \delta_H \leqslant 1$ and with the actual quantity determined by household demand. The model is thus completed by using PH_1 and PM_1 to calculate each family's demand and assuming that hospitals will supply this quantity.

Alternatively, the price response model may be evaluated with a supply-determined equilibrium by using the hospital supply equation

$$
\ln QH_1 = \ln QH_0 + \gamma_H \ln PH_1
$$

where γ_H is the elasticity of supply. The hospital rationing parameter (RH) is then defined by an equation analogous to (10). The individual demand equations and RH are then combined to determine the allocation of the rationed hospital care.

The price response model in which the quantities are constrained by supply can also be used to examine the case in which price controls are used to limit the price rise. The prices PM_1 and PH_1 are then determined by the price control agency instead of by equations (8) and (11). The corresponding supplies are then calculated with equations (9) and (12). The individual demand simulations yield rationing parameters RM and RH and the rationed allocation of services corresponding to the NHI plan, the controlled prices, and the quantities supplied.

The two alternative NHI options discussed in Section 3 have been reanalyzed with the current price response model. More specifically, the price response parameters δ_H and δ_M are both assigned the value 0.5; a 20 per cent decrease in the effective coinsurance rate (e.g., from 0.40 to 0.32) thus raises the gross prices by approximately 10 per cent and therefore also lowers the net price by about 10 per cent. For medical services, the total supply is assumed fixed—i.e., $\gamma_M = 0$. The equilibrium quantities of medical services are therefore supply-determined. For hospital services, a positive supply elasticity ($\gamma_H = 0.5$) is assumed. The same two alternative demand specifications as in Section 3 are again investigated. With the "moderate" demand elasticities ($\alpha_n = 0.5$, $\beta_m = 0.4$), the increase in demand exceeds the increase in supply and the allocation of hospital services is also supply-determined. Only with the "low" demand elasticities ($\alpha_n = 0.25$, $\beta_m = 0.2$) is there no excess demand and a demand-determined allocation.

The aggregate implications of these price response models are shown in columns 5 and 9 of tables 1 and 2. With the moderate demand elasticities, the total cost implications are quite similar to the previous analysis with supply elasticities of 0.8 and market-clearing prices. Total national spending under NHI-1 is $38.1 billion, in comparison to the earlier value of $37 billion; for NHI-2, the figures are $36.5 billion and $37.3 billion. Estimated costs to the government are also quite similar. The underlying price and quantity changes are, however, very different; price rises are greater and quantity increases are smaller. For NHI-1, total national spending increases by $14.8 billion to buy only $1.4 billion worth of additional services valued at original prices (i.e., quantity increases from 23.3 billion to 24.7 billion). With NHI-2, the extra spending of $13.2 billion induces only an extra quantity worth $2.5 billion at original prices.

Although the prices and aggregate quantities are quite different under the two models, for the two sets of assumptions examined here the distributional implications are approximately the same. Table 4 shows the distributions of benefits, direct out-of-pocket payments, and quantities for families with two adults and two children under the price response model and under the supply response model with $\gamma_H = \gamma_M = 0.8$. Although benefits and direct payments are lower under the price response model, the ratios of corresponding values under the two models is approximately constant. Similarly, quantities are some 10 per cent lower at each income level. It should, of course, be stressed that this result depends on the particular assumptions made for this comparison. With a more complex insurance structure (e.g., deductibles related to income) or different elasticities of demand and supply, the two different models of provider behavior may imply quite different distributional patterns.

TABLE 4 Distributional Aspects of NHI Plan 2: Comparison of Price Response and Supply Response Models

Income Class	Price Response Model			Supply Response Model		
	$\gamma_H = 0.5$	$\gamma_M = 0$		$\gamma_H = \gamma_M = 0.8$		
	Net Benefits	Direct Payments	Quantity	Net Benefits	Direct Payments	Quantity
	(1)	(2)	(3)	(4)	(5)	(6)
<$ 2,000	$945	$ 89	730	$968	$ 90	814
$ 2,000–	812	137	669	830	140	745
$ 3,000–	750	150	634	770	154	709
$ 4,000–	723	159	621	735	163	689
$ 5,000–	696	166	607	709	170	675
$ 6,000–	664	172	589	678	176	656
$ 7,000–	638	176	574	651	180	638
$ 8,000–	604	181	554	617	185	617
$10,000–	572	185	534	586	189	596
$12,000–	543	188	516	551	192	576
$15,000–	506	193	494	520	197	552
$25,000+	470	195	470	484	199	527
UDD Variables						
$\alpha = 0.0$	582	182	539	596	186	602
$\alpha = 0.5$	611	176	556	626	180	620
$\alpha = 1.0$	657	166	581	672	170	647
$\alpha = 1.5$	725	149	617	742	153	688
$\alpha = 2.0$	806	128	659	825	131	735

NOTE: All calculations use moderate demand elasticities and refer to families of two adults and two children.

5. CONCLUSION

The primary purpose of this paper has been to emphasize that any analysis of the effects of alternative national health insurance plans should take into account the effect of insurance on the prices and supplies of health services. An operational method was presented for combining a stochastic microsimulational model of household demand with aggregate supply and price determination equations.

The supply models used in this analysis are preliminary and can only be regarded as illustrative. Neither the traditional supply model in Section 2 nor the price response model in Section 4 can be eliminated as completely inconsistent with the data. More econometric research is therefore required to provide conditional estimates of the parameters of both models. We hope that the current evidence of the importance of these parameters will encourage others to continue work on these empirical issues.

NOTES

1. For simplicity, the actual calculations assume $E_m = \hat{E}_m$ in both subcases.
2. Although the independence assumption seems strong, there are several countervailing forces that may produce such independence. Some preliminary comparisons of convoluted "synthetic" family distributions and actual family distributions supported the assumption of independence.
3. This assumption for "typical" coverage is based on Reed (1969) and information supplied by the Department of Health, Education, and Welfare.
4. Notice that the simulation model in Section 1 permits specifying a separate set of deductibles, coinsurance rates, and MAX value for each of the 192 family demographic types and income classes.
5. Davis and Russel (1972) did provide some evidence of positive cross-price elasticities, but medical services in their study were limited to hospital outpatient care.
6. Actual costs in 1970 were $13.2 billion for hospital services and $10.1 billion for medical services. The calibration method described above does not yield these exact figures because of the nonlinearity of the insurance schedules. These dollar amounts refer to persons under age 65; see Cooper et al. (1973).
7. Columns 5 and 9 present results that will be discussed in Section 4.
8. These ideas are developed more fully in Feldstein (1970, 1974).
9. This model of price response is clearly a simplification that is used because no more specific hypothesis seems either theoretically or empirically superior.

REFERENCES

1. Acton, Jan Paul, "Demand for Health Care Among the Urban Poor, with Special Emphasis on the Role of Time," R-1151-OEO, The Rand Corporation, October 1972.
2. Cooper, Barbara et al., Medical Care Expenditures, Prices and Costs: Background Book (Washington, D.C.: Department of Health, Education, and Welfare, 1973).
3. Davis, K., and L. Russel, "The Substitution of Hospital Outpatient Care for Inpatient Care," Review of Economics and Statistics, 54 (May 1972), pp. 109–120.
4. Feldstein, M. S., "The Rising Price of Physicians' Services," Review of Economics and Statistics, 52 (May 1970), pp. 121–133.

5. _____ ,"Hospital Cost Inflation: A Study of Nonprofit Price Dynamics," *American Economic Review*, 61 (December 1971a), pp. 853–872.

6. _____ , *The Rising Cost of Hospital Care*, published for the National Center for Health Services Research and Development, Department of Health, Education, and Welfare (Washington, D.C.: Information Resources Press, 1971b).

7. _____ , "Econometric Studies of Health Economics," in M. Intriligator and D. Kendrick (editors), *Frontiers of Quantitative Economics*, II (Amsterdam: North-Holland, 1974).

8. _____ , B. Friedman, and H. Luft, "Distributional Aspects of National Health Insurance Benefits and Finance," *National Tax Journal*, 25 (December 1972), pp. 497–510.

9. Phelps, Charles E., and Joseph P. Newhouse, "Effect of Coinsurance: A Multivariate Analysis," *Social Security Bulletin*, 35 (June 1972), pp. 20–44.

10. Reed, Louis, *Private Health Insurance in the United States, 1968; Coverage and Benefits* (Washington, D.C.: Social Security Administration, Office of Research and Statistics, 1969).

12 ▌ COMMENTS

Barry R. Chiswick

Council of Economic Advisers and
National Bureau of Economic Research

Within the last few years there has been considerable interest in the adoption of national health insurance (NHI) in the U.S. Although the three letters NHI may have wide appeal, as with apple pie, there is substantial disagreement over which recipe is best. Legislative proposals range from the Long-Ribicoff mandatory catastrophic insurance to the virtual cradle-to-grave-universal-zero-out-of-pocket cost coverage of the Health Security Bill.

The various proposals, including the one to "do nothing," have elicited much discussion. Everyone seems to agree that NHI would increase the amount of services demanded and the price of a unit of service. Concern for the increased share of GNP devoted to the medical sector and the change in the distribution of income arising from NHI has led to a variety of collateral proposals to control units purchased and prices charged.

Part of the uncertainty about NHI is attributable to the difficulty economists

The views expressed in these comments, based on the version of the paper presented at the conference, are solely those of the author.

have in measuring magnitudes. We are quite good at measuring *directions* of change, but quite poor in measuring magnitudes. This is not unique to the health field—for example, it is now well established that a 10 per cent increase in the minimum wage will decrease the employment of teenagers, but by how much is far less certain. However, research on the impact of NHI has encountered additional handicaps. The data on current utilization are inadequate. Also, the economist's tools are designed for the analysis of marginal changes in a partial equilibrium model, whereas NHI would have such profound widespread effects that a model that allows for a variety of long-run interactions may be the best approximation.

These points indicate that measuring the impact of NHI is not an easy research topic. For some of the same reasons, however, the quantification of the impact is of vital concern. We know that NHI will influence the share of GNP devoted to the health sector. The magnitude of the change and what we get for it in terms of improved health will influence our view of the wisdom of NHI. A wrong decision with respect to NHI will be very costly. And, if an NHI is adopted, the political costs of reversing our policy may be substantial as new interest groups develop, even if it turns out that for the country as a whole NHI is economically inefficient.[1] In a world of uncertainty, the larger the cost of enduring a wrong decision and the greater the cost of reversing a decision, the greater the amount of resources that should be devoted to finding the correct decision, and the more we should appear to be risk averse.[2]

It is for these reasons that the Feldstein-Friedman paper, and the work of others, on estimating the impact of NHI is of considerable importance. Feldstein and Friedman correctly recognize that NHI has a direct impact on the demand for medical care and that this change in demand induces a supply response. It is the combined effects of the change in the demand curve and the movement along the supply curve for medical care that generate the change in the quantity and price of the units of medical care provided.

Feldstein and Friedman use a microsimulation model of household demand and an aggregate model of supply to predict the price and quantity of medical care services that would arise from alternative models of NHI. They prefer a microsimulation model because an "aggregate specification of demand behavior cannot capture the subtle differences in the response of demand to different types of insurance policies." There is truth in this statement.

An aggregate specification, however, may be better able to account for the effects, if any, of interactions in demand among individuals.[3] Although interacting individual demand may not be important for marginal changes, it may be important for a large nationwide change in the medical care system brought about by NHI. Also, the microsimulation model as formulated by Feldstein and Friedman—and any microsimulation model—embodies a variety of built-in behavioral assumptions. The authors assume, for example, that each family has the same price elasticity of demand, the income elasticity of demand for medical care is zero, the cross-price elasticity of demand for hospital and out-of-hospital care is zero, individual demand curves are independent of one another, etc. These are probably reasonably good assumptions. Unfortunately, by making these assumptions they cannot capture all the subtle differences in demand.

A priori, it is not clear that an aggregate model of demand would necessarily be a worse predictor than a microsimulation model. It would be interesting to know the extent to which the two procedures yield different estimates. If they generate essentially the same estimates, the aggregate model has the advantage of simplicity but the microsimulation model would provide predicted use rates for specific demographic groups. If the two procedures generate widely different estimates, the cause of the difference should be investigated. Unfortunately, we may not be able to determine which is a better predictor until after we have had some experience with NHI.

A preliminary answer could perhaps come from an analysis of our two current targeted NHI programs—Medicare and Medicaid. Using pre-1966 data on the utilization of health services by the aged, the poor, and all others, which of the two procedures more accurately predicts the current utilization pattern?

In their microsimulation model of household demand, Feldstein and Friedman estimate expenditures for hospital and out-of-hospital medical services by assuming a constant (gross price) elasticity of demand equation in the absence of insurance. By introducing modifications for deductibles and coinsurance, including zero per cent coinsurance beyond some level of expenditure, they are able to estimate the effect on demand of alternative models of NHI.

They explicitly include the parameter λ, which measures the nonmoney cost of medical care. The units for λ are not spelled out and I am troubled by the manner in which it is included. In equations (1) and (2), for example, for a zero per cent coinsurance, the market price, P_h, should have no effect on the demand for hospital care, yet the price variable is $\lambda P_h/(1 + \lambda)$. Since λ is (arbitrarily) assumed to be 0.1 in the computations, the price to the household is $0.09 P_h$, which is a function of P_h. It is not clear why the nonmoney cost to the household would be proportional to the market price.[4]

Unfortunately, we know very little about the role of nonmarket costs in the medical care field, and in others. With the growth of private and public insurance for out-of-pocket expenditures and the rise in the value of time, there has presumably been a substitution toward goods-intensive forms of medical care that economize on time. This suggests that the relative nonmoney cost parameter λ may not be constant but may decline in response to the expansion of insurance coverage for out-of-pocket expenditures. It would be useful if the microsimulation model allowed for this effect. It would also be interesting to see the effect of alternative specifications of the magnitude of nonmoney costs.

From economic theory we know that demand and supply curves are less elastic in the short run than in the long run. Using the very low demand and supply elasticities ($\alpha_h = 0.25$, $\beta_m = 0.20$, $\gamma = 0.2$), the simulation of the two NHI models predicts a modest 7 per cent increase in the quantity of hospital and medical care. However, prices increase by at least 40 per cent. For the long run we can expect a very large supply elasticity. Using an infinite supply elasticity and the Feldstein-Friedman "moderate" demand elasticities ($\alpha_h =$ 0.5, $\beta_m = 0.4$), the quantity of care provided increases by approximately 37 per cent in their simulation.

The long-run estimate of the increase in utilization is likely to be biased downward. With the subsidization of direct costs but not of time costs, we would expect a substitution of goods for time, and hence a decline in the parameter λ. By holding λ constant, Feldstein and Friedman ignore what may be an increasingly important source of increased demand for medical services.

Feldstein and Friedman present simulations of the distributional impact among income groups. They assume a zero income elasticity of demand, the same price elasticity of demand for all income groups, that λ equals 0.1 for all income groups, etc. Although these simplifying assumptions may be adequate if we are interested only in an aggregate simulation, they are clearly highly suspect if we focus on different income classes.

For example, the nonmonetary cost of a day of hospitalization is likely to be substantially higher for a professional than for a skilled craft worker, and the latter's time cost is likely to be higher than that of a domestic day worker. Hence, if λ falls with lower-income levels, NHI results in a larger relative decline in price for lower-income than for higher-income groups. Then, by assuming a constant λ, Feldstein and Friedman underestimate the increase in the utilization of services by low-income groups relative to higher-income groups. Thus, ceteris paribus, NHI would be more progressive in redistributing medical service to lower-income groups than would be indicated by Feldstein and Friedman's Table 3.

Feldstein and Friedman have made an important contribution in this paper by the explicit incorporation of nonmoney costs into the demand for medical care.

NOTES

1. The oil depletion allowance was but one example of an apparently politically irreversible policy.
2. K. Arrow and A. C. Fisher, "Environmental Preservation, Uncertainty and Irreversibility," *Quarterly Journal of Economics* (May 1974), pp. 312–320.
3. These interactions may be attributable to local styles of medicine, including bandwagon effects, and to the level and spread of information.
4. A positive nonmoney price, however, does play an important role, as indicated by the finite demand with "free" (zero per cent coinsurance) medical care. For the aged and the poor, an important component of the nonmoney price of medical care—the value of time—is very low. Does this explain the very large response to the introduction of Medicaid and Medicare?

Michael D. Intriligator

University of California, Los Angeles and
Human Resources Research Center,
University of Southern California

In their paper, Feldstein and Friedman (FF hereafter) use a microsimulation model of the health care system in order to study the effects of alternative national health insurance (NHI) proposals. These comments are organized into three sections. The first discusses the use of a microeconometric model as a tool for policy evaluation. The second summarizes the FF microeconometric model and compares it to the Human Resources Research Center (HRRC) microeconometric model of the health care system.[1] The third discusses the major conclusions of the FF and HRRC models with regard to NHI.

1. THE USE OF A MICROECONOMETRIC MODEL FOR POLICY EVALUATION

Figure 1 summarizes the procedure by which a microeconometric model could be used for policy evaluation in a wide variety of areas, including not only health but also education, transportation, housing, economic stabilization, and many others. It also specifies how it could be used in the particular application area treated by FF.

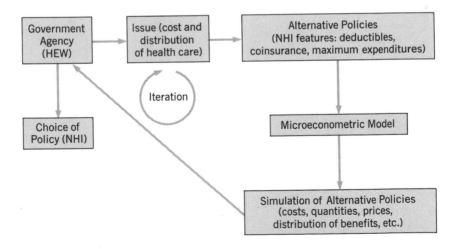

FIGURE 1 Use of a Microeconometric Model for Policy Evaluation

The procedure begins with a government agency responsible for policy in a particular area. For FF the agency is the Office of the Secretary of the Department of Health, Education, and Welfare (HEW). Responsible individuals in the agency identify a particular issue that is both of concern and subject to influence by the agency. For FF the issue is the cost and distribution of health care.

The agency individuals and/or model builders specify alternative policies that could affect the issue to be treated. In this instance, among the alternative policies are the various payment features of a NHI plan, specifically the levels of deductibles, coinsurance rates, and maximum net out-of-pocket expenditure for individuals or families.[2]

The alternative policies are analyzed and evaluated by use of a formal framework, which can take the form, as in FF, of a microeconometric model, involving interacting microsimulation and econometric models. The microsimulation portion of the structure facilitates both treatment of detailed features, such as changes in eligibility or differences in costs or benefits to different individuals, and treatment of distributional effect. The aggregate econometric portion of the structure facilitates treatment of macro interactions on markets, such as price/quantity determination in product markets and wage/employment determination in factor markets. FF use this interactive framework in relating demand, obtained from an aggregation of estimated demands via the microsimulation model, to supply, obtained from aggregate relationships, in order to determine prices.

The methodology used to evaluate the alternative policies is *simulation*. Each set of policies implies an alternative future course of relevant variables determined as a forecast of the estimated model, conditional on the particular set of policies. For FF the alternative payment features imply alternative values of total expenditure, cost to government, and quantity and price of medical and hospital care, as reported in their tables 1 and 2.

The simulations are then reported to the initiating agency, in this case the Office of the Secretary of HEW. If necessary, the entire process can be iterated by selecting related issues or other policies to derive new simulations. Eventually, the policy-makers select a particular simulation they desire and adopt the relevant set of policies implying this simulation. Of course, actually carrying out the adopted set of policies entails a complex process of legislative enactment, organizational development, budgetary appropriations, etc.

This procedure is quite general; it can be applied to a wide variety of policy-making situations. The future of policy evaluation could very well be based on this procedure, with close relationships being formed between policy-makers and model-builders. In effect, through the microeconometric model, the model-builders will be providing the policy-makers with a "wind tunnel" in which alternative policy configurations can be tested before actual use. Much of existing policy has been based on only the sketchiest idea about its immediate and primary effects and virtually no information concerning its delayed and secondary effects. The procedure outlined in Figure 1 could provide government agencies with needed guidance on important policy issues.

2. COMPARISON OF THE FF MICROSIMULATION AND HRRC MICROECONOMETRIC MODELS

The FF and HRRC models are two different microeconometric models of the health care system, both of which have been used for policy evaluation. A comparison of some of their more important structural components is presented in Table 1.

TABLE 1 Comparison of the Feldstein-Friedman (FF) Micro-Simulation Model and the Yett-Drabek-Intriligator-Kimbell (HRRC) Microeconometric Model

	Feldstein-Friedman (FF)	Human Resources Research Center (HRRC)

Population	Families: 192 types
	  16 family compositions
	  12 income categories
		Individuals
		  9 age
		  2 sex
		  2 race
		  3 income
		Nurses
		  6 age
		Physicians
		  11 age
		  14 specialty
		   5 professional activity
		   2 place of medical school training, domestic or foreign

Demand	Constant elasticity: $D = D_0 p^{-\epsilon}$
	  D_0: base quantity; p = net price;
	  ϵ: elasticity, assumed at "moderate" or "low" levels
		Constant elasticity: $D = D_0 p^{-\epsilon}$
		  D_0: base quantity; p = net price;
		  ϵ: elasticity, estimated for physicians and length of hospital stay

Supply	Constant elasticity: $S = S_0 p^{\gamma}$
	  S_0: base quantity
	  γ: elasticity, assumed at alternative levels: ∞, 0.8 or 0.2
		Quantity supplied determined from
		1. Numbers of physicians, nurses, and hospitals
		2. Demand for non-physician labor
		3. Production functions

Price Response	Either market clearing: P_t) or price response model: $$\frac{P_{t+1}}{P_t} = \left(\frac{NP_{t+1}}{NP_t} \right)^{1-\delta}$$ where N_p = net price	Adjustment of prices based on trend and excess demand: $$P_{t+1} = \alpha P_t + \beta(D_t - S_t)$$
Data Base	Over 300,000 federal government employees and dependents enrolled in Aetna "High Option" coverage in 1970	Over 130,000 responses from the Health Interview Survey, conducted by the U.S. National Center for Health Statistics in 1967.

An essential feature of a microsimulation model is a population (or populations) being simulated. In the FF study the population consists of families of 192 types, determined from family composition and income categories. These families determine demand for health services. In the HRRC Microeconometric Model there are three populations being simulated.[3] The first is a population of individuals demanding health services. This population is described by age, sex, race, and income characteristics. The second population is one of physicians supplying outpatient services. This population is described by age, specialty, professional activity, and training (domestic- or foreign-trained medical school graduates). The third population includes nurses assisting in the provision of outpatient and inpatient services. This population is described by age.

The demand specification of both models is of the constant elasticity type in which a demand curve is passed through a particular base quantity-price point by assuming that the price elasticity of demand is constant. In this instance price is net price—price times the coinsurance rate.[4] The base quantities are derived from historical data. In FF the elasticities of demand for physician and hospital services are assumed at two different levels, "moderate" or "low." In the HRRC study the demand elasticities are estimated through regression analysis and they differ, for example, for different specialties for outpatient services. Also, the demand for hospital services is treated somewhat differently in the HRRC study than in the FF study. Instead of estimating a single demand function for hospital services, separate demand functions are estimated for hospital admission and length of hospital stay.

The supply specification is radically different in the two models. In the FF model a supply function analogous to the demand function is postulated and is assumed to exhibit constant elasticity. Alternative assumptions are made about the value of this elasticity: ∞, 0.8, or 0.2. In the HRRC model, on the other hand, the quantities supplied of inpatient or outpatient services are determined from estimated production functions, using factor inputs that are determined both from input demand functions, dependent on wages, and from the simulated population of physicians.[5] Thus, supply in the HRRC model depends on simulated populations—of physicians, nurses and hospitals, factors not treated explicitly in the FF model. Explicit treatment of these factors, however, facilitates analysis of various policy initiatives, such as added training programs for physicians in medical schools, added nurse training programs, and hospital construction, that might be undertaken in conjunction with NHI. It might also be pointed out that such a supply specification must be based on the assumption of perfectly competitive markets for both inpatient and outpatient services, since it is only in such markets that supply functions of the type they treat exist. Such an assumption is both extreme and at considerable variance with previous analyses of these markets, which typically treat the relevant markets as ones of oligopoly, or monopolistic competition.

Because of the nature of their demand/supply specifications, FF do not have independent estimates of demand and supply. They therefore cannot directly treat disequilibrium phenomena in the relevant markets. This is a severe limitation given the existence of waiting lists, discussions of shortages, and rapid price increases in these markets, all of which suggest disequilibrium. FF postulate either a market-clearing model, wherein prices clear the markets, or a price response model, wherein price changes depend on changes in net price. In the HRRC model, on the other hand, wherein demand and supply are determined on the basis of fundamentally different considerations, disequilibrium phenomena can be treated directly. In this model, price in period $t + 1$ is the following function of price and excess demand in period t

$$P_{t+1} = \alpha P_t + \beta(D_t - S_t)$$

Thus, prices increase according to the trend rate $\alpha - 1$, with acceleration or deceleration around the trend rate depending on whether excess demand $(D_t - S_t)$ is positive or negative, respectively. If $\alpha = 1$, the price adjustment equation reduces to the usual tatonnement model, whereas if $\beta = 0$ (or $D_t = S_t$) the price adjustment equation reduces to a simple trend. Values of α are estimated from historical time trends. Alternative β's were considered and tested for sensitivity.[6]

Turning to the data, FF utilize data concerning over 300,000 families of federal government employees and their dependents who are enrolled in the Aetna "High Option" coverage. The HRRC study utilizes data concerning over 130,000 individuals from the 1967 Health Interview Survey, conducted by the National Center for Health Statistics. Although the FF data may be more precise, more complete, and available for greater numbers of individuals than the HRRC data, there is some question about its relevance. FF extrapolate from their data to national demands, but the behavior of federal employees who choose a particularly complete package of health insurance may not be representative of the behavior of the entire population. The HIS sample is a more representative sample of the entire population.

3. CONCLUSIONS REGARDING THE TWO MICROSIMULATION MODELS

There are two major conclusions that FF draw from their model: First, they conclude that supply, particularly the price elasticity of supply, is of major importance in calculating effects of NHI on prices, quantities, cost to the government, etc. Second, they conclude that the demographic composition of the population is of major importance in evaluating distributional effects. Their conclusions, in qualitative form, are apparent from a simple supply-demand diagram wherein the effects of a NHI-induced shift in demand depend on the elasticity of the supply schedule and the extent of the shift in demand depends on the family composition of the population. The quantitative counterparts of this diagrammatic observation are summarized in the tables in the FF paper.

There are five major conclusions of the HRRC study. First, demographic information and prices are not nearly so effective in explaining demand for health services as demographic information, prices, and health conditions.[7] The health status of the population, as well as such NHI features as coinsurance, etc., determine demand for health services.

The second conclusion of the HRRC study is the importance of the distribution of the population for the composition of health services provided. Thus, a "bulge" in the number of women of child-bearing age has a significant effect on demands for the services of pediatricians and obstetricians, two of the physician specialties explicitly treated in the HRRC model.

The third conclusion of the HRRC study is the importance of the foreign medical graduates (FMG's), based on a simulation study that exploited the capability of the model to track separately physicians trained domestically and those trained abroad. The FMG's are important components of the health care system, especially for hospital staffs, and the number of FMG's is more susceptible to policy choices, especially in the short run, than the numbers of physicians trained domestically. In fact, the most critical factor influencing the supply of physicians in the short run is the net migration rate of FMG's. A more liberal policy toward FMG's could play a significant role in meeting the demands created by NHI. There are, however, indications that a less liberal policy will be pursued over the next several years. This policy could have profound effects on the supply of physician services.

The fourth conclusion of the HRRC study is the fundamental importance to NHI outcomes of the productivity of physicians and other labor inputs in producing outpatient and inpatient services. Thus, the HRRC study found, as FF did, that supply is of major importance to NHI outcomes, but it treated explicitly the determinants of supply—manpower and productivity.

The fifth major conclusion of the HRRC study is the importance of organizational factors. Changing the mix of practice settings (e.g., a shift from solo to group practices) and changing the mix of institutions (e.g., types of hospitals) can be of considerable significance in evaluating the impact of NHI.

CONCLUSION

Feldstein and Friedman and the Human Resources Research Center have developed microeconomic models of the health care system that exhibit some similarities (e.g., in the specification of demand) but differ in both certain structural components (e.g., population, supply, price adjustment) and in the nature of their conclusions. Both are pathbreaking studies, however, in the application of formal analyses to the study of policy issues, specifically the application of microeconometric models to the study of features of national health insurance.

NOTES

1. The HRRC microeconometric model of the health care system, developed by Donald E. Yett, Leonard J. Drabek, Michael D. Intriligator, and Larry J. Kimbell, was first conceptualized in "The Development of a Microsimulation Model of Health Manpower Demand and Supply." See *Proceedings and Report of Conference on a Health Manpower Simulation Model,* Vol. 1 (Washington, D.C.: Bureau of Health Manpower, Department of Health, Education, and Welfare, December 1970), pp. 9–172.

    Elements of the model and comparisons with the HRRC macroeconometric model were presented in "Health Manpower Planning: An Econometric Approach," *Health Services Research,* 7 (1972), pp. 134–147.

    Components of the model were presented in "A Microsimulation Model of the Health Care System in the United States: The Role of the Physician Services Sector," paper presented at the 5th Conference on Optimization Techniques, Rome, May 1, 1973, published in R. Conti and A. Ruberti (editors), *5th Conference on Optimization Techniques, Part II* (Heidelberg: Springer-Verlag, 1974), and in "A Microsimulation Model of the Health Care System: The Role of the Hospital Sector," paper presented at the TIMS meetings, Tel Aviv, 1973, published in *Applied Mathematics and Computation,* 1 (1975), pp. 105–130.

    An overview of the model was presented in "A Microeconometric Model of the Health Care System in the U.S.," paper presented at the Econometric Society Meetings, New York, December 29, 1973, published in *Annals of Economic and Social Measurement,* 4/3 (1975), pp. 407–433.

    The complete model will be published as *A Forecasting and Policy Simulation Model of the Health Care Sector: The HRRC Prototype Microeconometric Model* (Lexington, Massachusetts: Lexington Books, 1977).

    All publications are by the four authors listed above.
2. For another treatment of NHI, using a macroeconometric model, see D. E. Yett, L. Drabek, M. D. Intriligator, and L. J. Kimbell, "Econometric Forecasts of Health Services and Health Manpower" in M. Perlman (editor), *The Economics of Health and Medical Care* (London: Macmillan, 1974). This paper identifies and treats several different features of alternative NHI plans, including not only payment features (coinsurance, deductibles, etc.) but also training and reorganization features, such as the expansion of medical schools and the development of health maintenance organizations (HMO's), respectively.
3. In addition, there is a population of hospitals in the HRRC microeconometric model.
4. FF also appropriately treat nonmonetary costs in their specification of demand functions.
5. Production function estimates are adopted from Larry J. Kimbell and John H. Lorant, "Production Functions for Physicians' Services," paper presented at the Econometric Society Meetings, December 1972. Demand functions for aides were derived from estimates in Michael D. Intriligator and Barbara H. Kehrer, "A Simultaneous Equations Model of Allied Health Personnel Employed in Physicians' Offices," in M. Perlman (editor), *The Economics of Health and Medical Care* (London: Macmillan, 1974).
6. The β's are the only coefficients of the HRRC microeconometric model that are not explicitly estimated. They constitute fewer than 1/10 of 1 per cent of the parameters in the model.
7. Health conditions are used in the demand functions, but they are not maintained in the population simulation of the HRRC microeconometric model.

12 ‖ REPLY

Martin Feldstein and Bernard Friedman

The comments of Chiswick and Intriligator suggest to us that we did not adequately emphasize the role of *stochastic* microsimulation. Although our model and the HRRC model discussed by Intriligator are both described as "microsimulation" studies, ours alone uses a *stochastic* simulation of *individual* behavior. The HRRC model might better be called a "detailed" or "disaggregated" macrosimulation model since no allowance is made for variations in individual experience within demographic groups.

The stochastic simulation method is particularly important for studying the effects of different insurance structures. Changes in deductibles, in upper limits, and in coinsurance rates affect the mean costs and benefits of insurance in complex and nonlinear ways that depend on the *distribution* of health expenditures and not just on the mean of that distribution. We see no adequate method of comparing, say, a $200 deductible and a $400 deductible without a model that contains information on the proportion of expenses below $200 and between $200 and $400. We therefore feel that the HRRC model cannot be used to analyze the types of policy alternatives with which we are concerned. Similarly, we do not understand Chiswick's remark that "it is not clear that an aggregate model of demand would necessarily be a worse predictor than a microsimulation model."

The two alternative specifications of supply and price response are very aggregate and very simple. Greater disaggregation would clearly be desirable if reliable parameter estimates were available.[1] We see no reason, however, to provide a stochastic model of supplies behavior.

Although we made no attempt to deal with the time path of the system's response to a change in demand, it is not true that we do not "directly treat disequilibrium phenomena in the relevant markets," as Intriligator says. In Section 4 we explicitly consider the possibilities of excess demand, describe a "supply-determined" equilibrium, and, in Equation (10), posit a model of rationing behavior.

Chiswick correctly points out that our simulations assume no cross-elasticities of demand, no income elasticity, and the same price elasticities for all individuals. Although we obviously agree with Chiswick that these are reasonable assumptions, they should be borne in mind in considering the specific empirical results. These restrictions are, of course, not inherent in the microsimulation method. Equations (1) and (2) explicitly allow for cross-elasticities of demand. The first sentence in Section 1 indicates that separate demand equations can be specified for each income and demographic group. The original simulations prepared as part of a study for the Department of Health, Education, and Welfare did use these features to examine the implications of alternative income elasticities and different sets of demand parameters.

Finally, we recognize that our treatment of the nonmonetary costs of health care was only a first attempt at a difficult problem. We are grateful to Chiswick for suggesting ways to extend and improve our specification.

NOTE

1. We had previously studied the data in the 1967 Health Interview Survey and concluded that although it is very valuable for certain purposes, the information on prices paid is so poor as to invalidate an estimated demand equation.

Index

Death rates: predicted, percentage deviation between actual and (1967–69; table), 390. *See also* White females; White males

Demand. *See* specific types of health insurance

Disability:Medicare and, 377, 378 (figure), 379–381; in price elasticities estimates model, 267. *See also* Hospital days

Distortion, risk and, in welfare analysis, 27

Education: in price elasticities estimates model, 266; as variable in health care demand among the poor, 177, 188

Elasticities: in children's health care demand (table), 242; consumption, in children's health care (table), 240; of expected value of dependent variables (table), 182; perfectly elastic supply of medical services, 13; of physician utilization by the elderly, by region (table), 415; of supply, welfare analysis of changes in coinsurance rates and, 3–4; wage income (table), 277. *See also* Price elasticities estimates

Elderly, the. *See* Medicare

Employed individuals, price elasticities estimates and medical care demands of, 280

Employee equilibrium in Tiebout-type model, 76

Employee share, optimal, in imperfect mobility model, 89–91

Employer-choice equilibrium in Tiebout-type model, 76–77

Employers, choice of group health insurance by, 92–93

ENT diseases, prevalence of, in children (table), 220

Equilibrium: conditions of, in preventive medicine-health insurance joint demand model, 46–47; displacements of, 47–51; employee, in Tiebout-type model, 76; employer-choice, in Tiebout-type model, 76–77; general, in imperfect mobility model, 91; supply response model and equilibrium solution, 511, 512 (figure), 513 (figure), 514–515. *See also* General equilibrium

Equilibrium prices, 4

Error structure, in children's health demand system, 226–27

Estimation: children's health model, 227, 228 (table), 229–30, 231 (table), 232–233,

234–235 (table), 236–237 (table), 238–240; estimating equation for medical price variables (table), 152; of health care demand among the urban poor, 178–179, 180–183 (tables), 184–189; ordinary least squares, of health care demand among urban poor (table), 196; ordinary least squares, of office visits by age groups (table), 418–419; reimbursement insurance, 132–133. *See also* Price elasticities estimates

Expected utility: criterion of welfare as, 7; evaluating change in, 4

Expenditures: Canadian health care, 447, 448–450 (tables), 451; Canadian medical, 468, 469 (table), 470–471 (table), 472, 473–475 (tables), 476–477, 478 (table), 479–480

Family size in price elasticities estimates model, 266

Family unit heads, recalculating price elasticities estimates for, 298, 299, 300, 301–304 (tables), 305, 306–307 (table), 308–309

Fees, fee-setting dynamics, 337–338. *See also* Loading fees; Physician-fee inflation

Feldstein-Friedman (FF) microsimulation model, 505–510, 534, 535 (table), 536–538

Females. *See* White females; Working mothers

Financing of health insurance, welfare analysis of changes in coinsurance rates and, 3

Fixed levels of medical services, 15

Fringe benefit plan: binary variables of (table), 99; of group health insurance, 74–75

General equilibrium: in imperfect mobility model of group health insurance, 91; model of, net welfare changes expressed by means of, 3

Gross receipts, indexes of average, per active fee-practice physicians (table), 474

Group health insurance, 73–114; comments on, 110–114; data on, 93–94; difference between union and employer choice in, 92–93; empirical variables in, 94–97; as fringe benefit, 74–75; fringe benefit plan binary variables (table), 99; illustrative calculation of price and income elasticity

Mothers, children's health care and non-working, 236–237 (table)

National health insurance, 505–540; analyzing two plans of, 515–516, 517 (table), 518, 519 (table), 520, 521 (table), 522; comments on, 529–534, 535 (table), 536–540; implications of Medicaid and Medicare for, 416–417 (*see also* Medicaid; Medicare); microsimulation model of, 505–510, 533–538; price response model of, 523–526, 527 (table); supply response model of, 511, 512 (figure), 513 (figure), 514–515, 521 (table), 527 (table). *See also* Canadian national health insurance

Noncontributory union group health insurance, 104 (table), 105–106 (table)

Nonunionized groups, group health insurance for (table), 103

Nonworking mothers, children's health care and, 236–237 (table)

Nonwage income in price elasticities estimates model, 266

Normative model for Medicare assessment, 367–370

Office visits: by age, 393 (table), 396 (table); by the elderly, by health status and income (table), 413; equations of, 292–294 (table); by income, welfare status and age (1969; table), 396; ordinary least squares estimates of, by age group, 418–419 (table); per capita, by age and income (table), 393; percentage of, by income (table), 398; per person for various levels of income, insurance and health status (table), 281; price elasticities estimates and, 275, 276 (table); in price elasticities estimates for family unit heads, 308–309; price and income elasticities and, 279

Optimal employee share in imperfect mobility model, 89–91

Output and price equations, in physician-fee inflation model, 327–328

Overconsumption, model based on, 27

Own-price: in price elasticities estimates model, 264–265; price elasticities estimates for family unit heads and (table), 302

Parents: children's health and preferences and health attitudes of, 226; working mothers' demand for children's health care, 234–235 (table)

Payoffs, altering, of random experiments, 36

Physician-fee inflation, 321–362; comments on, 354–362; cost equations in model of, 325–327; demand equations in model of, 323–325; empirical results of study, 331, 332–333 (table), 334 (table), 335–338; implications of, for policies, 338–341; model and variable specifications of, 323–331; reimbursement and wage variables in, 341–344, 345 (table), 346–347

Physician-population ratio, 267

Physicians: Canadian, expenditures for, 468, 469 (table), 470–471 (table), 472, 473–475 (tables), 476–477, 478 (table), 479–480; use of, by the elderly, by region (table), 415; use or nonuse of, price elasticities estimates and, 270–273, 274 (table)

Poor, the. *See* Medicare; Urban poor

Population-beds ratio, 267

Population-physician ratio, 267

Predictions: of health care demand among the urban poor, 170–171; percentage deviation between actual and predicted death rates (1967–69; table), 390

Preventive-medicine health-insurance demand, 35–71; basic model for, 45–51; comments on, 66–71; concepts relevant to, 38–39, 40 (figure), 41 (figure), 42–43, 44 (figure); model of, with consumption affecting health prospects, 51–57

Price changes: effects of, on consumption model of health care among the poor, 168–169; in formal model of health care demand among the poor, 198–201; insurance, as equilibrium displacements, 49–50

Price elasticities: of demand, illustrative calculations of, 97–98; travel time, for ambulatory care (table), 183

Price elasticities estimates, 261–320; amount of medical services demanded conditional on some being demanded, 276, 277 (table), 278–280, 281 (table); comments on, 313–320; data statistics on, 286–287 (table); demand for care from unemployed individuals and, 268–270; hospital admissions and, 270–273, 274 (table); model of, 262–268; office-visit equations with interactions in, 292–294 (table); overall, 281, 282 (table), 283 (table), 284–285; price equations and, 295–296 (table); recalculating, for family unit heads, 298, 299, 300, 301–304 (tables), 305, 306–307 (table), 308–309; summary estimates, values used for, 283; time equations used for, 287–288 (table); utilization equations used for, 289–290 (table)

Price equations: effects of proportion covered by third parties on (table), 334; in physician-fee inflation study, general specifications of, 332–333 (table); in physician-fee inflation model, output and, 327–328

Price response model of national health insurance, 523–526, 527 (table)

Prices: equilibrium, 4; estimating equations for variables in (table), 152; in health care demand among the urban poor, 173–175; income elasticity of demand and, in group health insurance, 97–98; marginal, price elastiticies estimates and (table), 282; in model specification of children's health, 223–224. *See also* Cross-price; Fees; Medical prices; Own-price

Public policy: children's health and, 241, 242 (table), 243–244. *See also* National health insurance

Quality of medical services, Medicare and, 397, 398 (table), 399

Race: coverage under supplementary insurance program by (table), 434; health care among urban poor and, 178, 188–189; predicted Medicaid distribution by (table), 407; in price elasticities estimates model, 267. *See also* White females; White males

Random factors: in demand, 3; health data as, 4

Red Hook population, selected characteristics of, 171–172

Region: coverage under supplementary insurance program by (table), 434; elasticities of physician utilization by the elderly by (table), 415; in price elasticities estimates model, 268

Reimbursement insurance, 115–162; comments on, 156–162; comparative statics for coinsurance, 126–131; comparative statics of, for maximum coverage, 120–125; demand for coverage in, 133, 134–135 (table), 136–137; demand for maximum coverage in, 137–138, 139–140 (table), 141–142 (table), 143–144 (table), 145; estimation of, 132–133; observed coinsurance rates for, 145, 146–147 (table), 148–149, 150 (table), 151 (table), 152 (table), 153; physician-fee inflation and, 341–344, 345 (table), 346–347

Revenue: indexes of average gross receipts per active fee-practice physicians (table), 474; of physicians, usual fees vs. average, 330–331. *See also* Fees; Medical prices; Prices

Risk: changes in, as equilibrium displacement, 50–51; distortion and, in welfare analysis, 27; risk adjustment to marginal welfare change, 17

Risk aversion, 41–42

Room and board prices: price elasticities estimates and, 278–279; in price elasticities estimates for family unit heads, 308

Selection, adverse, in Tiebout-type model, 78–79

Self-perceived health status, 267

Sex: health care demand among urban poor by, 178, 189; in price elasticities estimates model, 267

SIC code binary variables (table), 99–100

Statics: in reimbursement coinsurance demand, 126–131; in reimbursement insurance, for maximum coverage, 120–125

Stochastic dominance, 38, 39, 40 (figure), 41 (figure)

Subsidized health care for urban poor, tradeoffs of, 192–193

Supplementary medical insurance, coverage services under, by health, welfare status, region and race (table), 434

Supply: general formula for welfare effects taking explicit account of, 13–15; inelasticity of, in welfare analysis, 6, 18–19. *See also* Medical services

Supply response model, 511, 512 (figure), 513 (figure), 514–515, 521 (table), 527 (table)